D1716261

Emerging Trends and Innovations in Privacy and Health Information Management

Cristina Albuquerque
University of Coimbra, Portugal

A volume in the Advances in
Healthcare Information Systems
and Administration (AHISA) Book
Series

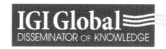

1-12-21
LN
$231.00

Published in the United States of America by
    IGI Global
    Medical Information Science Reference (an imprint of IGI Global)
    701 E. Chocolate Avenue
    Hershey PA, USA 17033
    Tel: 717-533-8845
    Fax: 717-533-8661
    E-mail: cust@igi-global.com
    Web site: http://www.igi-global.com

Library of Congress Cataloging-in-Publication Data

Names: Albuquerque, Cristina Maria Pinto, editor.
Title: Emerging trends and innovations in privacy and health information
    management / Cristina Albuquerque, editor.
Description: Hershey, PA : Medical Information Science Reference, [2019] |
    Includes bibliographical references.
Identifiers: LCCN 2018054552| ISBN 9781522584704 (hardcover) | ISBN
    9781522584711 (ebook)
Subjects: | MESH: Health Information Management--trends | Privacy | Delivery
    of Health Care--trends
Classification: LCC R858 | NLM W 26.5 | DDC 610.285--dc23 LC record available at https://lccn.
loc.gov/2018054552

This book is published in the IGI Global book series Advances in Healthcare Information Systems and Administration (AHISA) (ISSN: 2328-1243; eISSN: 2328-126X)

British Cataloguing in Publication Data
A Cataloguing in Publication record for this book is available from the British Library.

All work contributed to this book is new, previously-unpublished material.
The views expressed in this book are those of the authors, but not necessarily of the publisher.

For electronic access to this publication, please contact: eresources@igi-global.com.

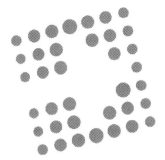

Advances in Healthcare Information Systems and Administration (AHISA) Book Series

ISSN:2328-1243
EISSN:2328-126X

Editor-in-Chief: Anastasius Moumtzoglou, Hellenic Society for Quality & Safety in Healthcare and P. & A. Kyriakou Children's Hospital, Greece

MISSION

The **Advances in Healthcare Information Systems and Administration (AHISA) Book Series** aims to provide a channel for international researchers to progress the field of study on technology and its implications on healthcare and health information systems. With the growing focus on healthcare and the importance of enhancing this industry to tend to the expanding population, the book series seeks to accelerate the awareness of technological advancements of health information systems and expand awareness and implementation.

Driven by advancing technologies and their clinical applications, the emerging field of health information systems and informatics is still searching for coherent directing frameworks to advance health care and clinical practices and research. Conducting research in these areas is both promising and challenging due to a host of factors, including rapidly evolving technologies and their application complexity. At the same time, organizational issues, including technology adoption, diffusion and acceptance as well as cost benefits and cost effectiveness of advancing health information systems and informatics applications as innovative forms of investment in healthcare are gaining attention as well. **AHISA** addresses these concepts and critical issues.

COVERAGE

- Measurements and Impact of HISA on Public and Social Policy
- Pharmaceutical and Home Healthcare Informatics
- Management of Emerging Health Care Technologies
- Rehabilitative Technologies
- Decision Support Systems
- Clinical Decision Support Design, Development and Implementation
- IT security and privacy issues
- Role of informatics specialists
- Medical Informatics
- E-Health and M-Health

IGI Global is currently accepting manuscripts for publication within this series. To submit a proposal for a volume in this series, please contact our Acquisition Editors at Acquisitions@igi-global.com or visit: http://www.igi-global.com/publish/.

Titles in this Series

For a list of additional titles in this series, please visit:
https://www.igi-global.com/book-series/advances-healthcare-information-systems-administration/37156

Mobile Health Applications for Quality Healthcare Delivery
Anastasius Moumtzoglou (P&A Kyriakou Children's Hospital, Greece)
Medical Information Science Reference • ©2019 • 327pp • H/C (ISBN: 9781522580218)
• US $265.00

Intelligent Systems for Healthcare Management and Delivery
Nardjes Bouchemal (University Center of Mila, Algeria)
Medical Information Science Reference • ©2019 • 377pp • H/C (ISBN: 9781522570714)
• US $245.00

Human Rights, Public Values, and Leadership in Healthcare Policy
Augustine Nduka Eneanya (University of Lagos, Nigeria)
Medical Information Science Reference • ©2019 • 311pp • H/C (ISBN: 9781522561330)
• US $225.00

Contemporary Applications of Mobile Computing in Healthcare Settings
R. Rajkumar (VIT University, India)
Medical Information Science Reference • ©2018 • 259pp • H/C (ISBN: 9781522550365)
• US $205.00

Handbook of Research on Emerging Perspectives on Healthcare Information Systems ...
Joseph Tan (McMaster University, Canada)
Medical Information Science Reference • ©2018 • 641pp • H/C (ISBN: 9781522554608)
• US $355.00

Big Data Analytics in HIV/AIDS Research
Ali Al Mazari (Alfaisal University, Saudi Arabia)
Medical Information Science Reference • ©2018 • 294pp • H/C (ISBN: 9781522532033)
• US $215.00

For an entire list of titles in this series, please visit:
https://www.igi-global.com/book-series/advances-healthcare-information-systems-administration/37156

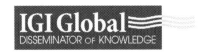

701 East Chocolate Avenue, Hershey, PA 17033, USA
Tel: 717-533-8845 x100 • Fax: 717-533-8661
E-Mail: cust@igi-global.com • www.igi-global.com

Table of Contents

Section 1
Health Information Management: Emerging Trends, Challenges, and Impacts

George Leal Jamil, Informações em Rede Consultoria e Treinamento
*   Ltda., Brazil*
Leandro R. Santos, IN3 Inteligencia de Mercado LTDA, Brazil
Liliane C. Jamil, Independent Researcher, Brazil
Augusto P. Vieira, Independent Researcher, Brazil

Uma V., Pondicherry University, India
Jayanthi Ganapathy, Anna University, India

Joana Vale Guerra, University of Coimbra, Portugal

Section 2
Innovation, Privacy, and Inclusion: Critical Approaches and Recommendations

Detailed Table of Contents

Section 1
Health Information Management: Emerging Trends, Challenges, and Impacts

Chapter 1

> *George Leal Jamil, Informações em Rede Consultoria e Treinamento Ltda., Brazil*
> *Leandro R. Santos, IN3 Inteligencia de Mercado LTDA, Brazil*
> *Liliane C. Jamil, Independent Researcher, Brazil*
> *Augusto P. Vieira, Independent Researcher, Brazil*

It was observed, in these last years, the consolidation of the market intelligence (MI) concept as a source of competitive results in several strategic ways, impacting decision-making and entrepreneurship. This article intends to explore the conceptualization of the MI process, observing specially its application in Healthcare sector under the emergence of new technologies. Approaching the healthcare market, a framework for an intelligence system for marketing decisions was discussed and it is now evaluated with the contribution of information architecture and new technologies concepts. The review formerly produced is updated regarding the focus of the MI system under the influences and potentialities for emerging technologies application, through a lemma of "digital transformation" (DT), validating and expanding market intelligence background towards new dynamism and application in Healthcare contexts.

Health-care systems aid in the diagnosis, treatment and prevention of diseases. Epidemiology deals with the demographic study on frequency, distribution and determinants of disease in order to provide better health-care. Today information technology has made data pervasive i.e. data is available anywhere and in abundance. GIS in epidemiology enables prompt services to mankind or people at risk. It brings out health-care services that are amicable for prevention and control of disease spread. This could be achieved when epidemiology data is modeled considering temporal and spatial factors and using data driven computation techniques over such models. This chapter discusses 1) the need for integrating GIS and epidemiology, 2) various case studies that indicates the need for spatial analysis being performed on epidemiologic data, 3) few techniques involved in the spatial analysis, 4) functionalities provided by some of the widely used GIS software packages and tools.

The widespread use of digital technology allows for a number of transformations in the organization of work which renders the importance of professional and expert knowledge more open to challenges. The digital age is impacting and changing many aspects of professional development, therefore must be examined in its effects on reshaping healthcare professions and its implications on professional autonomy and discretionary judgment. To achieve this goal, advantages and disadvantages will be highlighted about the usage of electronic health record software to the healthcare professional's autonomy and discretionary power. The increased use of digital technologies is deeply affecting most professional occupations, transforming their identities, structures, and practices. In recognizing the challenges and opportunities to professional work of the digital transformation is underlined the importance of trying to understand how to remain professional in different digital environments and how to work in contexts with ambient surveillance.

Chapter 4

Marta Freitas Olim, Diaverum, Portugal
Sónia Guadalupe, University Coimbra, Portugal
Fernanda da Conceição Bento Daniel, University Coimbra, Portugal
Joana Pimenta, Diaverum, Portugal
Luís Carrasco, Diaverum, Portugal
Alexandre Gomes da Silva, University of Coimbra, Portugal

This chapter discusses the standardization of instruments and typologies in social work assessment and introduces, from a multidimensional perspective, a new standardized instrument evaluating the level of complexity associated with the social intervention process in a sample of chronic kidney disease (CKD) patients. The authors evaluated the matrix's metric properties by internal consistency and defined a rating index through the best cutoff points, using receiver operator curve and Youden Index. Matrix construction and validation used focus groups of experts in blinded classification of 100 CKD patients and indicator weighting. The matrix shows good internal consistency and reliability (Cronbach's alpha = .742). Cutoff points indicate three levels of complexity classification. The matrix is a good instrument to identify the complexity associated with the social intervention process in the area of Nephrology, and is a relevant contribution to the social information management of social workers, the health teams and the administration of health units.

Section 2
Innovation, Privacy, and Inclusion: Critical Approaches and Recommendations

Chapter 5

Pradeep Nair, Central University of Himachal Pradesh, India

The reason for considering ICT-based communication platforms, especially mobile phones, as the most efficacious media tool to interconnect health care providers, practitioners and other stakeholders to a substantially large number of consumers in the healthcare system is that the mobile phone subscribers in India has reached to 1,013.23 million in the third quarter of 2018. The prices of smartphones have also come down by 11 percent with a demand for 4G devices capturing 6 percent of smartphone unit demand in India. Hence, it is an appropriate time to understand that the future of healthcare business in India lies with mobile based healthcare services. This chapter explores some of the significant innovations taking place in mobile healthcare business in India and examines the emerging approach of integrated health care ecosystems to provide quality health services to everyone where and when it is required.

Chapter 6

In this chapter, the author discusses the contribution of technological achievements and ICT applications to prevent or reverse frailty in elderly people and to promote active and healthy aging. After a theoretical and political reflection about the issues associated to a new paradigm of aging in current societies, the author underlines the potentialities of technology as a complementary mechanism to achieve alternative and innovative responses as well as integrated and multidimensional policies and actions.

Chapter 7

In this chapter, the author develop a sociological analysis of the role played by professional management of information about patients' end-of-life (EoL) processes in palliative care (PC). Thus the author will thus highlight the processes by which PC professionals manage private health information about patients in the frame of this type of care. Thus the author will show how managing information about prospective EoL trajectories by healthcare professionals is one of the major challenges in their daily work in PC wards. The author verifies that, in these contexts, patients and their families and members of the healthcare teams tend to have different experiential and personal careers in their relation with disease, the organization of care, and EoL trajectories, whose confrontation at the level of interaction produces complex effects in social processes that occur in daily activity contexts of PC.

In health promotion discourses, access to medical care is presented as a universal remedy. As a result, ethical considerations are often limited to the issue of equitable access. Yet focusing on access to healthcare hides the issue of access to data needed for scientific development. Putting into place a system for saving lives involves population health monitoring and is founded on scientific rationality. This chapter refocuses political attention from medical intervention to what makes it possible. In doing so, the underlying ethical issue shifts from a concern with universal access to healthcare—considered a right from an equity standpoint—to a discussion of the options and consequences of a type of government based on science. The author puts forward the idea that it is not because it is technically and scientifically possible to do something that it should be done. To illustrate this argument, the chapter discusses the example of The Lancet's project on stillbirths (2011-2030) taken up by the WHO.

Chapter 9
Healing Cultural Personae With the Media Dream: Using Jungian
Compensation to Foster ICT Coherence 212
    Stephen Brock Schafer, Pacific Rim Enterprises, USA

Issues of cultural morality and health in a mediated reality of simulated illusion may be addressed with Jungian principles. The psychological dynamics of interactive images projected as media images correspond with psychological dream images as defined by Carl G. Jung. Therefore, images in the media mirror patterns of energy and information in what Jung called the collective unconscious. Dream dynamics may be used to address global political hacking, cyber warfare, and neuromarketing with ICTs.

Preface

The use of technological advancements in the management of healthcare services and health information poses currently unprecedented and complex issues about the suitability and boundaries of the ongoing changes. The discussion around the preservation of privacy and confidential data of patients stands side by side the debate about innovation, effectiveness and quality of healthcare. Patients' data and big data - to be used for example for scientific experiments – are today easier to collect and store and must be handled consciously and responsibly. Therefore renewed questions emerge around the processes and tools to manage larger amounts of health information and to assure its confidentiality, trust and security.

Additionally, the progressive statement of a "salutogenesis" paradigm (Antonovsky, 1979; Lindström & Eriksson, 2005; Mittelmark et al., 2017) shifts the expectations of the patients, the conceptions of care and the role of health professionals, as well as the structure of healthcare services. Health becomes today mainly a lifestyle. Personal health choices may even surpass and hinder medical authority and collective interests. Innovative technological applications are allied with the desire to increase and monitor a state of permanent health and wellbeing. At the same time, the possible connections and boundaries between Science, technology, politics and healthcare stands up as the background of a necessary reflection. The book *Emerging Trends and Innovations in Privacy and Health Information Management* identifies and discusses, under a multidisciplinary focus, these diverse and interconnected poles of the equation and the critical *equilibrium* between them.

The introduction of increasingly advanced technical innovations and devices, both in the way health information is collected, stored and screened, and in the treatment and prevention of diseases, changes in fact the way healthcare itself is thought, structured and managed. The implications in the management of health services and in the actions and gestures of healthcare professionals are, under this scope, profound and well known. Functionality, speed, efficacy, anticipation, precision and non-invasive intervention become principles of a medical practice increasingly more technical and adaptable to the unexpected. Technological innovation applied to healthcare creates the conditions for these changes to take place, but it does not fail to pose renewed analytical challenges, in particular on the possible balance between quality and effectiveness. The various theoretical and empirical contributions to the book reflect on the plural dimensions of these debates, which will be resumed, systematized and deepened in the conclusive part of the volume.

The book consists of nine chapters and is structured in two sections. The first section—Health Information Management: Emerging Trends, Challenges, and Impacts—aggregates four chapters which discuss and justify the relevance and challenges of information management for the effective and accountable realization of the purposes of healthcare systems. The contributions that are assembled in this first part of the book present thus new forms of health information management using technology, but also reflect on the challenges to be faced and the impacts generated, both within health teams and in the redefinition of the concept of health care itself.

Some of the challenges to be faced, in addition to the associated costs and access to the technology and innovations required to enter an age of digital health for all (people, groups and regions), are related to privacy issues, to the relationship between health, science and politics, and to the warranties of cohesive and inclusive digital societies and services. These challenges are addressed in the second section of the book—Innovation, Privacy, and Inclusion: Critical Approaches and Recommendations—consisting of five chapters. The various contributions assume, on the subjects referred above, a perspective both critical and engaged in alternative ways of reflection.

In the conclusion, the editor highlights, systematizes and deepens, the discussion about the main structuring analytical pillars of the book, addressed, in different ways, in the various chapters that compose it: 1) a new understanding of healthcare in a digital era; 2) healthcare and technological innovation; 3) science, ethics, and technics; 4) information management, accountability, confidence, and security.

BACKGROUND OF CURRENT DEBATES

Critical Shifts in the Healthcare Paradigm

The preservation of health and the neutralization of pain are assumed in modern societies as basic principles of a "good life". The state of "complete well-being" is in fact the guiding principle embodied in the World Health Organization's (WHO) own definition of health[1] and determines not only a demanding standard of care, but also a multidimensional attention to the various health plans of well-being (physical, emotional and social) and their articulation. Already Hippocrates (460-370 BC), considered the father of Western medicine, called "good health" or "*physis*" (φύσις) the state of *equilibrium* between different dimensions and factors. Like this "good health" would be not a static and acquired condition, but rather the result of a continuous process. In other words, a virtue of personal growth and development.

The inclusion of this perspective in the WHO definition, surpassing a concept of mere absence of disease and the associated biomedical paradigm, was a turning point in a renewed understanding of healthcare and inherently in the structuring of health policies and services (Jambroes et al., 2016). The requirement associated with the notion of "completeness" actually restores the etymological roots of the concept of health[2], and the inherent ideas of "perfection" and "purity", placing greater ambition in the actions and processes for its realization (Huber, 2014). It is, therefore, an intentionally affirmed ideal that at the same time guides actions and constitutes itself as the scope of what is still necessary to accomplish.

The idea of continuity (taking care of health and preventing disease permanently) is thus associated with the notion of state (to be healthy). In parallel, the narrative associated with the conception of healthcare is transformed. Not only in terms of the relationship between health professionals and patients - the autonomy of the individual in the active choice of health care and in the appreciation of the results to see materialized - but also in the way health services themselves are structured and articulated. Currently, the person is not only responsible for maintaining positive lifestyle choices across life, but also for preserving and controlling their own health. To this extent the responsibility for healthier options became a sort of public moral, guiding the rudder of personal and collective options. The conception of active and healthy aging (EC, 2018; WHO, 2015), for example, is based on this assumption.

The importance and role of the patient in the healthcare system is thus reconfigured under a principle of healthfulness. The person is no longer only the object of action of health professionals, but also a consumer of healthcare, determining how and where to be cared for. Under this scope, the subjective or personalized dimension of health constitutes as a central element of the ongoing paradigmatic shift. Already in the mid-1940s, Georges Canguilhem in the famous book, in later editions prefaced by Michel Foucault, "The Normal and the Pathologic" (1989 [1943]), endorsed the argument that the categories of normal and pathological are not objective scientific concepts. Likewise he underscored the idea that the feeling and expectations of health are essentially defined by the individuals, according to their functional needs and particular prevailing conditions, and not by the physician. Doctor and patient are, therefore, conceived as partners in the construction of what must be repaired and in the identification of what the patient aspires to in terms of well-being and health.

Actually, as Auffray, Charron, and Hood (2010) underline, the medicine "of the future" (or we could say already "the medicine of today") is P4, videlicet predictive, personalized, preventive and participatory (Hood & Auffray, 2013). Patient's self-awareness becomes a central guiding principle. However, this "subjectivation" of healthcare poses fundamental questions. In particular, those regarding the difficulties of objective and accountable evaluation of the care provided and the difficulties of delivering continuous and "tailor-made" health care solutions.

Several voices also argue the disadvantages of the absolute neutralization of pain, whether from a philosophical or religious perspective, or from a political and social focus. Philosophically several thinkers emphasize the centrality of suffering and the acceptance of death, and of the inadequacies of life, as essential mechanisms of self-discovery and personal development. It is enough to recall the Nietzschean notion of '*große Gesundheit*' ("great health") and its relation to a broad sense of life.

In a religious perspective, the admission of suffering is very linked with the unquestionable acceptance of the will of a Supreme Being. Pain is thus, under this perspective, a mechanism of improvement and sacrifice (sometimes self-inflicted) for a greater good, the divine recognition after life; the last proof of Job's faith. This conception generated over the years numerous conflicts and paradoxes in the relationship between religion and medical-scientific advances. It is enough to recall the reaction of some members of the Church against vaccination. For example, in 1772, the Reverend Edmund Massey in the well-known sermon "The Dangerous and Sinful Practice of Inoculation" classified the vaccines as "diabolical operations". Several others, from diverse religions, have pronounced in the same way.

In political and sociological terms, the suspicious of medical control over body and mind are not new. It is enough to recall the questioning around the concepts of pathologic and normal by Canguilhem (1943), the notion of bio-power developed by Michel Foucault (1976), or the ones of normality and deficiency by Irving Zola (1982), among others. It is denounced, under these theoretical ideas, the development of absolute moral judgments oriented by a specific health conception that determines collective lifestyles and influence personal choices. A sort of absolutist conception of health parameters and healthy life habits tends thus to be strengthened and erected as a moral requirement of self and hetero appreciation. Consequently healthier life choices, from recycling to nutrition, become the basis to found and evaluate personal and collective responsibility. The results of scientific discoveries are also engaged to serve as the uncontested background for choices, policies or practices. The example of the tobacco consumption is paradigmatic. Exceeding the discussion about the malefic effects to the individual's health and the possible impacts on people around, the tobacco consumption became in current societies essentially a political and moral issue. The mirror of a responsible active health across life emerges also in the consumption of gymnasiums and sports, alternative medicines, natural treatments, "healthy" nutrition, psychotherapies, rejuvenation programs, etc. All these options do not fail to advocate a more or less shared, albeit personalized, sense of well-being and health, achieved and preserved. A sort of lens of appreciation of oneself and others under the focus of perfection and harmony. The increasingly intricate technological innovations applied to healthcare treatment, monitoring and prediction can in fact increase and profound these lenses. The final chapters of the book (in the second part) discuss this possibility and its implications.

The desideratum of a "complete state of well-being" has become indeed increasingly easier to achieve with medical-pharmacological developments over the last century, in parallel with the scientific-technical findings applied to healthcare. However, if these evolutions allow to respond to an ancestral aspiration of the human being - to live always more and better - they also put in the forefront of the debate questions about how health care is provided and the ethical and deontological issues involved.

The concept of health and well-being, as already emphasized, has evolved over time, and in different spaces, revealing not only differentiated values, but also expectations and forms of achievement more or less aligned with the scientific and technological developments. To that extent discussing health issues and preventing and treating diseases is not only a philosophical and humanistic query, but also a political, scientific and social issue that requires a serious debate about the relationship between means and ends.

Health is a fundamental right of human beings[3]. Failures in its achievement jeopardize the realization of other rights, including social and labor rights. Health and freedom, of being, of acting and of deciding, have in fact an essential link. The conditions of effectiveness and preservation are actually revealed as a principle of action and comparability between individuals and nations (for example, under the Human Development Index). It is also a priority in the 2030 Agenda for Sustainable Development (objective 3), both in terms of universal access to quality healthcare, and in the support to scientific research to combat epidemics, develop vaccination programs and promote development policies in a broadest sense.

Technical and scientific innovation and achievements in the field of disease treatment, prevention, and monitoring of health information have produced increasingly positive results in preserving the lives of a large number of people, although with significant differences in distinct parts of the world. The difficulties of access to the most advanced technology, considering the costs still involved, or even the accessibility, in certain regions, to training in new therapeutic and surgical techniques, remain a fact. Nonetheless, technical advances themselves can help to progressively minimize this inequality. For example, improvements in robotics and tele-surgery have enabled surgical interventions thousands of kilometers away since the second half of the 1980s. Likewise, the possibility of training and follow-up of surgeries or remote consultations (telemedicine and telehealth) has increased the accessibility of certain populations (isolated and/or dependent) to healthcare, as well as the exchange of experiences and knowledge between the world's leading specialists, universities and surgical centers, and the regions, professionals and services with greatest difficulties in accessing advanced training.

However, a long path still remains to be traveled in order to ensure a higher quality of life after surgery and during treatment, as well as in situations of dependency and chronical diseases. In fact, since the discovery of penicillin by Alexander Fleming, in 1928, the control of the majority of infectious diseases has become possible, but the control and follow-up of chronic diseases are still an important challenge for health professionals and healthcare services today.

Passionate discussions are also ongoing concerning the use of genetic heritage for research and precision medicine, the pharmacosurveillance processes, or the safety and privacy margins of medical information and the way it is, and can be used. Between the effectiveness of treatment and the pursuit of cure, often requiring the sharing and use of patient's medical information (between professionals and for scientific research purposes), and the preservation of privacy, autonomy, informed choices and intimacy of people, the boundaries are not always linear and the consensus are difficult to establish. The use of genetic material to control certain diseases or to promote human enhancement is, at this level, exemplary.

Also, the type and amount of information that is requested to patients (which must be based on principles of necessity and suitability), how it is collected and safely stored and the purposes for which it is intended (sometimes associated with external parameters, for example information for insurers), presuppose the definition of boundaries and compromises occasionally unstable, although currently very regulated. The definition of norms and directives of data protection is very relevant and contributes to create a climate of accountability and confidence on healthcare systems and professionals. Recognizable and shared norms is in fact one of the fundamental basis of confidence in modern societies (Messu, 2017; 2018). Patients trust that the personal information they share with health professionals is confidential, and even deontological and legally privileged. They assume an assumption of confidence. Confidence in health professionals, confidence in the results of science and medical treatments, confidence in the responsible use of data and information collected (Checkland, Marshall, & Harrison, 2004; McKinlay & Marceau, 2002; Porter, Morphet, Missen, & Raymond, 2013; Zheng, 2014). The unveiling of intimacy, the vulnerability of a totally naked body, the voluntary "reduction" to a manipulated medical object presupposes thus, in the other face of the "contract" between patients and health professionals, the possibility to be healed and the confidence that the "denudated vulnerability" stays in the boundaries of healthcare facilities and in the frame of patients' personal autonomy. Therefore, trust in healthcare systems and professionals goes over the mere existence of regulations. It is also anchored in the complex relationships between patients, families and professionals in healthcare organizations. Relationships that truly influence and are influenced by a particular conception of health and health care delivery, and the consequent mutual expectations and exigencies, both of healthcare professionals and patients.

Different rationalities can in fact be mixed in the hospital environment, leading to a certain confrontation, often dilemmatic, of arguments about how to care for certain patients. For example, in the name of personal convictions, some people refuse the appropriate professional gesture. A paradigmatic case is the refusal of vaccination. Another is the rejection of blood transfusions because of religious or moral convictions. And many other examples could be presented. In these cases a clear conflict arises between medical rationality, which governs the organization of healthcare itself, and what we might call the existential rationality that guides the patient. It is mainly a conflict between systems of values. On the one hand, the values adopted by the medical profession and embodied in the Hippocratic Oath: "the utmost respect for human life". The basis of a system built, unified, generalized and used as the foundation of professional ethics. On the other hand, the values assumed by citizens who access health services and carry their cultural, religious or moral values. A system of values and autonomy that, according to the same Oath, must also be respected: "I will respect the autonomy and dignity of my patient"[4].

Beyond this dilemma—which requires a complex reflection on what is framed, in the face of life and death issues, in the generic principles of "autonomy" and "dignity"—conflicts between personal convictions and collective interest can also emerge. For example, the conflict among personal refusal of vaccination[5] and the right to be collectively protected against transmissible or eradicated diseases. The anti-vaccination supporters claim, namely, the illegitimacy of State intrusion into individual autonomy. Policymakers underline the utilitarian rule of the greatest good for the greatest number, under the focus of Stuart Mill's "harm principle" which advocates the possibility of interference in individual freedom when it comes to prevent harm for others (Hussain, Ali, Ahmed, & Hussain, 2018). The debate is not simple and has been raising new developments and passionate discussions over the past decade. Nevertheless, some of these debates are permeated by moralizing and pseudo-scientific conceptions, which tend to obscure the most important pillars of the analysis. For example, the relation between freedom and security, or between private and public interests.

Emerging Trends in Privacy and Health Information Management

Currently health services are under great pressure. Between the necessary reduction of costs, and guarantees of sustainability, and the demonstration of results, both in terms of treatment success and decrease of the recovery times, and in terms of the volume of patients assisted under the assumption of management by objectives.

The Report "ICTs and the Health Sector. Towards Smarter Health and Wellness Models" (OECD, 2013) underlines that the sustainability of healthcare systems is profoundly associated with their capacity and will to be innovative, participatory, preventive and personalized, developing intelligent models of care and services namely by using adequately technological applications and devices (Albuquerque, 2016). Technological innovation (both in the field of surgical and diagnostic techniques and in the field of health facilities management) is thus a crucial investment and a differentiating factor for investors and patient-consumers.

A more effective way of managing health services and collected information, for example through the use of technologies, may allow greater accessibility, proximity and quality of services provided. The critical element under this scope is related to the preservation or not of personalized and empathic attention in the relationship between health professionals and patients. A more technological and digital environment does not necessarily has to be a "dehumanized" environment. The balance between technique and personal relationship is thus the essential element to be preserved.

In fact, new opportunities emerge from the connection between technological development, cutting-edge scientific research, and health care. Innovative solutions make it possible to profoundly transform patients' relationship with health services (at a time when services themselves dematerialize). Data collected via any digitally-based activity allows for more efficient management and sharing of information, but also for better understanding and anticipation of recurrent and chronic health problems (many of which are rooted in socio-economic contexts and stem from styles and life choices to be studied and monitor). Big data and data analytics allow for example to identify and interpret repetitive or anomalous patterns of variables in certain groups or in a given region and/or frame of time. Likewise, they can inform medical and policy decisions, allowing not only to compare regularities and risk factors, but also to recommend preventive treatments, to generate prospective scenarios and to strategically identify possible obstacles or opportunities to the implementation of new solutions. This way, not only medical intervention but also public health policies can be more targeted and monitored, producing clear gains in terms of health promotion and disease prevention.

Likewise, the access to quality health care at any time and place (Kvedar, Coye, & Everett, 2014) by the use of telemedicine (use of technologies to deliver healthcare services in a remote way) and telehealth technologies (consumer-oriented use of technologies allowing remote health monitoring and teleconsultation), or the use of mobile devices and electronic medical records, transform radically the bases of accessibility to health care and the parameters of response effectiveness. Both in time, assuring greater speed and immediacy and in space, with no need to physically travel long distances, and in information mining, screening and registration, increasingly dematerialized and easily interchangeable between professionals and services.

The more easily accessible information actually can enhance enormously the quality of care and a more efficient management of resources. However it puts also the issues associated with the guarantees of confidentiality, privacy and information security in the first line of analysis. The privileged use of the information provided in the context of a clinical relationship (confidentiality) and the right of the patient to decide by what means and with which objectives the information concerning him / her health is shared (privacy) requires, in counterpoint, the warranty of processes of information protection (Brodnik, Rinehart-Thompson, & Reynolds, 2012).

The issues of information security is an old concern of health systems, However they have been compounded by dematerialization processes and the use of increasingly sophisticated electronic recording systems. The mechanisms for protecting and guaranteeing limited access to registered information are also evolving, both from a technical and regulatory point of view. Nevertheless, in one and another domain paths are always unfinished and require constant revision and vigilance.

The various regulations seek to strike a balance between the necessary accesses of health professionals to reserved information *versus* the protection of individuals' privacy. All the professionals who work with health information are obliged to respect data confidentiality. However the security of data is more than a matter of health professionals' responsibility or of mere legal regulations. It is necessary to assure continuously more sophisticated data protection mechanisms which imply, for health services, large and regular investments. It is necessary also, and mainly, a continuous and profound reflection about the changes ongoing and the balances between a certain conception of healthcare and the means to achieve it. The book Emerging Trends and Innovations in Privacy and Health Information Management intends to be a contribution to this necessary and pertinent debate.

SCOPE AND STRUCTURE OF THE BOOK

The book, as already mentioned, is composed of nine chapters distributed by two sections. Multidisciplinary contributions (from technology, engineering, sociology, social work, anthropology, nursing and medicine), both from academy and professional fields, are aggregated covering vast and diverse reflections on management of medical-scientific information, namely through the use of technological innovation.

Assuming an original contribution to the reflection on the current innovations in the field of health and health information management and privacy, the book is focused in particular on the substantive issues that these innovations may entail or trigger. In other words, it is not a technical description book of emerging technological innovations, but rather a set of perspectives from different academic areas to understand what is changing in health information availability, screening and register, the implications it may entail and the recommendations to be weighed in today's rapidly changing scenarios.

In the first section of the book—Health Information Management: Emerging Trends, Challenges, and Impacts—the first two chapters focus on exploring the idea that appropriate information management—using the possibilities and advantages of technological processes and devices—is essential for good decision-making and planning, especially considering health-related issues. The next two chapters seek to discuss the impact, at a mezzo level, of new forms of health information management within the framework of health institutions and, in particular, in the performance of health teams and professionals.

In the first chapter of the book, "Approaching Information Architecture for a Market Intelligence System Based on Emerging Technologies," the authors George Jamil, Leandro Henrique Rocha dos Santos, Liliane Carvalho Jamil e Augusto Alves Pinho Vieira underline the importance of information management as a strategic element planning and decision-making in organizations. They argue that learning to manage the large volume of information available requires renewed strategies of articulation between data, information and knowledge for which new technologies have a very relevant role to play. An inadequate information management, or its dispersion or disorganization, has impacts on the decision processes and their tactical and strategic adequacy. The chapter focuses on the exploration and updating of the so-called market intelligence cycle, powered by new technologies and specifically applied to the Healthcare sector. As the authors emphasize, the market intelligence process is anchored in the systematic provision of knowledge for strategic marketing planning and application in the context of an organization respecting its specificities and rationalities. In this sense, the authors explore the concept of "information architecture" as a conceptual background that gives consistency to the definition of a marketing intelligence process. This process can help organizations, in particular in the healthcare context, to better define the structuring and strategic use of information and to solve emerging problems. Knowledge allows understanding current developments, enabling complex decision-making, and setting scenarios and predictions. However, this knowledge, especially in a rapidly changing world, is difficult to manage. Functions of gathering, registering, sharing and valuating knowledge, along with other tasks associated with the main field of interest of an organization are particularly pressing. Thus the authors recommend - assuming that these evolutions are unfinished and still unstable - the development of managerial skills such as information architecture. This can lead to a more mature period where data, information and knowledge can become integrated assets to manage and to contribute, in a controlled and coordinated way, for the strategic management of the organization. The chapter also contributes to present results for further theoretical researches as well as its application, namely in the healthcare services' processes and decisions.

V. Uma and Ganapathy Jayanthi present, in the second chapter, "Spatial-Temporal Hot Spot Analysis of Epidemic Diseases Using Geographic Information System," a process of epidemiological evaluation using a technological tool of geographic information, the Geographic Information System (GIS). The rising of the population and of the available information is becoming increasingly difficult to administer, especially in a country like India. The authors therefore advocate the importance of use adequately technological tools to increase the quality of health services provided, the adequacy of health policies and the empirically based orientation of preventive measures. Epidemiological studies describe the distribution of diseases and the risks of their spread in a particular group of people, so, the spatial-temporal understanding of their distribution provides important insight about the prevailing geographical location of a disease and its variation, as well as about the different location of factors, spatially and over time. Understanding patterns of geographical distribution of diseases is an important asset to health professionals by assisting them in disease control and understanding of prevention factors. Thus, as the authors emphasize, epidemiological studies based on GIS - Geographic Information System - are gaining increasing technical and scientific relevance. This software stores and crosses spatial distribution data allowing to compare its temporal characteristics. It can therefore make a relevant contribution to the control of certain diseases and their dissemination using the methods of geo-referencing, area estimation, migration of population, disease mapping, detection of areas of interest, and integration of spatial and temporal clusters. The complex algorithms produced can be used to construct prediction, monitoring or risk assessment solutions in epidemiological studies. To illustrate the application of the software, the authors present several case studies and identify the concepts, methods and tools used in the Geographic Information System. Future research directions in this field already point to machine learning techniques, ensuring the predictability of disease outbreaks added to the current capacity of raster and vector operations for better information extraction and exploration of data.

The chapter of Joana Vale Guerra, "Digital Professionalism: Challenges and Opportunities to Healthcare Professions," discusses the implications of digital technologies in the reconstruction of "professionalism" in health care contexts. It advocates the idea that technologies transform professional practices by changing knowledge-based narratives and traditional caregiving processes. The transposing to a digital or digitized work paradigm is also associated with meeting the objectives and guidelines associated with new public management. The entrepreneurialisation of health care, a relatively recent process in the Portuguese context, actually produces and strengthens this movement. Access to digital platforms for recording and accessing data has long been a standard practice, although not without dilemmas. The adoption of management principles, emphasizing measurable production, creation of new management structures, incentive to competition and creation of performance indicators have generated, as the author defends, the bases for the transformation of the health services management model with multiple and differentiated impacts in health professionals' practices and patients' roles and expectations. The New Public Management also emphasizes a specific role for managers, requiring improvements in terms of economic efficiency and productivity, and advocating management by objectives and results. The chapter seeks thus to identify and discuss the reforms and strategies of the health policy that the professionals assumed, and how. In particular the processes of adaptation to a new organizational environment on the one hand, potentiating efficiency and effectiveness, and on the other hand the potential for generating forms of control and management that emphasize economic rationalization. These processes of professional adequacy end up being defined not by a decision of the professionals, but mainly by organizational management objectives, which poses important questions about the cohesion in health services, and thus on the relational quality of the care provided. The chapter identifies the two sides of this question - managerial objectives and relational quality - adopting a theoretical reflection anchored in the sociology of the professions and using, as an example, the application of rationalized and digital procedures in the management of the national network of long term integrated care.

The last chapter of the first section, "The Matrix of Complexity Associated With the Process of Social Intervention with Chronic Kidney Disease Patients," authored by Marta Freitas Olim, Sónia Guadalupe, Fernanda da Conceição Bento Daniel, Joana Pimenta, Luís Carrasco and Alexandre Gomes da Silva, seeks above all to advocate the need for scientifically validated and homogenized records of information to mainstream the analysis among the different healthcare professionals and generate a greater possibility of effective and quality decision making. The authors use as an example the work done by one of the professionals of the multidisciplinary health teams in Portugal, the social worker. They advocate the argument that it is necessary for the elaboration of adequate social diagnoses, namely with patients with chronic kidney disease, to use complex, uniform and data-intensive information collection instruments. Considering a global health concept, the social dimension and its evaluation is particularly important. So improving the quality of the social diagnostic and monitoring processes will necessarily impact on the overall quality of the healthcare provided. The complexity of patients' social situations rarely emerges from linear and fragmented statistics derived from records based on isolated variables. In close complementarity with clinical and prognostic diagnosis, social diagnosis should be expressed through methods that recognize this complexity and that can be used and understood by other health professionals. The use of typologies allows the expression of perspectives on consensual realities, using a reference construct, thus delineating the contours of a given situation by dismantling the professional jargon that makes difficult to construct a common narrative, aggregator of multiple "reference universes". Thus, the chapter focuses essentially on the development and validation of a new standardized instrument that assesses the level of complexity associated with the process of social intervention with patients with chronic kidney disease - the Matrix of Complexity Associated with the Process of Social Intervention - with the purpose of constructing an index to be used by social workers. As the authors argue, the systematization of information in a classification index favors team and administration decision making, since social (initial) evaluation and systematic or periodic social reassessment not only provide relevant information on individual situations, but also over a given population.

The second section of the book—Innovation, Privacy, and Inclusion: Critical Approaches and Recommendations—is centered on the reflection about the impacts and challenges in an age of digital health for all (people, groups and regions). The main themes worked out in the five chapters of this second part are related essentially to privacy issues, to the relationship between health, science and politics, and to the possibilities and warranties of cohesive and inclusive digital societies. The various contributions assume a perspective both critical and propositional, showing the new possibilities open by technological innovation and discussing possible "dangers" and alternative ways of reflection.

Under this scope, Chapter 5, by Pradeep Nair, "The Emerging Concept of an Inclusive mHealth Ecosystem in India," emphasizes the opportunity for more universal connection and access to health care, quickly, effectively, and with quality, through the use of mobile communication. Assuming that the possession and use of mobile phones is relatively widespread throughout the Indian population, the author argues that the use of this technological tool can contribute to greater equity and accessibility to healthcare. This is particularly important in India, as the author points out, because of the strong population growth and the country's difficult health services' coverage, which would require a huge economic investment. The mobile communication allows, in fact, from the author's perspective, not only an adequate and rapid response (ensuring synchronous and fast communication) to the doubts and health problems of the populations, but also, an easier collaboration between several healthcare providers and stakeholders, an efficient connection between "all the information highways of the country" and a better articulation between "health plans and policies into an integrated ecosystem". Thus, as advocated throughout the chapter, mobile communication technologies are not only essential for the future of India healthcare delivery and for the constitution of health ecosystems, but also for the affirmation of inclusive and patient centered health. In addition, the dissemination of information can help to control epidemics by promptly identifying shared symptoms in one or more regions and by releasing hospitals from large population demands and outbreaks of contamination. The author provides also some examples of projects that use mhealth - such as the kilkari, the ananya, the citizen health information system and the mpedigree - and highlights the challenges that integration between health services and professionals can still pose in Indian society. The need of a structural change, in particular in the field of care culture, is therefore essential to change the design and delivery of health care and to produce positive impacts on the welfare and development of the country, thus aggregating social, economic and scientific value.

Cristina Pinto Albuquerque, in the sixth chapter, "The Contribution of Technologies to Promote Healthy Aging and Prevent Frailty in Elderly People," presents the advantages and possibilities associated with the use of technologies and ICT devices to promote positive and healthy ageing, and to the prevention, or minimization, of frailty in elderly people. The use of technological innovation (robotics; domotics; telehealth, etc.) can play, as it is argued across the chapter, an important role allowing real decision possibilities (for example stay home) for elderly people and preventing or controlling frailty. This perspective of intervention in the older ages is coupled with a new research and political interest in innovative experiences that can guide an evidence-based definition of the main priorities for current public health and ageing policies. Several international orientations sets clearly the commitment to "develop age-friendly environments, to align health systems to the needs of older populations, to develop sustainable and equitable systems for providing long-term care (home, communities, institutions), and to improve measurement, monitoring and research on Healthy Ageing". The author underlines, in this perspective, the opportunities open by the application of technologies to support elderly or dependent people: networking and social participation; autonomy and mobility; learning and education, among others. However, the possible obstacles and unexpected effects are also evinced. In fact, technologies can, on one hand, increase the possibilities to minimize social exclusion but, on the other, they can enlarge the possibilities of "digital divide". Additionally the guaranties of safety for elderly people are associated with their capacity to control the technological devices and to the evaluation of their reliability. Thus, as it is underlined, innovative applications must respect privacy and be conceived as pertinent from the elderly people' point of view. Likewise technology cannot be conceived as a panacea to solve all the problems of care systems, or the issues associated with adverse aging problems and inadequate lifestyles and conditions across life. The author presents also, concerning these possible obstacles, some recommendations and reflects around possible solutions.

The seventh chapter, "Managing End-of-Life Information in Palliative Care: Between Discord and Conceptual Blends," authored by Alexandre Cotovio Martins, focuses on the understanding of different ways of perceiving (by the patient, family and health professionals) and managing the information regarding the end-of-life moment in palliative care. Under these conditions, health professionals try to combine conceptual and material structures (notably the physical signs on the bodies of patients close to death) that allow the articulation of different rationalities and reduce the diversity of perceptions of the actors involved. Using this "translation" processes health professionals intend to avoid, in the perspective of the author, the creation of unrealistic expectations and the emergence of certain situations of discord over the trajectories of death and related care procedures. Assuming a micro analysis of the way data concerning dying patients are managed the author discusses thus the quality of care in palliative services. To illustrate the analysis he presents the results of a study carried out in some palliative care services in Portugal. In this study the project team observed that different conceptions of end-of-life processes can affect greatly the interaction between the terminal patients, their families and professionals. These different rationalities have also impacts in the management of patient's terminal care and can engage associated conflicts of interpretation which demands the continuous explanation by health professionals of what is going on, namely the progressive "signs of death" in the patient's body.

The next two chapters focus mainly on a critical reflection on how scientific and medical information is worked out and used to frame a particular sociopolitical message on health, the adequate lifestyle and the standards it seeks to standardize, as well as on the possibilities of manipulation or "collective healing" with the use of digitized information.

That way, Samuel Beaudoin, in Chapter 8, "The Hidden Face of Medical Intervention," presents a critical perspective on the monitoring of information as a power anchored in a scientific rationality that becomes political. The example of reproductive health and the reduction of stillbirths as if it were a scientific imperative is in fact, from the author's perspective, a project that implies a certain way of governing people. Biomedicine thus becomes a project of transformation of man's relationship with himself, with illness, with suffering and with death. The project to change the world - "the best science must lead to better lives" - transposed to the medical-scientific discourse is, in this perspective, mainly political. Under this scope, the author presents, as an example, The Lancet global research project on stillbirths. The chapter seeks to reveal the "debates surrounding equitable access to health care and reveal what is hidden in medical intervention" and the shifts in the interconnection between politics, ethics and science. As the author underscore "The first shift aims to refocus political attention from medical intervention to what makes it possible. The second is a shift in ethical focus from the issue of equitable access to a discussion of the options and consequences of a type of government based on science. The third shift is an invitation to reexamine the processes of knowledge production, moving from unlimited data production to an ethic of research restraint". Following the discussion on solutions and recommendations, the author presents also a third argument concerning the future of research and suggesting that the unlimited production of data on the human body and life hides the failure of progress, which is the very justification for universal coverage.

In the last chapter of the book, "Healing Cultural Personae With the Media Dream," Stephen Brock Schafer defends the perspective that at present times the Information and Communication Technologies (ICTs) are changing the psychological parameters of the human reality. Indications of a mediated and simulated reality by the intervention of the media and digital society have impacts on collective health and require new research and development. The psychological dynamics of interactive images projected as media images correspond, in the perspective advocated by the author, to the psychological and structural dynamics of the dream images, in Carl G. Jung's approach. If this is true, images in the media reflect patterns of energy and information in what Jung called the collective unconscious. Research and discussion on the psychological influence of the media is already ancient, however only recently the research has focused on the neurobiological nature of its influence. The author defends, under this assumption, the perspective that it is possible to reverse and reconstruct these influences, contributing to the preservation of the human autonomy of thought and decision. Computational biofeedback can help, in this regard, to the healing, generation and maintenance of a global culture of consciousness.

In the conclusion, the editor highlights, systematizes and deepens, in a final concluding chapter, the discussion about the main structuring analytical pillars of the book: health conception, innovation, technology, and healthcare quality, health information management and ethical concerns. To this extent, Cristina Pinto Albuquerque seeks to highlight some of the great changes taking place in the field of health by the use of new technologies—surgery 4.0, precision medicine, genetic engineering and human enhancement, devices for continuous monitoring of health status, etc.—and discuss possible resistances to innovation in healthcare. In this context, she advocates the idea that many of the current resistances to innovations in the field of treatment and prevention of disease stem not from the potentially associated technical risks, but of moral dimensions. Under this scope, a deeper debate is required on the relationship between science and ethics and between science and politics. A debate that goes on for the second pillar of the debate. The author seeks, at this level, to reflect on the health care provided, the rationales in confrontation, especially in increasingly multicultural contexts, and on the ways information can be managed in the interconnection between ethical concerns and the economic and managerial pressures of healthcare systems today.

The book constitutes thus a relevant contribution and reflective asset for multiple professionals and stakeholders. The target audience is large and composed of professionals and researchers working in the field of health, social intervention, information management in health care facilities, communication sciences, administrative sciences and management, sociology, computer science, and information technology. The various chapters provide relevant theoretical frameworks and some of the latest empirical research findings in a large scope of health information management. They are written for professionals who want to improve their understanding of the potentialities of technology and innovation to change healthcare management practices, medical practices and health care procedures. The various multidisciplinary contributions also promote the reflection on new ways to protect confidentiality and privacy of patients, as well as the ethical and social associated constraints, and give insights to support executives concerned with the management of expertise, knowledge, information and organizational development in different types of healthcare environments.

Cristina Albuquerque
University of Coimbra, Portugal

REFERENCES

Albuquerque, C. (2016). Social Care and Life Quality of Frail or Dependent Elderly: The Contribution of Technologies. *International Journal of Privacy and Health Information Management*, 4(1), 12–22. doi:10.4018/IJPHIM.2016010102

Antonovsky, A. (1979). *Health, stress and coping*. San Francisco: Jossey-Bass.

Auffray, C., Charron, D., & Hood, L. (2010). Predictive, preventive, personalized and participatory medicine: Back to the future. *Genome Medicine*, 2(8), 57. doi:10.1186/gm178 PMID:20804580

Brodnik, M. S., Rinehart-Thompson, L. A., & Reynolds, R. (2012). *Fundamentals of Law for Health Informatics and Information Management*. Chicago: AHIMA - American Health Information Management Association.

Canguilhem, G. (1989). *The normal and the pathological*. Cambridge, MA: The MIT Press, Zone Books. (Original work published 1943)

Checkland, K., Marshall, M., & Harrison, S. (2004). Re-thinking accountability: Trust versus confidence in medical practice. *Quality & Safety in Health Care*, 13(2), 130–135. doi:10.1136/qshc.2003.009720 PMID:15069221

Connick, R. M., Connick, P., Klotsas, A. E., Tsagkaraki, P. A., & Gkrania-Klotsas, E. (2009). Procedural confidence in hospital based practitioners: Implications for the training and practice of doctors at all grades. *BMC Medical Education*, 9(1), 2. doi:10.1186/1472-6920-9-2 PMID:19138395

European Commission (EC). (2018). Innovation Partnership on Active and Healthy Ageing (EIP on AHA) (2018-2020). Brussels: EC.

Foucault, M. (1976). *Histoire de la sexualité: La volonté de savoir* (Vol. 1). Paris: Les Éditions Gallimard.

Hood, L., & Auffray, C. (2013). Participatory medicine: A driving force for revolutionizing healthcare. *Genome Medicine*, *5*(12), 110. doi:10.1186/gm514 PMID:24360023

Huber, M. A. S. (2014). *Towards a new, dynamic concept of Health. Its operationalisation and use in public health and healthcare, and in evaluating health effects of food* (Unpublished Doctoral dissertation). School for Public Health and Primary Care CAPHRI, Maastricht University, Maastricht.

Hussain, A., Ali, S., Ahmed, M., & Hussain, S. (2018). The Anti-vaccination Movement: A Regression in Modern Medicine. *Cureus*, *10*(7), e2919. doi:10.7759/cureus.2919 PMID:30186724

Jambroes, M., Nederland, T., Kaljouw, M., van Vliet, K., Essink-Bot, M.-L., & Ruwaard, D. (2016). Implications of health as 'the ability to adapt and self-manage' for public health policy: A qualitative study. *European Journal of Public Health*, *26*(3), 412–416. doi:10.1093/eurpub/ckv206 PMID:26705568

Kvedar, J., Coye, M. J., & Everett, W. (2014). Connected health: A review of technologies and strategies to improve patient care with telemedicine and telehealth. *Health Affairs*, *33*(2), 194–199. doi:10.1377/hlthaff.2013.0992 PMID:24493760

Lindström, B., & Eriksson, M. (2005). Salutogenesis. *Journal of Epidemiology and Community Health*, *59*(6), 440–442. doi:10.1136/jech.2005.034777 PMID:15911636

McKinlay, J. B., & Marceau, L. D. (2002). The end of the golden age of doctoring. *International Journal of Health Services*, *32*(2), 379–416. doi:10.2190/JL1D-21BG-PK2N-J0KD PMID:12067037

Messu, M. (2017). Confiance et vitimisation. In M. Messu & C. Albuquerque (Eds.), *Confiance et Barbarie. Pour une anthropologie renouvelée de l'action* (pp. 95–150). Paris: L'Harmattan.

Messu, M. (2018). *L'Ere De La Victimisation*. La Tour d'Aigues: Éditions de l'Aube.

Mittelmark, M. B., Sagy, S., Eriksson, M., Bauer, G., Pelikan, J. M., Lindström, B., & Espnes, G. A. (Eds.). (2017). *The Handbook of Salutogenesis*. Cham: Springer. doi:10.1007/978-3-319-04600-6

OECD. (2013). *ICTs and the Health Sector.Towards Smarter Health and Wellness Models*. Paris: OECD Publishing; doi:10.1787/9789264202863-

Porter, J., Morphet, J., Missen, K., & Raymond, A. (2013). Preparation for high-acuity clinical placement: Confidence levels of final-year nursing students. *Advances in Medical Education and Practice, 4*, 83–89. doi:10.2147/AMEP.S42157 PMID:23900655

WHO. (2015). *World Report on Ageing and Health*. Luxembourg: World Health Organization.

Zheng, H. (2015). Losing confidence in medicine in an era of medical expansion? *Social Science Research, 52*, 701–715. doi:10.1016/j.ssresearch.2014.10.009 PMID:26004490

Zola, I. K. (1982). *Missing Pieces: A Chronicle of Living with a Disability*. Philadelphia, PA: Temple University Press.

ENDNOTES

[1] 'Health is a state of complete physical, mental and social well-being and not merely the absence of disease or infirmity' (WHO, 1948).

[2] Etymologically the notion of health seems to indicate above all the association with an idea of totality, cohesion, strength and wholeness of beings. The medieval root of the concept refers to an idea of perfection with mystical and religious basis. If we look at health concepts in several languages, the notion of integrity seems to be evident. In the Latin root languages, health (saúde, santé, sanidad) derives from the words *salus*, attribute of the integers, and the connotation of "pure, immaculate" and "correct, true", and *salvus*, which indicated the preservation of physical integrity of the subjects. The word "são" (Portuguese) refers thus not only to the idea of absence of disease but also to the conception of holy or perfect, without blemish. The relation with the Greek term holos is also evidenced, which refers to the idea of totality. For example, the term health is associated, in its archaic constitution - Healeth - with the present concept of healed, treated. In Scandinavian variations, the concept refers mainly to the idea of wholeness or completeness. In Swedish, for example, health is hälsa, referring to the Greek notion of holos. It should also be noted that all the words in this semantic family derive from the old Germanic term höl, which means not only wholeness but also - in the hölig root which gives rise to the contemporary word "holy", which means - "sacred."

3   The Alma Ata Declaration (1978) places health as a fundamental human right by emphasizing the connection between health inequalities and socio-economic inequalities. The same idea is underlined in the "Health for All by the year 2000" Declaration (1981) and in the "Ottawa Charter for Health Promotion "(1986). In the 8th Global Conference on Health Promotion (Helsinki, 2013), the need to create the conditions for the realization of health ideals through a shared and integrated "health in all policies" approach, is accentuated.

4   Particularly interesting is the recent transformation of the Hippocratic Oath reflecting a new understanding of the medical profession and of medical ethics and deontology. In 2017 a new wording was endorsed by the World Medical Association. The central shift is the emphasis on patient autonomy - "I will respect the autonomy and dignity of my patient". Comparing the versions of 1948 and 2017 interesting insights emerge revealing a new way of conceiving healthcare in a changing axiological and political context. The 1948 version states: "I will maintain the utmost respect for human life from the time of conception"; "Even under threat, I will not use my medical knowledge contrary to the laws of humanity"; "I will maintain by all means in my power, the honor and the noble traditions of the medical profession, my colleagues will be my brothers ". In the 2017 version: "I will maintain the utmost respect for human life"; "I will not use my medical knowledge to violate human rights and civil liberties, even under threat"; "I will foster the honor and noble traditions of the medical profession". The UNESCO Declaration on Bioethics and Human Rights, adopted by UNESCO's General Conference on 19 October 2005, adds an important reflection on societal changes and even on global balances brought about by scientific and technological developments. To the already difficult question posed by life sciences - How far can we go? - other queries must be related to the relationship between ethics, science and freedom "(http://www.unesco.org/new/en/social-and-human-sciences/themes/bioethics/bioethics-and-human-rights). It is particularly relevant the introduction of patients' perceptions and expectations about healthcare and scientific developments in the creation of the Declaration.

5   The anti-vaccination movement acquires currently many followers in Western countries. Many parents are refusing to vaccinate their children due to differentiated reasons: scientific (the fear of associated diseases); ideological and legal (vaccines are only a business of large laboratories; they put in question the liberty of citizens in healthcare concerns) or religious (control of diseases is against the will of God). The "scientific fear", especially against the measles, mumps and rubella vaccine (MMR), is very associated with the publication (in 1998), by the prominent British journal The Lancet, of Andrew's Wakefield study that claimed the causal relationship between the vaccine and the autism

syndrome in some children. Even if the results were false - as some researchers proved after - the study produced a very severe reaction concerning vaccination. In fact the reaction against vaccines is very ancient. In 1772, Reverend Edmund Massey in his well-known sermon "The Dangerous and Sinful Practice of Inoculation", classified the vaccines as "diabolical operations". In the 19th century when vaccines became mandatory in England the Anti-Vaccination League was formed, defending the arguments of liberty protection against the invasion of the State in the private sphere of citizens' decision. Currently the anti-vaccination movement continues active questioning – against all kinds of scientific evidences about the conquests of modern medicine - the advantages of vaccination. In Pakistan, for example, many children continue to die because Taliban banned and killed health workers under the argument that vaccination was a strategy to do espionage and control.

Acknowledgment

The editor would like to acknowledge the help of all the people involved in this project. Without their support, this book would not have become a reality.

First, our sincere gratitude goes to the chapter's authors who contributed their time and expertise to this book.

Second, the editor wishes to acknowledge the valuable contributions of the reviewers regarding the improvement of quality, coherence, and content presentation of chapters. We highly appreciate their double task.

Most special thanks to Professor Michel Messu for his personal support and magnificent contribution to the reflection and discussion about the book contents' and the Final Remarks.

Finally, the Editor would also like to acknowledge the support of IGI Global and specially Ms. Jordan Tepper's invaluable help in the course of the editorial process.

Cristina Albuquerque
University of Coimbra, Portugal

Section 1
Health Information Management:
Emerging Trends, Challenges, and Impacts

Chapter 1
Approaching Information Architecture for a Market Intelligence System Based on Emerging Technologies

George Leal Jamil
https://orcid.org/0000-0003-0989-6600
Informações em Rede Consultoria e Treinamento Ltda., Brazil

Leandro R. Santos
IN3 Inteligencia de Mercado LTDA, Brazil

Liliane C. Jamil
Independent Researcher, Brazil

Augusto P. Vieira
Independent Researcher, Brazil

ABSTRACT

It was observed, in these last years, the consolidation of the market intelligence (MI) concept as a source of competitive results in several strategic ways, impacting decision-making and entrepreneurship. This article intends to explore the conceptualization of the MI process, observing specially its application in Healthcare sector under the emergence of new technologies. Approaching the healthcare market, a framework for an intelligence system for marketing decisions was discussed and it is now evaluated with the contribution of information architecture and new technologies concepts. The review formerly produced is updated regarding the focus of the MI system under the influences and potentialities for emerging technologies application, through a lemma of "digital transformation" (DT), validating and expanding market intelligence background towards new dynamism and application in Healthcare contexts.

DOI: 10.4018/978-1-5225-8470-4.ch001

INTRODUCTION

When the actual corporative scenario is observed, it is possible to understand how information management, as an essential strategic process, has been challenged. Business environments are overloaded with disorganized data and information contexts, spread throughout the organization and productive chain. This fact underlines the reason for usual lack of consistency for strategic and tactical decisions, such as critical marketing planning, where a mistake can lead to a risky situation, as an error in product offer, misinterpretation of customer needs or definition of incoherent prices which can result in financial losses or opportunistic chances for competitors. Based on a former work, this chapter updates the view for market intelligence (MI) cycle under the emergence of new technologies, aiming to improve understanding in the case of Healthcare sector.

Market intelligence process focus on the systemic supply of knowledge for strategic marketing planning and subsequent execution in one organization. In this case, we choose healthcare industry, as the sector to be reasoned for the MI update comprehension. Market movements signals how Healthcare, along with its obvious attributes on being directly related to our lives, is interesting to study as a technology-driven and intensively competitive scenario, where knowledge has been applied for millennia, in attempt to adequate quality levels to final offer of services. Information architecture, as presented in Jamil *et al.* (2014), is a conceptual background that can perfectly provide substance for a marketing intelligence process definition, as this knowledge generating business cycle can help companies solve emerging problems for their strategic marketing planning.

As a methodological approach, the chapter initially presents a literature review of fundamental and recent concepts to develop the understanding of information architecture and marketing intelligence. This analysis is made from contributions of different scientific areas aiming to relate intelligence basis to information and knowledge management systems. After this review, a summary overview of concepts behind emerging technologies is developed, allowing for a further discussion around its application for MI results in Healthcare context. With this approach in mind, it was possible to produce a result that can base further researches and works through theoretical improvement on MI relations to technology and to its application in this sector and others, serving as a contribution for scholars and practitioners.

THEORETICAL BACKGROUND

In this section, concepts will be discussed to form the fundamental base for market intelligence system theoretical background. This section is structured approaching first the basic descriptions, then information architecture, completed by an overview of emerging technologies and its possible application in corporative, marketing arenas and contexts. This aims to produce a solid base to develop the reflections around an updated view of MI cycle and how it is applied, for instance, for Healthcare processes and decisions.

Basic Concepts

As main elements for knowledge production, thinking a potential knowledge management process, concepts of data, information and knowledge, itself, must be addressed, along with its possible management in one organizational context. According to Davenport and Prusak (2000), Tuomi (2000) and Jamil (2005), data is regarded as a signal or value, directly measured, calculated or collected from an automatic source, or through a human intervention. Usual quantities, as number of events (number of cars in one road, for example), temperature and other physical units, metrical system, etc. are amongst the endless set of examples of data. These are simple items, easy to get, store and transfer, although they lack meaning, not providing valuable decision capabilities, denoting eventual incompleteness. As a development of data concept, information is regarded as a collection of correlated data plus a context, identifying where or how it was generated. It provides a better condition for deciding, but offers more complexity as gathered data must be treated or processed, forming a standardized, based collection to result in useful information. Information increases decision capabilities but demands additional work to be observed and applied as a coherent set.

Speaking about a possible cyclic fashion, data is collected or generated automatically or in a more spontaneous way in several human transactions and interactions. Information became opportune, as data producers are more interested on understanding the complete picture where data was collected or generated. An interesting provocation arises when we think about automatic systems, of various sources and provisions, produce data and data sets intensively, as in some "industry 4.0" solutions. As this happens, information and knowledge are opportune concepts and relations to be studied.

Knowledge allows maximum perception of a scenery evolution, for example, enabling more complex decisions and even prediction capabilities (Davenport, 2000; Akbar, 2003; Jamil, 2005). But on the other hand, knowledge is difficult to manage, understanding it as a process composed of functions such as gathering, registering, sharing and valuating knowledge, along with other tasks related to specific organizational interests (Choo, 2003; Kearns & Lederer, 2003). For that snack price example, its evolution, related to estimate demand, is a more complex study, which results in the knowledge about its variation, demand and consumption.

Information systems are defined by O´Brien & Marakas (2008) and Stair & Reynolds (2009) as sets of interrelated components that are applied to perform several informational functions as collect, process, share, publish, store and control information, reaching the perspective of knowledge creation. This definition contributes to those practiced by Turban, Rainer & Potter (2007), when authors evaluated how information technology projects can be sought as systemic tools, not only operational implements. These concepts result in one approach on how IT application is an infrastructure implemented to produce knowledge in one organizational chain, specified by an information system design, motivations and projects (Davenport, 2000; Choo, 2005; Nonaka, 2008; Celaschi, 2017).

Several authors have been working on knowledge management (KM) concept. Here, it is possible to refer to Nonaka (2008), where the author describes KM as a process designed to deal with the generation, storage, dissemination, usage monitoring and valuation of knowledge in any organizational activity (Clark Jr., Jones & Armstrong, 2007; El-Bashir, Collier & Sutton, 2011). This way, we have the first overlook for the conception of market intelligence cycle, defining MI as a process which can be understood as a typical instance of knowledge management specific for strategic marketing applications (Jamil, 2014).

As a contextual delimitation, these concepts can be gathered to relate IT resources as constituents for an essential infrastructure platform to build information systems (Kearns & Lederer, 2003; Jamil, 2005) and usage on managerial systems solution (Clark Jr., Jones & Armstrong, 2007; Nonaka, 2008; Kimball & Ross, 2010) to support corporative decisions. In this case, organizational intelligence, as it was studied by Huber (1990), can be fostered by "advanced information technologies", defined as an organizational action designed to cyclically produce knowledge for decisions. It is possible to relate new, emerging technologies for this purpose, as to produce the relationship focused by this chapter, to market intelligence under information architecture background.

At this point, it is opportune to refer that IT resources offers, depending on a coherent system design and overall conditions for its application, alternatives to develop and implement intelligence functions for organizations (Davenport & Prusak, 2000; Jamil, 2005; Clark Jr., Jones & Armstrong, 2007; El-Bashir, Collier & Sutton, 2011). Information system design fundamentals and its associated processes, such as knowledge management and strategic planning integration, can be, thinking this way, decisive to implement these functions for an organization and as an integrative project where emerging technologies can be applied through a disciplined, guided and reliable base, encompassing information architecture principles, which will be discussed in the following.

Information Architecture (IA)

Producing a fundamental context from two or more powerful conceptual background can result in a multidisciplinary base to promote comprehension on objective themes. Information Architecture (IA) is so an interesting and opportune contextualization where this level can be reached. Architecture is a scientific field which apply design principles, considering esthetical and functional aspects of constructions, taking into considerations user interests, social and environmental repercussions, cultural and historical influences and constructive factors (RIBA, 2014; RAIC, 2014; IAB, 2014). It is a classical, broad area of scientific knowledge whose most known results are those of remarkable, artistic, useful, cultural and social propositions that cooperate with civil construction techniques and projects. These fundamental aspects of Architecture form a first level of relationship with information management, making it possible to study IA as the intention, need and plan to produce optimal, esthetical, rationalized and efficient blueprints of information processes and artifacts in one organization life cycle (Jamil, 2014).

Information architecture appears as a continuously debated concept, recently explored by academic and practical area, which conceptual definitions and delimitations are still in discussion, some related to software design applications, interface design, operational issues, etc. which is considered important, but only a part of a possible conceptualization for information architecture (Jamil *et al.,* 2015). First remarkable provocations around an IA concept arose when Richard Saul Wurman, a renowned architect, argued about the need for modelling structures that allowed the overall perception and productive control of information, reaching to a basic level of management. This anxiety about the information uncontrolled proliferation increased, as it is still something apparently easy to produce, difficult to store in an organized way and difficult to control, with the inclusion of systems, data generator devices (as those entitled as "internet of things" or "cloud systems", among many others). "Controlling" anything is also a critical issue, becoming focus of several studies not approached here, which take into consideration the dilemma around limitations, restrictions, management and improvement, as perceptions of the control concept itself. It has been applied to managerial contexts, among many others, in this aspect of doubt, contraposing needs, desires and impossibilities on controlling information and other organizational assets.

Wurman´s worries still challenge researchers and market professionals, as data has increased its relevance as a strategic item, resulting in a more complex demand for information management and control. Information architecture was defined as a background that promotes a logical arrangement, providing methods for various information-related functions as identification, classification, mapping, storage organization, systematic access, among many others, with positive implications for several critical organizational areas, as information systems design and plans – Stair & Reynolds (2008) –, information technology specifications – Turban, Mc Lean & Wetherbee (2002), Lucas Jr. (2005) or Turban, Rainer Jr. & Potter (2007) – and, as for an objective for this study, helping to define market intelligence cycles and its related process Choo (1996), Jamil (2001), Choo (2005) and Nonaka (2008). Other authors also refer to information architecture approaching information usage, for organizational tasks, such as decision or risk management processes, which can be depicted by IA principles and methods application (Leidner & Elam (1995); Marchand, Kettinger, & Rollins (2001); Inmon, Strauss & Neushloss, G. (2008)).

There have been efforts on detailing IA, as Dillon (2002), who presented a dual view of information architecture, identifying the tactical, user related information architecture as small IA. This specific view of IA relates so to its immediate usage, answers from automated systems for immediate decisions, notification of events to interested users and so on. On the other hand, big IA relates to a wider view of information architecture, where it relates to its strategic management, provision for complex decision-making, planning and overall structuration of a complete organization from its general coordination point, observing, this way, a more complex context where information was produced, adopted, acquired and registered. A stricter way to conceptualize it, perhaps, should be citing it as micro and macro information architecture contexts, tuning these conceptualizations to other fields, such as strategy or information systems, with similar analysis and denominations.

This view was also supported by Bailey (2002), where operational aspects for information, as finding, navigating, storing and updating, were enunciated as elements, which compose the needed architectural plan or project, reaching its application. Morville & Rosenfeld (2009) defined information architecture in four different ways: (1) It is a "structural design of shared information environments"; (2) In web services context "organization, labeling, (prepare for) search and navigation systems"; (3) The "art and science of shaping information products and experiences to support usability and findability", and (4) IA as an "emerging discipline and community of practice focused on bringing principles of design to the digital landscape". This last definition enlightens the fact that IA is a recent, dynamic, innovative field that must be studied and developed. Those four elements of definition also base the works of Information Architect Institute (IA Institute, 2014). The powerful work from Morville and Rosenfeld depicts how information conception demands a thorough study, this way encompassed by a wide contextual concept, such as information architecture, resulting in a view that involves other scientific bases, such as Design, Process, Production management, Projects, etc. and permits the multidisciplinary and dynamic view for this consolidation.

Completing this study for IA conceptualization, Covert (2014) states that IA is "a set of concepts that can help anyone do anything to make sense of messes caused by facts related to the main object, as misinformation, disinformation, not enough, too much information". From this point of view, it is possible to understand that Wurman´s motivations over the need for information architecture are still present, and facts as those categorized as "Big Data" (Mc Kinsey, 2011; Ohata & Kumar, 2012; Park, Huh, Oh & Han, 2012; McAfee & Brynjolfsson, 2012; Budford, 2014) suggest that information is easier and faster to be produced these days, generating even the perception of an "information overload". A first relationship to emerging technologies, this way, is presented, reinforcing this article intention on advancing former observations regarding the association with these innovative implements to information architecture.

Consolidating these definitions, the following set of definitions for IA was revised, from Jamil *et al* (2015):

- It is a functional, application-related concept.
- It is always exercised also in function of information usage – retrieval, application, etc. – by an end-user. This way, it is an actor-involved conceptualization.
- IA relates to information classification, correlation and documentation for usability purposes.
- As Architecture can be understood as a discipline for illustrating building projects, information architecture has potentialities, in a wider and more complexity than the simple construction of information systems maps, although it is one of its results.
- It is a conceptual platform for its own planning, as it offers structures for information management, represented by standardized symbols, methods, professional profiles, among many other resources.
- Its organizational contributions are precisely related to processes and subsystems which store, classify, identify (allowing posterior optimal and safe retrieval) and define forms of usage for any information.

As a managerial maturity level, as one organization evolves, information architecture adoption encompasses several abilities, competences and aspects which result in more capabilities for one organization as to deal with information in a wider and contextualized way, resulting in a strategic continent that will favor competitive advantage around its applications (Jamil, 2014).

Before we advance to market relations, a brief overview about some of the emerging technologies has to be developed, completing the intended theoretical background.

An Overview for Emerging Technologies

It would be very ambitious to consolidate and discuss emerging technologies in one section of a chapter, alone, as this topic seems to be undelimited at this moment. Market providers and commercial players, along with practitioners, exert a powerful pressure over academic studies these days, as scientific discussion is still trying to cope and understand the implications and goals of some of these technologies, as they could be applied in corporative and organizational usual processes. Here, we inserted just some limited, objective exerts which allow the reader to merely understand names, expressions and themes related to these technologies, in order to observe their application in Healthcare context for market intelligence supporting services.

This analysis starts with the simple although powerful set of tools called "Analytics." It was stated, in Jamil (2018), as a process regarded to produce knowledge from internet interactions, supported by IT infrastructure and tools. According to (Jamil & Magalhães, 2015), as data is produced massively in such systems and environments, more contextual knowledge can be produced, defining new contexts for its usage, dynamically. A special attention is paid to modern strategic and marketing systems, which can produce fast reactions to costumers' interests and provocative interactions, composing productive and motivational answers, as analytical tools where dynamism is the main support, evolving the customer relationships to a higher level of power. These systems, nowadays, provide infrastructural base for several platforms, such as a simple e-mail service to a customized market-driven insurance selling system, where the user potentially wants a more reliable and continuous perception of value in his or her interactions. They are found and implemented through e-commerce websites, mass commerce web services, associative sites, social media and, mainly, through mobile systems "apps", enabling a wide capability on collecting and objectively analyzing to provide immediate customer behavior comprehension.

This way, analytics can, in a superficial level, create profiles on how customers can, for instance, react in a campaign, announcement or behave, as a typical member of a group of users, regarding any business proposition, really differing internet-based services from old physical, traditional ones, as analytical prospections can be done quickly, answering to users´ potential needs or, eventually, predicting future behaviors (Chau & Xu, 2012; Choo, 2005; SAS, 2014; Doneria, Vinodani, 2017; SAS, 2017).

Another related service or resource, which is characteristic for our observation about new tools to build a new context for IM processes is Big Data. As seen from El-Gayar & Timsina (2014), big data methods are applied to both structure and then provide analysis from structured and unstructured data sets, improving overall condition to obtain results about interactions in different medias. This way, Big data services can be applied through contents available in an open scope of registered, which covers from formal information systems – as Accounting, Control or Supply chain – where, usually, quantitative data is stored and processed through social media, blogs, instant messengers and several other data sets, where posts and informal publications, along with audio and video are registered by users (Johnson, 2012; Hoffman, 2013; SAS, 2014; Gallos et al.,2017). Relating those contents is still a challenging process, as it remains difficult to find reliable sources originated by the same person or agent, but there is a recognition of fast-evolving field, as it has been shown by video and audio processing, including the implementation of machine learning and deep learning algorithms, where contents are being tested and, effectively, learned (Vayena, Blasimme & Cohen, 2018).

Big data main outcomes will produce results as to identify customer interactions with a service, prediction analysis, knowledge creation and dynamic profiling, leading to a wider and deeper context for comprehension around business and systems phenomena. In marketing processes, for example, it will allow an expansion of learning and servicing, enabling the implementation of automated answering and interaction systems – known as chatbots or simply bots – that offer a trend for replacing human repetitive and exhaustive tasks, as similar situations that happened some years ago, with "call centers" business adoption.

Considering the "harder" side, an overlook of physical implementations, it is opportune to cite the simple but easy to implement RFID-based systems (Ngai, 2010). Basically, it consists on a capsule or implement that associates a tiny memory resource, a battery and an antenna, which allows a continuous sending of identification code, serving as a piece of registering which can be instantaneously perceived by a reader or decoder, serving to implement fast recognition systems. Its main application is on routine processes, such as those related to supply chains dispatch, stock control, basic registering and several others, efficiently reaching huge and complex systems in ports, docks and airports – luggage, load and vehicles (Liukonnen, 2012). As a basic communication component, RFID implements can easily integrate to any system, providing what can be called the basics for an IM cycle, as to identify each component, part or assembled composition that must be associated with decision. Overall, it is another piece of hardware which allow data generation continuously (Jamil, 2015).

One comprehensive evolution of RFID connectors, implementations and systems is Internet of things implementations, or IoT, as it is generally called. IoT resources enable not only systemic identification, but also provide a versatile, semi or complete autonomously connection through internet wide range of communications and interactions, serving to build the main structure of what can be regarded as an intelligent system (Sun et al., 2012; Yunbiao, 2016). Adding the flexibility of internet-based applications, IoT systems is a context where new devices, smart or intelligent apparatus, are being conceived, as it does not only collect and / or stores data, but also can issue and receive commands from human operators or from other IoT devices, connected through an array. These implements are on the realm of new implementations of artificial intelligence projects, encompassing solutions of machine and deep learning, under automated algorithms.

One peculiarity along the IoT systems, this way, is to consider that the "end-user point", or the final contact with the user has plenty capability of processing and interaction, resulting in new possibilities, as to offer smart devices in replacement of static old ones (Turber & Smiela, 2014). One thermometer, for example, could send a message to one hospital pharmacy asking to provide anti-thermal medicine to one patient who was sampled with fever for the second time in a previewed sequence of tests. So, this is an evolutionary concept, which transforms the data collection / provision point to a higher-level of knowledge storage and retention, with future potentialities on building and developing more interconnected knowledge regarding a phenomenon being monitored.

Artificial intelligence is not a new or emerging topic (Lunin & Smith, 1984), but the alternatives to bring it to customers and end user interactions are becoming remarkably available nowadays. This way, it is possible to implement it in an easier way in customer-oriented software and machinery in information systems projects, reaching the way of the mobile "apps" platforms (Skansi, 2018). As an evolution of its opportune offer in markets, artificial intelligence is translated into products through two main evolutive propositions: machine learning and deep learning.

Machine learning is an implementation which aims to produce artificial intelligence by "learning from humans" (Balasubramaniam, 2018) through code programming or training from several different ways – repetitive procedures, as the industrial automatic systems or even sampling signals from a production line and developing a statistics-based model which aims to reproduce all operative tasks. Machine Learning promotes artificial intelligence as to allow machines to repeat and operationally optimize what human operators do. As to deep learning, it is possible to understand an expressive development, as machines, equipped with algorithms that allow them to store a codification of inter-relations of facts and knowledge domains, "learn", modelling and storing relations developed with these observations from the real field (Malik, 2017).

Simply speaking, artificial intelligence reaches customer relations scenario through a series of facilities, such as answering avatars in e-commerce systems, interactive structures in services of massive commercialization companies, information in public services systems, prediction of behaviors for human operators or events, like weather conditions and so forth. As these systems are available in states where they are "learning" progressively, reaching higher level of standards recognition every day, it is perceivable how they are advancing with human interactions, generating expectations that they will replace humans for repetitive tasks and services, in a new wave of technology insertion in the market.

Other areas which are experiencing a fast evolution and have plenty potential to be implemented in solutions for the market, specially speaking about Healthcare, are visual recognition and processing systems, commercially characterized as "virtual reality" or "augmented reality" resources and cognitive computing. Virtual reality proposes to generate a hypothetical view for some phenomena or context, based on data and information previously collected. This new scenario is hypothetical, it does not exist indeed, can be generated for training, simulation or other teaching purposes (as in games, for example). Augmented reality, on its way, intends to offer an expanded view of a real scenario, composing an additional picture of something that is real. Both are related to video implements such as special screens, eye glasses or panels, which translates data and information to visual contents to be processed and lived by users.

As the technology and its bases advance every day, other services and resources are launched, put available in the market. Together with powerful players, such as information technology and consulting companies, new corporations who develop interesting technologies can offer promotions and new implements in the market, which can extend this list in the future. Here, just a glance of technologic implements that allows us to advance our analysis in this chapter was discussed.

Intelligence and Its Relation to a Market Systematic Approach

At a first glance, intelligence concept can be detailed from several contributions from fields like Information Science, Management, Strategic planning, Information Systems, Information technology among many others. For instance, one of the latest and most discussed observations is "business intelligence", which comes from conceptions around information technology resources application in corporative decisions that can be reviewed with the influence of emerging technologies (Kimball & Ross, 2010, El-Bashir, Collier & Sutton, 2011). The opportune review will be held in the last section of this chapter, as cases are discussed. As presented by Jamil (2018), this concept has been expanded with big data analytics actions and implementations.

As presented in Inmon, Strauss & Nishloss (2008), business intelligence systems and associated processes are structured around elements identified as data warehouses (as complex organizational data collections, a gathering of associated and related databases) and other data collectors, such as data mining programs and infrastructures. For Kimball & Ross (2010), the function of information providers must be defined as a high-level component being responsible for the service effectively connected to business intelligence solutions. As an architectural element for information management, it is opportune to define BI as a context where these classical and new tools and methods can be defined and studied, allowing the intended development (Yonce *et al.*2018).

For Cao, Zhang & Liu (2006), in another perspective, business intelligence is built by the composition of such set of technologic tools, together with ontological procedures (or engineering, as called by the authors) in order to perform in a high-level knowledge generation and application for an enterprise environment, resulting in a "intelligent system", this way encompassing emerging technologies, such as information management-oriented like analytics and big data (Boncea et al., 2017; Yonce et al., 2018). Observing intelligence concept, it is valuable to understand it as composed in a context where knowledge, information and data are managed for decision making with the help of an integrated set of technologic infrastructures. Opportunely, there is a cyclic, process principle in the business intelligence application, through its continuous organizational usage, which produces knowledge. This cyclic structuration is one of the basic principles around the concept for MI process.

Artificial intelligence is an expression formerly announced by the researcher John McCarty in a conference at the Dartmouth College in 1956. This pioneer conceptualization helped define a discipline sometimes related to philosophy or, alternatively, understood as a computational engineering support for automated or robotic system. This area evolved independently or applied with several other associated topics (as Computing Science, for example), with an extensive discussion that is also driven by numberless informal citations, movies, articles, stories and theories that analyze how a computer system, understood as a group of computers, software and infrastructure, can gather information and knowledge about a reality, and based on stored rules and process fundamentals, take decisions, learn another set of rules or simply inform anyone about an important event.

As stated before, nowadays, artificial intelligence domain is more defined, exactly by the introduction of machine learning – towards repetition and imitation of human behaviors – and deep learning – an effective level of learning, that guides implementations of knowledge domain developments which, by its turn, enables an automat to produce decisions, develop situational memory and create its own logical and knowledge relationships (Russel & Norvig, 2009; Buch, Ahmed. & Maruthappu, 2018).

There are two important fundamentals in artificial intelligence context that can be considered for our conceptualization. First, it is a cyclic, continuous process, where "learning" can occur by the accumulative storing of situations, risks, problem solutions and several other ways a machine, or group of machines, equipped with the correct and adequate infrastructure, can develop an organized perception of the reality (Jamil, 2015). The second aspect relates on how this learning can be implemented. It is usual that artificial intelligence systems are coded to operate with a base of rules, defined as mathematical and algorithms that can be added, upgraded, with new conceptions developed from the real world (Buch, Ahmed. & Maruthappu, 2018).

One last scenario which cooperates to this definition for intelligence cycle is given by Competitive Intelligence process, as structured in SCIP (2011) and by Kahaner (1998) and Miller (2002), where a process of data and information collection, towards a provision of a strategic answer to a planning session or intervention is produced. It is a continuous process, so configuring an organizational continuum that has the goal to provide better decision support, specifically for strategic levels in any organization.

Concluding, market intelligence (MI) process was discussed by Weiss and Verma (2002), aligned with a definition of a marketing information system (MIS). This approach helps define MI process as applicable to a practical decision context and will be the focus for our case discussion in the following, observing the planning moment of strategic marketing actions. Also, from Marketing information systems (MISs) literature, as defined by Kotler & Keller (2008) and Laudon & Laudon (2009) it is possible to find an explanation on how these components can be implemented together in order to process data and information to be applied for complex decisions in Marketing planning studies.

Other works that validate the conceptualization of market intelligence as a process which provides continuous deliver of knowledge for strategic marketing planning, are Schiffman & Kanuk (2007), Kotler & Keller (2008), Leidner & Elam (1995) Clark Jr., Jones & Armstrong (2007) and Ferrel & Hartline (2010), in several decision scenarios, related to strategy to tactics under marketing conceptions. In one example, Markovitch, Steckel and Yeung (2005) researched how variations in stock prices could impact ways that executives can take decisions in the corporative world, calling this application of knowledge to study effects and implications of stock variations as "market intelligence", extending our conception to this other aspect, but reinforcing its cyclic structure proposition.

In the next section, we advance to decision cases scenario, where a review of a previous study – Jamil *et al.* (2016) will be held, considering emerging technologies.

Marketing Intelligence System Design Issues: A Technology-Based Review for Healthcare

In this conclusive section, the market intelligence cycle will be rethought, observing information architecture principles, to understand opportunities to apply some of the emerging technologies described above, using Healthcare examples and cases.

Initially, to explore market intelligence cycle in this simulated context, it is important to review the conceptual proposition. MI process can be defined as the process detailed in the figure 1.

Based on these definitions, market intelligence process is defined as the following continuous process, in a cycle definition (Jamil, 2014; Jamil, 2015):

Phase I: Pre-cycle Market analysis:

- **Aggregated chain value conception:** Enables to understand precisely how the organizational arrangement where the MI cycle will occur and has its results applied.
- **Data and information diagnosis:** To identify where business sector contents of data and information can be found, as a mapping component that represents what is available for the process design.
- **Knowledge requirements:** To conceive, initially, what are the main contents of knowledge demanded for typical market decisions.

Figure 1. Market intelligence cycle (Source: Author)

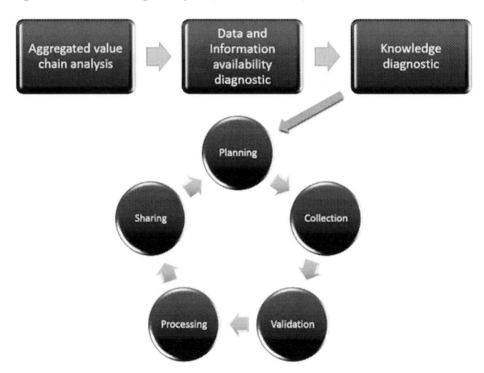

Phase II: MI process cycle (modeling and implementation):

- **Planning:** As a start / stop point of every cycle, it is a step of planning next cycle execution based on auditing success and failures of the last cycle execution.
- **Collection:** It is the automated or manual gathering of data and information from organizations of the sector analyzed, from sources indicated by the mapping effort in the first phase.
- **Validation:** Correction of data and information collected, as those sources can produce different or mistreated contents that must be leveled to become understandable as similar for cyclic analysis.
- **Processing:** Usage of business rules, logic modeling, statistical and mathematical analysis applied to data and information to produce specified knowledge contexts.
- **Sharing:** Results of the processing are delivered, presented, transmitted to interested market players for further application in their decision scenarios, through training sessions, social and technological implementations.

After this presentation, it is important to state, initially, that market intelligence cycle was proposed to adhere to information architecture principles, where data and information are dealt – collected, generated and produced, along with its processing – to reach the intended decision-context results. Overall, emerging technologies can be studied in several different and integrative scenarios, recurring to the cases previously discussed in Jamil (2014), as it follows.

Associating Market Intelligence, Information Architecture, and Emerging Technologies

Data collection turns out to be a critical and diverse process in this new paradigm, where emerging technologies, such as big data and analytics allow to gather its contents from several sources (Gallos et al., 2017). For example, demographic analysis, taken from public and institutional information services, can describe population composition, characteristics and habits, allowing medium and long-term strategies to be designed in order to answer public events, such as epidemic surges (flu outbreak, for example) and social or demographic seasonal events, such as bad weather (heatwaves, blizzards, etc.) associated diseases, defining a typical profile of one population. With this description in mind, one Healthcare unit, as a clinic or hospital, can design policies and plans to enable its logistics and management towards answering more predictable events in the future. Hiring skilled personnel, scheduling resources application and availability, optimized financial planning, among several other actions can be planned, enabling forecasts and control of resources, in a dynamic strategic design.

Other tools to collect data can be integrated to surgical planning, as internet of things sensors, to be provided to follow patients with different degrees of needs and demands by the Healthcare professional staff. If some event, which demands detailed analysis, such as detection of a disease progression, demands, according to patient profile, the intervention of a specialist, he or she can be immediately invoked by the sensor, directly. It is important to notice that a well-designed routine can demand this professional intervention, according with the sending of a logistics robot with specific medicine to the patient room and, overall, provide information update to Healthcare unit managers, informing about the development of this specific treatment.

The main difference from other static implementations is that IoT resources can be programmed to be efficient in reaction and producing all the related, interconnected actions, automating several steps of Healthcare work, providing fast and standardized actions and answers, when they are recommendable (according to unit´s standards, under regulatory requirements). These implementations allow also communication with formal and routine procedures and systems, as, for example, those applied for stock management, professional payroll, etc. RFID tags and its associated installations can be implemented, enabling communication with automated robots, for example, in the surgery room or in the medicine warehouse, optimizing resources and time.

Visual support for simulations, with augmented reality, can allow doctors to expand their evaluation of clinical and surgical situations, adding auxiliary functions for their critical decision-making. Integrating special exams, as X-rays, tomography and MRIs, for example, in a visual context, could enable a more detailed comprehension, for a medical doctor, about the health status of one patient. Along with cognitive computing, a better way to treat some condition, including the risk and collateral implications, can improve control for one specific treatment, also bringing optimization of resources. It is important to mention that, at this time, surgical robots are becoming increasingly applied in Hospitals, in an initial and irreversible way for Healthcare services.

Infrastructure can also be a base for new services in Healthcare organizations. For instance, "cloud"-resident and associated information systems can produce a distributed or shared environment where information can be collected and spread easily, according with corporative, legal and governed standards. This way, a digital transformation which can result in a high-performance, global arrangement of corporative bases that can allow a patient to be answered instantaneously and without interruption in different places, can adhere completely to information architecture definitions (Tadeu et al., 2018). This architecture, by its turn, is an adequate situation to implement a market intelligence system, which will analyze data collected from events related to patients – clearly without intervening with any problem regarding safety or privacy – and produce dynamic results for marketing strategies which provide services for a patient as he or she was in his hometown. These dynamics can result in a marketing optimized scenario, where value is positioned to the customer in a transparent way, at the same time when data and information is processed to produce knowledge that will offer conditions for services optimization.

This last system could be efficiently connected to those devices, approached in the first paragraphs of this section, IoT and RFID, to compose an architecture to attend tougher problems in real-time, depending on characteristics of each patient and the Healthcare center specialty.

Data analysis is another aspect that can be both proposed and generated through these systems, encompassing the actuation of deep learning-based answering machines and apparatus. In the future, some of the Healthcare basic services could be designed to be offered by "bots", presented in semi-human features, as robotized call-centers or service centers. These structures can allow a first level answer to patients, as to clarify basic doubts on taking a medicine, testing for some basic symptoms (as to send this patient to be observed by a specific doctor) or, maybe, to be in contact with an automated robot for a small, controlled and remotely supervised intervention. A science-fiction scenario is coming to real offer, as artificial intelligence is now at the operational point, exactly demanding applicable policies and practices to become an efficient service in complex organizations, as Hospitals, clinics and research institutes.

A function always desired by strategic marketing is forecasting or predicting customer movements, toward possible offers in the future. Anticipating customer needs is one of the main wishes of marketing planners, as these professionals will attempt to position value offers as to fulfill customer needs at the same moment these demands are noticed. In Healthcare, patient needs can be critical, as we can find in situations where demographic signals – aging, economy factors, migration, etc. – can pose various problems for organizations to serve customers efficiently. Also, a demand on managing correctly all events regarding to the progress of customers health, promote a reasonable condition to evolve market relationships, resulting in a potential branding strategy and longer customer transaction processes, retaining negotiations around value offers. These are typical projections usually done by marketing managers.

In here, when all emerging technologies can be well deployed, integrating a scenario where customers services are identified since the beginning, or, eventually, even before it starts, as some predictions can be developed, long-term relationships can be produced as when technology is offered for long-term relations. For instance, when following a patient who is facing a genetic disease, reliable exams can be offered to his or her relatives, in order to provide a careful and prompt answer to any manifestation regarding a possible occurrence of that problem. Information management can be, this way, associated to risk management plans for customers, providing an anticipation of health problems, based on statistical and market intelligence-processed knowledge.

Finally, as it is usual for Healthcare providers, there are numberless regulatory issues when serving patients, as reporting diagnostics and associated treatments. One of the main reasons usually found in these relations, is to inform governmental and regulatory organizations about any event, allowing reaction to occurrences that demand risk plans to be implemented, as endemic processes, for example. Data and information collected and provided by information systems and market intelligence processes, as they are tuned to an architectural plot, structured through information and knowledge design patterns, could serve those governmental organizations, as an integrative part of the Healthcare administrative system, improving overall control and management.

This exercise of thinking about organizational integration through platforms and business models which considers information architecture-oriented market intelligence processes, enable a fair and stable design of informational services, which will produce reliable bases to receive new technological implementations. When one organization tries to define plans and policies to implement new technologies, as those detailed as "emergent" – IoT, Virtual reality, Augmented Reality, Cloud and cognitive computing, artificial intelligence, chatbots, among several others – a support of a robust design, as that provided by architectural plans, is essential. With that knowledge regarding information classification, processing and systemic analysis, along with its functionalities, processes as market intelligence can be benefitted from technology implementations with safer and risk-controlled specifications.

One severe and frequent mistake, to be avoided by the adoption of information architecture disciplines for systematic implementations, is to devote main attention on technology itself, naively believing that it, alone, will solve problems, produce a new scenario for competitive advantage innovative positioning and, at the end, promote a new strategic level. Technology is regarded as an essential component of any strategic array, but it demands a fair and stable base, as the one proposed by information architecture designs and principles, to produce desired successes associated to manageable plans and policies. In Healthcare environments, we have a stricter demand, imposed by required regulatory specifications, of transparent, governable and safe systems, projects and plans, answering correctly and precisely to these regulations and law codes, leveraging the organization to a trustable classification by authorities and patients.

RECOMMENDATIONS AND CONCLUSION

We had, in last years, several waves of technological offers that sometimes helped to develop management theoretical background accepted at that time, other times confronted the actual scenario, proposing a rupture. This happened with the introduction of personal computing in corporative environment, where, for example, guided companies to install "one computer in each desk where a work is being done". After some years of huge investments in computers, auxiliary devices and peripherals and software, along with internal education, some mistakes and risks emerged, as those related to information management – privacy, update, storage, etc. Some time later, the trend of connecting those machines in networks, where there would be more concentration, central management, storage (data bases) and handling of data could produce reliability and correctness regarding versioning and ownership prevailed, leading to another path of investments and associated managerial problems and risks.

Enterprise resource planning and other automated information systems, centralization and decentralization dilemma, data warehouse as a "medicine" for mistakes on internal competing information systems, video and audio sharing techniques, safety and privacy issues, among many others, produced also impacts, mainly regarding doubts on how to produce plans and policies and how to manage those solutions effectively in long-term periods, as robust managerial support. The lack of stable technology produced this undesirable level of indecision, implicating also in unstable conditions to promote the higher-level of management support and evolution desired by companies and other organizations which invested. Pioneering, a trend always related to courage and innovation is increasingly related to immaturity and undesirable level of uncertainty in planning abilities for business people and organizations.

Mobility and internet-based systems evolution proposed also a new level of working, still being dominated and focuses by several organizations. It implicated even in business model redesign, both offering a new level of competition, introducing innovative relations in internal (organizational structure, decision processes, etc.) and external (productive chain, customers) that must be learned and exercised by companies "on the fly", as implementations occur. As undeniable innovative solutions, with new business models, these plots on redefinition of functions and communication also posed threats and risks not yet completely dominated by organizations. Changes were rapidly implemented and taking an organization completely, where, sometimes, the organization was not fully configured or prepared to take this route of "being mobile".

This scenario can occur again with the fast introduction of emerging technologies. As organizations became more able to deal with new offers by market, proposing longer periods for testing and adequacy of new technologies in their workplaces, technology offers advance, with decreasing costs (promise, indeed) and new standards for adoption. This, again, proposes a pioneering posture which will result in a "Blue Ocean" strategy and associated operation to leaders, becoming their actions to define new markets. Unfortunately, it is not different, in this promised fashion of establishing a naïve relationship of pioneering to innovative and, this way, to market leadership. Innovation is, always, one of the main economic engines of human history, but it brings associated level of risks and conflicts which are not facts to reject innovation propositions, otherwise must be inserted in plans and managerial postures and actions.

This way, processes like "mobile organizations", "industry 4.0", "automated customer-oriented processes" are considered a no return way. Yes, this is a strong trend, a market standard to be planned, tested, adapted and finally adopted by companies and organizations, such as governments. Several signals and fundamentals, for example, cost management, production levels, optimization, automation of repetitive functions, regulatory burdens, unfeasible legal standards and several others are among pressures which demand such a level of automated services and processes in organizations. So, robotic, automated, industrial and digital transformation implements are here to stay and change our way to propose review for classical systems and corporative arrays, but also implement new organizations (Tadeu *et al.*, 2018).

What is strictly recommendable for managers is to address carefully their organizational plans and policies, check if they comply with ethics of governance and regulatory definitions, in a first level, not incurring in the risk of proposing a disruptive new level of work that offers risk to be illegal or not precisely adjusted to acceptable standards.

In the following, organizational strategies must be assessed and reviewed, as it is a normal action, inserted and predicted in strategic planning processes. This must be considered even when the adoption of a new system, level, business model or other organizational design is to be implemented, as the organization, in its new design will attempt to get away from a previous level and structure – which must be precisely known and configured. Planning abilities, with openness to new technological implementations, are needed more than ever, reviewing strategic and tactical planning principles and methods.

Additionally, professional skills must also be reconsidered, but taking previous experiences into account, getting all former experiences on conducting technology to increase performance, reduce costs and redefine processes as to avoid repetition of old mistakes and risks evidences. This leads to a recommendable attention to human resources preparation and development, considering that students, at their earlier ages will be increasingly exposed to new technologies, at home, leisure and basic education, becoming heavy technology users before they are professionals to be hired, in many ways, by companies.

Interestingly, themes such as information architecture, a soft and apparently classical way to consider a turbulent context, as it happens with information management, can bring and present a design-oriented principle to be adopted by organizations in order to a reliable planning level, presenting a more consistent managerial condition to deal with information processing. As information can be conceived as a relation concept, which connects data to knowledge, users to systems, usage to organizations, proposing one architectural relationship for information can produce a comprehension on how to connect all these parts in predictable and well related associations, mapping needs, interests and sources of assets to its usage by organizations.

Associating information architecture to market intelligence produces a good case to evaluate how emerging technologies can improve simple, but essential, functions, as data collection and storage, allowing companies to understand information production and needs, associating criteria to classify and validate this information for demanding decision instances, as strategic marketing planning capabilities. Designing a system, based on a process, for critical usage, as it happens in Healthcare services is challenging, but exposes a platform where emerging technologies can be implemented in safer and more robust way.

Concluding this article, a strong recommendation is stated, considering this new wave of technology as unfinished, unstable and, moreover, demanded and opportune for companies: developing managerial skills, considering management supportive models, such as information architecture is a recommendation which can lead to a more mature level, where data, information and knowledge can become assets to be managed, positioned and associated to organizational efforts in a controlled way, not corresponding to restrictions, but allowing the needed coordination to conduct one organization through these wonderful but risky series of market offers and trends.

FURTHER RESEARCH DIRECTIONS

Market intelligence is still a topic that demands applied research as to achieve a more mature level for its comprehension. With this purpose, we present here some suggestions to develop the study of MI, taking into consideration this text achievements and the next step for the development of the present study. First, the application of quantitative techniques and methods, to evaluate how market intelligence processes are successful in commercial and market cases is one topic that will help verify its actual state of the art, leading to an understanding for the best opportunity to improve emerging technologies opportunities in its configuration and processing.

Other field for observation is to study how these emerging technologies will be really applicable for managerial processes in the following. For example, there is a trend that some artificial intelligence platforms to be offered through internet, by information management providers. If this trend is confirmed, AI services could become cheaper and with standardized access to be included in MI cycle processing for commercial and strategic sectors. To better understand this potential evolution, keeping the observation on technology offer is essential.

Other arena are the business processes and their related business model configurations. Marketplaces, SaaS, Signature, On-demand, Platforms and many other business model types are being adopted by strategic planners for different markets and businesses. As these models turn to a strong trend in some markets, as marketplaces are nowadays almost a standard for transportation of people and load, this can become another relevant factor to influence on emerging technologies adoption for market intelligence cycle processing (Jamil & Berwanger, 2019; Anunciação & Esteves, F. M., 2019).

With these dynamics, MI cycle and its services present a strong potential relationship to emerging technologies and their conditions to be successfully implemented, as those provided by business models. With correct application of scientific methodology principles, this is an arena for continuous learning in the forthcoming years.

REFERENCES

Abubaker, H.; Dugger, J. C. & Lee, H. (2015). Manufacturing Control, Asset Tracking, and Asset Maintenance: Assessing the impact of RFID technology adoption. *Journal of international information and technology management, 24*(2), 35-54.

Akbar, H. (2003). Knowledge Levels and their Transformation: Towards the Integration of Knowledge Creation and Individual Learning. *Journal of Management Studies, 40*(8), 1997–2021. doi:10.1046/j.1467-6486.2003.00409.x

Anunciação, P. F., & Esteves, F. M. (2019). Challenges to Business Models in the Digital Transformation context. In *Handbook of Research on Business Models in Modern Competitive Scenarios*. Hershey, US: IGI Global. doi:10.4018/978-1-5225-7265-7.ch011

Avram, G., Bannon, L., Bowers, J., Sheehan, A., & Sullivan, D. (2009). Bridging, Patching and Keeping the Work Flowing: Defect Resolution in Distributed Software Development. *Computer Supported Cooperative Work, 18*(5-6), 477–507. doi:10.100710606-009-9099-6

Balasubramaniam, S. (2018). Artificial Intelligence. DAWN. *Journal for Contemporary Research in Management, 5*(1), 12–18.

Bird, C., Nagappan, N., Devanbu, P., Gall, H., & Murphy, B. (2008). Does distribute development affect software quality? an empirical case study of Windows Vista. *Communications of the ACM, 52*(8), 85–93. doi:10.1145/1536616.1536639

Boncea, R., Petre, I., Smada, D., & Zamfiroiu, A. (2017). A Maturity Analysis of Big Data technologies. *Informações Econômicas, 21*(1), 60–71. doi:10.12948/issn14531305/21.1.2017.05

Buch, V. H., Ahmed, I., & Maruthappu, M. (2018). Artificial intelligence in medicine: Current trends and future possibilities. *The British Journal Of General Practice: The Journal Of The Royal College Of General Practitioners, 68*(668), 143–144. doi:10.3399/bjgp18X695213 PMID:29472224

Cao, L., Zhang, C., & Liu, J. (2006). Ontology-based integration of business intelligence. *Web Intelligence and Agent Systems. International Journal (Toronto, Ont.), 4*, 313–325.

Celaschi, F. (2017, May-August). Advanced design-driven approaches for an Industry 4.0 framework: The human-centered dimension of the digital industrial Revolution. *Strategic Design Research Journal, 10*(2), 97–104. doi:10.4013drj.2017.102.02

Chau, M., & Xu, J. (2012). Business intelligence in blogs: Understanding consumer interactions and communities. *Management Information Systems Quarterly, 36*(4), 1189–1216.

Choo, C. W. (1996). The knowing organization: How organizations use information to construct meaning, create knowledge and make decisions. *International Journal of Information Management, 16*(5), 329–340. doi:10.1016/0268-4012(96)00020-5

Choo, C. W. (2005). *The knowing organization: how organizations use information to construct meaning, create knowledge and make decisions (2nd ed.).* Oxford: Ed. Oxford University Press. doi:10.1093/acprof:oso/9780195176780.001.0001

Clark, T. D. Jr, Jones, M. C., & Armstrong, C. P. (2007). The dynamic structure of management support systems: Theory development, research, focus and direction. *Management Information Systems Quarterly, 31*(3), 579–615. doi:10.2307/25148808

Davenport, T. H., & Prusak, L. (2000). *Working knowledge: how organizations manage what they know* (2nd ed.). Harvard Business Press.

Doneria, K., & Vinodani, S. (2017). Marketing Emerging Technologies: A Business to Business Perspective Strategic Overview, Opportunities and Challenges. *Amity Global Business Review, 12*(2), 15-19. Retrieved from http://search.ebscohost.com/login.aspx?direct=true&db=bsu&AN=128325994&lang=pt-br&site=ehost-live

El-Bashir, M. Z., Collier, P., & Sutton, S. G. (2011). The Role of Organizational Absorptive Capacity in Strategic Use of Business Intelligence to Support Integrated Management Control Systems. *The Accounting Review, 86*(1), 155–184. doi:10.2308/accr.00000010

El-Gayar, O., & Timsina, P. (2014). Opportunities for Business Intelligence and Big Data Analytics In Evidence Based Medicine. In *Annals of 47th Hawaii International Conference on System Science.* IEEE. 10.1109/HICSS.2014.100

Ferrel, O. C., & Hartline, M. (2010). *Marketing Strategy.* South Western College Publications.

Gallos, P., Minou, J., Routsis, F., & Mantas, J. (2017). Investigating the Perceived Innovation of the Big Data Technology in Healthcare. *Studies in Health Technology and Informatics, 238,* 151–153. Retrieved from http://search.ebscohost.com/login.aspx?direct=true&db=mdc&AN=28679910&lang=pt-br&site=ehost-live PMID:28679910

Hoffman, L. (2013, April). Looking back at the big data. *Communications of the ACM, 56*(4), 21–23. doi:10.1145/2436256.2436263

Huber, G. P. (1990). A theory of the effects of advanced information technologies on organizational design, intelligence and decision making. *Academy of Management Review, 15*(1), 47–71. doi:10.5465/amr.1990.4308227

IA Institute – Information Architecture Institute. (2014) *Recommended reading.* Retrieved from http://iainstitute.org/en/learn/education/recommended_reading.php

Inmon, B., Strauss, D., & Neushloss, G. (2008). *DW 2.0: The Architecture for the Next Generation of Data Warehousing*. Morgan Kaufmann.

Instituto de Arquitetos do Brasil (IAB). (2014). Retrieved from http://www.iab.org

Jamil, G. L. (2001). *Repensando a TI na empresa moderna*. Rio de Janeiro: Axcel Books do Brasil.

Jamil, G. L. (2005). *Gestão da Informação e do conhecimento em empresas brasileiras: estudo de múltiplos casos*. Belo Horizonte: Ed. Con / Art.

Jamil, G. L. (2018). *Market intelligence as an information system element: delivering knowledge for decisions in a continuous process in Handbook of Research on Expanding Business Opportunities with information systems and analytics*. Hershey, PA: IGI Global.

Jamil, G. L., & Berwanger, S. G. (2019). Choosing a Business Model: Entrepreneurship, Strategy and Competition. In *Handbook of Research on Business Models in Modern Competitive Scenarios*. Hershey, PA: IGI Global. doi:10.4018/978-1-5225-7265-7.ch001

Jamil, G. L., Jamil, L. C., Vieira, A. A. P., & Xavier, A. J. D. (2015). Challenges in modelling Healthcare services: A study case of information architecture perspectives. In G. L. Jamil, J. P. Rascão, A. M. Silva, & F. Ribeiro (Eds.), *Handbook of Research on Information Architecture and Management in Modern Organizations*. Hershey, PA: IGI Global.

Jamil, G. L., & Magalhães, L. F. C. (2015). Perspectives for big data analysis for knowledge generation in project management contexts. In G. L. Jamil, *S.M. Lopes, A.M. Silva et al.* (Ed.), *Handbook of research on effective project management research through the integration of knowledge and innovation*. Hershey, PA: IGI Global. doi:10.4018/978-1-4666-7536-0.ch001

Jamil, G. L., Santos, L. H. R., Lindgren, M. A., Furbino, L., Santiago, R., & Loyola, S. A. (2011). Design Framework for a Market Intelligence System for Healthcare Sector: A Support Decision Tool in an Emergent Economy. In M. M. Cruz-Cunha, I. S. Miranda, & P. Gonçalves (Eds.), *Handbook of Research on ICTs and Management Systems for Improving Efficiency in Healthcare and Social Care*. Hershey, PA: IGI Global.

Johnson, J. E. (2012). Big data + Big Analytics + Big opportunity. Financial & Executive, (July/August), 51-53.

Kanaher, L. (1998). *Competitive Intelligence: How to gather, analyse, and use Information to move your business to the top*. New York: Touchstone Books.

Kearns, G. S., & Lederer, A. L. (2003). A resource based view of IT alignment: How knowledge sharing creates a competitive advantage. *Decision Sciences*, *34*(1), 1–29. doi:10.1111/1540-5915.02289

Kimball, R., & Ross, M. (2010). *Relentlessly Practical Tools for Data Warehousing and Business Intelligence*. John Wiley and sons.

Kotler, P., & Keller, K. (2005). *Marketing Management* (12th ed.). Prentice Hall.

Laudon, K., & Laudon, L. (2009). *Management Information Systems* (11th ed.). Prentice Hall.

Leidner, D., & Elam, J. J. (1995). The impact of executive information systems on organizational design, intelligence and decision making. *Organization Science*, *6*(6), 645–664. doi:10.1287/orsc.6.6.645

Liukkonen, M. (2015). RFID technology in manufacturing and supply chain. *International Journal of Computer Integrated Manufacturing*, *28*(8), 861–880. doi:10.1080/0951192X.2014.941406

Lucas, H. C. Jr. (2005). *Information technology: strategic decision making for managers*. Hoboken, NJ: John Wiley and Sons.

Lunin, L. F., & Smith, L. C. (1984). Artificial Intelligence: Concepts, Techniques, Applications, Promise. *Journal of the American Society for Information Science*, *35*(5), 277–279. doi:10.1002/asi.4630350504

Malik, J. (2017). What Led Computer Vision to Deep Learning? *Communications of the ACM*, *60*(6), 82–83. doi:10.1145/3065384

Marchand, D., & Davenport, T. (Eds.). (2000). *Mastering Information Management*. New York: Financial Times Prentice Hall.

Marchand, D., Kettinger, W., & Rollins, J. (2001). *Making the invisible visible: how companies win the right information, people and IT*. Wiley.

Markovitch, D. G., Steckel, J. H., & Yeung, B. (2005). Using Capital Markets as Market Intelligence: Evidence from the Pharmaceutical Industry. *Management Science*, *51*(10), 1467–1480. doi:10.1287/mnsc.1050.0401

McAfee, A., & Brynjolfsson, E. (2012). Big data: The management revolution. *Harvard Business Review*, *90*(10), 60–68. PMID:23074865

Miller, S. (2002). Competitive Intelligence - an overview. *Competitive Intelligence Magazine*, *14*(3), 43-55. Retrieved from http://www.sci.org/library/overview.pdf

Ngai, E. W. T. (2010). RFID technology and applications in production and supply chain management. *International Journal of Production Research*, *48*(9), 2481–2483. doi:10.1080/00207540903564892

Nonaka, I. (2008). *The knowledge creating company*. Harvard Business Review Classics.

O'Brien, J., & Marakas, G. (2008). *Management Information Systems*. Irwin: Mc Graw Hill.

Ohata, M. & Kumar, A. (2012). Big Data: A Boom for Business Intelligence. *Financial Executive*, (September).

Pfleeger, S., & Atlee, J. (2009). *Software Engineering: Theory and Practice* (4th ed.). Prentice Hall.

RAIC – Raic Canada. (2014). Raic / Irac Architecture Canada. Retrieved from https://www.raic.org/

Royal Institute of British Architects (RIBA). (2014). Retrieved from http://www.architecture.com/Explore/Home.aspx

Russel, S., & Norvig, P. (2009). *Artificial intelligence: A modern approach* (3rd ed.). Prentice Hall.

SAS. (2014). *SAS Enterprise Miner – SEMMA*. Retrieved from http://www.sas.com/technologies/analytics/datamining/miner/semma.html

SAS. (2017). *What is Analytics?* Retrieved from https://www.sas.com/en_us/insights/analytics/what-is-analytics.html

Schiffman, L., & Kanuk, L. (2010). *Consumer behavior*. Prentice Hall.

SCIP. (2011). Strategic and Competitive Intelligence Professionals. *What is competitive intelligence,* Retrieved from http://www.scip.org/content.cfm

Skansi, S. (2018). *Introduction to Deep Learning: from logical calculus to artificial intelligence*. New York: Springer-Verlag. doi:10.1007/978-3-319-73004-2

Sommerville, I. (2010). *Software Engineering* (9th ed.). Addison Wesley.

Stair, R., & Reynolds, G. (2009). *Principles of information systems*. Course Technology.

Sun, Y., Yan, H., Lu, C., Bie, R., & Thomas, P. (2012). A holistic approach to visualizing business models for the internet of things. *Communications in Mobile Computing*, *1*(1), 1–7. doi:10.1186/2192-1121-1-4

Tadeu, H. F. B., Duarte, A. L. C., Chade, C. T., & Jamil, G. L. (2018). *Digital Transformation: Digital Maturity Applied to Study Brazilian Perspective for Industry 4.0. In J.L.G. Alcaraz et al. (Eds.), Best Practices in Manufacturing: Experiences from Latin America*. Cham, Switzerland: Springer Nature AG.

Tuomi, I. (2000). Data is more than knowledge: Implications of the reversed knowledge hierarchy for knowledge management and organizational memory. *Journal of Management Systems*, *16*(3), 103–117.

Turban, E., Mc Lean, E., & Wetherbe, J. (2002). *Information technology for management: transforming business in the digital economy* (3rd ed.). Hoboken, NJ: John Wiley and Sons.

Turban, E., Rainer, R. K. Jr, & Potter, R. E. (2007). *Introduction to information systems*. Hoboken, NJ: John Wiley and Sons.

Turber, S., & Smiela, C. (2014). A business model type for the internet of things. In *22nd European Conference on Information Systems (ECIS 2014), Tel Aviv, Israel.*

Vayena, E., Blasimme, A., & Cohen, I. G. (2018). Machine learning in medicine: Addressing ethical challenges. *PLoS Medicine*, *15*(11), 1–4. doi:10.1371/journal.pmed.1002689 PMID:30399149

Weiss, S. M., & Verma, N. K. (2002). A System for Real-time Competitive Market Intelligence. In *Proceedings of the eighth ACM SIGKDD international conference on Knowledge discovery and data mining* (pp. 360-365). 10.1145/775047.775100

Yaoguang, H., & Rao, W. (2008). Research on collaborative design software integration on SOA. *Journal of Advanced Manufacturing Systems*, *7*(1), 91–99. doi:10.1142/S0219686708001152

Yonce, C.; Taylor, J.; Kelly, N. & Gnau, S. (2017). BI Experts´ perspective: Are you ready for what´s coming in Analytics. *Business Intelligence Journal, 22*(3), 36-42.

Yunbiao, S. (n.d.). Internet of Things: Wireless Sensor Networks. *IEC White Paper*. Retrieved from http://www.iec.ch/whitepaper/pdf/iecWP-internetofthings-LR-en.pdf

ADDITIONAL READING

Albescu, F., & Pugna, I. B. (2014). *Marketing intelligence: The last frontier of business information technologies. Romanian Journal of Marketing, 3*(July-September), 55–68.

Chen, H., Chiang, R. H. L., & Storey, V. C. (2012). Business intelligence and analytics: from big data to big impact. MIS Quarterly, 36(4), 1165-1188.

Courtney, M. (2013). Puzzling out Big Data. Engineering & Technology, 7(12), 56-60.

Hoffman, L. (2013, April). Looking back at the big data. *Communications of the ACM, 56*(4), 21–23. doi:10.1145/2436256.2436263

Kremer, M., Mantin, B., & Ovchinnikov, A. (2013). Strategic consumers, Myopic retailers. Darden School of Business at University of Virginia. Retrieved from http://www.darden.virginia.edu/web/uploadedFiles/Darden/Faculty_Research/Research_Publications/Ovchinnikov_StrategicConsumer_MyopicRetailers.pdf

Mahrt, M., & Scharkow, M. (2013). The value of big data in Digital Media research. *Journal of Broadcasting & Electronic Media, 57*(1), 20–33. doi:10.1080/08838151.2012.761700

Schuchmann, D., & Seufert, S. (2015). Corporate Learning in Times of Digital Transformation: A Conceptual Framework and Service Portfolio for the Learning Function in Banking Organizations. *International Journal of Corporate Learning, 8*(1), 31–39.

Schwab, K. (2017). *The fourth industrial revolution.* London, UK: Crown Business.

Westerman, G., Bonnet, D., & McAfee, A. (2014). The nine elements of digital transformation. *MIT Sloan Management Review, 55*(3), 1–6.

KEY TERMS AND DEFINITIONS

Artificial Intelligence: Scientific field which aims to study perspectives of computers and automated systems application to replace humans in repetitive operations.

Big Data: Collaborative analysis done from structured (formally, predictable and formatted) and unstructured (posts, informal communication, social media usage) data regarding one specific topic.

Information Architecture: Systematic way to produce design-oriented artifacts, such as plans and project specifications towards information management.

Information Systems: Set of organizational components, aggregated to process data and information aiming to produce knowledge.

Information Technology: Scientific field dedicated to study and promote science-based technologies to process information towards its application.

Knowledge: Content produced from data and information, which retains the most valued experience of an event or phenomena.

Marketing: Set of managerial disciplines applied to add value to a service or product.

Market Intelligence: A cyclic process to provide knowledge from collected data and information in one productive array, for strategic marketing decisions.

Chapter 2
Spatio–Temporal Hot Spot Analysis of Epidemic Diseases Using Geographic Information System for Improved Healthcare

Uma V.
ⓘ https://orcid.org/0000-0002-7257-7920
Pondicherry University, India

Jayanthi Ganapathy
Anna University, India

ABSTRACT

Health-care systems aid in the diagnosis, treatment and prevention of diseases. Epidemiology deals with the demographic study on frequency, distribution and determinants of disease in order to provide better health-care. Today information technology has made data pervasive i.e. data is available anywhere and in abundance. GIS in epidemiology enables prompt services to mankind or people at risk. It brings out health-care services that are amicable for prevention and control of disease spread. This could be achieved when epidemiology data is modeled considering temporal and spatial factors and using data driven computation techniques over such models. This chapter discusses 1) the need for integrating GIS and epidemiology, 2) various case studies that indicates the need for spatial analysis being performed on epidemiologic data, 3) few techniques involved in the spatial analysis, 4) functionalities provided by some of the widely used GIS software packages and tools.

DOI: 10.4018/978-1-5225-8470-4.ch002

INTRODUCTION

Health-care systems focus on prevention, diagnosis and treatment of diseases. With the increase in population, the amount of medical information that the health-care administrators should handle is exponentially increasing. So, in order to provide better health-care facilities to human beings it is necessary that health-care systems are to be integrated with technology. This chapter will clearly explain the need for innovative technologies in handling medical data.

Epidemiology data describes distribution of disease and risk of the disease spread among a given population. The space – time modeling of such data gives insights about spatial variation of disease and risk factors causing such diseases in various spatial locations through time. Epidemiological studies based on GPS technology is a research area which is gaining importance wherein the space time data histories are used for epidemiologic analyses (Meliker et al., 2011). Spatial and Temporal factors of epidemiology data have its significance in various applications like hotspot detection of Kalaazar disease in the Vaishali district (Bihar), India (Bhunia et al., 2013). Epidemiology data collection methods include investigation on symptoms of disease, epidemiologists survey records, death rate, etc. These data are employed in geo-epidemiology analysis for disease mapping. One such notable application is use of geo-statistical analysis methods for disease mapping (Giorgi et al., 2008). Hence, analysis of epidemiological data can contribute towards development of better health-care systems.

Geographic Information System is software system that stores and manipulates spatial and a-spatial data. In addition, spatial and temporal characteristics of epidemiology data can be modeled using GIS. Scientific methods can be applied to understand the distribution of epidemiologic data which can help in controlling the disease spread by forecasting the disease progression. One such application was proposed for controlling the mumps disease using Spatio-temporal analysis (Yu et al., 2018). Several scientific methods employed in epidemiology applications are geo-referencing, area estimation, migration of population, disease mapping, detection of area of interest of disease, and integration of spatial and temporal clusters (Zulu et al., 2014; Kirby et al., 2017).

Recent study on endemic disease (Srinivasa Roa et al., 2018) was made to explore the use of GIS tools and spatial autocorrelation methods using spatial statistics Getis-Ord Gi*. Data mining techniques were applied to classify endemicity level using patterns generated by Self Organizing Map (SOM). The objective of this chapter is to bring insight about the need for GIS in epidemiological studies. This chapter also highlights the significance of spatial analysis in finding the distribution of diseases which would help the health-care professionals in controlling the diseases. This chapter also presents details about the scientific methods and tools involved in GIS.

In the second section, an introduction to health information management and its importance in epidemiology is presented. Third section explains the basic concepts in GIS, its applications, future directions with respect to forecasting. Fourth section explains case studies on hotspot analysis that has been performed over epidemiological data collected from various sources. Fifth section presents case studies with respect to epidemiological data analysis. Sixth section presents some of the spatial analysis and modeling techniques that can be used. Seventh section explains some of the GIS software that is used widely. The chapter concludes by providing some future research directions. Finally, the related terms are listed for better understanding of this chapter.

BACKGROUND: HEALTH INFORMATION MANAGEMENT AND EPIDEMIOLOGY

Health Information is the data pertaining to patient's medical history, their symptoms, diagnosis, treatments and outcomes. This clinical information helps in delivering healthcare services and plays an important role in making health-care related decisions. Health information management is practice of acquiring, analyzing and storing digital medical information. Managing and analyzing this data is very much essential as with the modern means of data acquisition like remote sensing the medical data is ever increasing. Artificial intelligence based clinical decision-making systems are prevalent nowadays. These expert systems entirely depend on the amount of facts that are stored. Managing this huge data is crucial for better diagnosis and prognosis of diseases. So, health information management is very much essential to improve the health services. Health information includes epidemiological data as well.

Epidemiology is the scientific study of the extent of diseases with respect to time, location and methods to control them. Geographical epidemiology deals with the study of origin of diseases whereas Spatial Epidemiology deals with the study and analysis of distribution of diseases with respect to location. So, epidemiology involves analysis of disease information pertaining to patients with respect to location and time.

In order to analyze the relationship between the diseases and locations, epidemiologists usually use the geographical maps. Geographic Information System (GIS) can capture the epidemiological data referenced with location coordinates over a period of time. It helps in visualization of information using maps. The spatial analysis techniques used in GIS can help the epidemiologists in knowing the relation between the diseases and environmental factors which would help them in making health-care related decisions.

The basic terms that are related to epidemiology and their definitions are presented at the end of this chapter.

MAIN FOCUS OF THE CHAPTER

Geographic Information Systems (GIS)

Geographic information system captures, stores, analyses and displays geographical data. The geographical data is otherwise called as spatial data or geo spatial data. GIS works on location data expressed in forms such as latitude, longitude, ZIP codes, etc. The data about population for specific locations like city or state can be represented in maps using different colors based on the population density. Overlaying of different layers of spatial data such as education, transport, income can be done on this map thus providing additional dimensions of analysis.

Analysis can be performed for finding the areas that are statistically significant. The power of GIS is harnessed by decision making systems in making vital decisions. Nowadays, GIS plays an important role in managing transport, tourism, etc. Also, the visualization of data in mapped format using GIS enables easier communication of information. Various analysis is done on the spatial data which could aid in prediction of disasters like earthquakes, volcanoes, landslides, forest fires etc. The spatial analysis also helps in identifying the crime hotspots, epidemiological hotspots etc. so that it enables planning of precautionary activities.

The two types of GIS formats are raster and vector data. Raster data is made up of pixel values that represent the geographical data. Raster data can be discrete or continuous. Discrete raster data are used in representing land cover whereas, continuous raster data are used in representing gradual changes like temperature etc. Vector data is not pixel values. Points, lines and polygons representing geographical data form vector data. The level of detail provided by vector data is easier to comprehend. Points can be used to represent a place like city. Rivers, Roads can be represented using lines. Polygons can be used to represent regions like forests, agricultural lands etc. Based on the application for which the data is used the data can be represented in the form of raster or vector.

The good description of data enables effective spatial analysis. Spatial analysis enables exploration of sequence of events, the association between the events thereby enabling prediction of events which could help in effective management and planning. So, the epidemiological data when analyzed spatially and temporally can help in identifying the presence of diseases, its distribution over time. Further analysis can help in predicting the likelihood of the disease outbreak in other locations. This would help the health care professionals to take remedial steps so that people can be protected from the infectious diseases.

There are many spatial analysis software packages available. The GIS software packages are explained briefly later in this chapter. The understanding of the terms related to GIS is essential before exploring the relation between epidemiology and spatial analysis. So, the basic terms that are related to GIS is explained at the end of this chapter to enable the naive reader to get acquainted. Having understood the basics of Epidemiology and GIS, Figure 1 shows the conceptual framework in which GIS and machine learning integration is presented. The framework also explains our perspective used in approaching GIS for health care.

We now explain the applications of GIS followed by the future of GIS and the role of machine learning.

Applications of GIS in Healthcare: Evidence Based Study

GIS have numerous applications in health care. By collecting relevant epidemiological information, GIS with strong analytical performance would help in making decisions.

Figure 1. Conceptual framework of GIS and machine learning integration

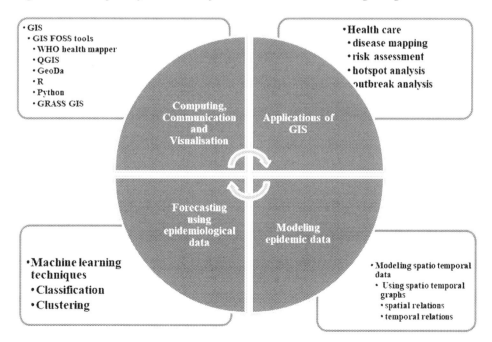

1.   The increased prostate cancer levels in California's intensely agricultural Central Valley have been analysed (Myles Cockburn et al. 2011). The relations between environmental pesticide/fungicide exposure and prostate cancer have been studied. It was found that increased risk of prostate cancer was observed among persons living around homes in agricultural areas exposed to pesticides.

2.   According to an analysis published in Journal of Transport and Health by Erika Ikeda et al. (2018), shorter distances to school and neighbourhoods have resulted in higher rate of prevalence of obesity among school children. The analysis was performed using GIS.

3.   The effectiveness of the Short Interval Additional Dose approach in vaccination drives have been studied by WHO, Rotary International, US CDC and UNICEF using geo-spatial data.

4.   Currently, the ESRI (Environmental Systems Research Institute) has over 5,000 health care clients worldwide who are using GIS in decision making.

5.   GIS has played a significant role in gaining insights about Ebola virus and assessing the disease spread in Africa.

6.   Myanmar in 2017 has decided to build policies to enable powerful use of geospatial data and technologies in monitoring and controlling maternal, new born death and diseases like malaria.

7.   In a recent study, Maps created using GIS software were used in visualising the health disparities in South Miami as compared to North Miami. This helped in understanding the difficulties faced by under-served communities and providing better health care facilities.

The above stated facts stand as a testimony that over the last several years, the growth in sophistication and ease of use of geographic information system (GIS) software has paved the way for wide deployment of GIS in health care world-wide.

Issues and Future of GIS

Now, to have more accurate decision making, GIS should be augmented with knowledge about the nomadic patterns of people, natural hazards and other disease breeding grounds. These factors can help in providing much needed vaccinations for diseases such as Polio, West Nile virus and malaria. So, the migration of tribes can be mined based on the travel patterns and this inferred knowledge can provide more precise and timely reports. Similarly, forecasting of natural disasters by time series analysis can also help in providing health care to people by proper health care planning. The breakdown of various diseases can be forecasted based on the breeding grounds. Geo spatial tools therefore when ensemble with machine learning approaches can provide the base for proper health care management.

Solutions and Recommendations: Machine Learning in Prediction of Disease Outbreak

Machine learning approaches help in detecting patterns in data and use the patterns in forecasting future data. In performing cluster analysis like hotspot analysis various clustering techniques are being used. K-Means clustering algorithms are applied in clustering the hot spots. Machine learning algorithms provides better predictions by understanding even the social determinants. Machine learning approaches namely linear regression, Random forests and Neural networks performed better in detecting patterns in the data for prediction. Seligman et al. (2018) highlighted the strengths and limitations of the machine learning approaches. Linear regression performed better in prediction among linear relationships. Random forests have better prediction rate by handling outliers and missing data well. Neural networks achieved non-linear learning, but generalization was difficult to achieve in the absence of large samples of data. In performing skin cancer classification, a deep learning algorithm was trained on almost 130,000 clinical images of skin lesions. The algorithm performed on par with 21 board-certified dermatologist (Esteva et al., 2017).

Huge amounts of epidemiological data are necessary for the machine learning algorithms to perform well. In the presence of large amounts of data, storing and manipulating abilities of GIS, Machine learning approaches can help in learning patterns. Thus, it is clear that machine learning approaches are expected to be the major trend dominating epidemiology in the next decade. But, in this chapter we are not further exploring how machine learning concepts can be integrated with GIS as we feel that it is beyond the scope of this chapter.

The next section explains hotspot analysis, a type of spatial analysis that can be performed using various GIS software packages. It is explained by considering various case studies.

GIS AND EPIDEMIOLOGY

Geographical Information system (GIS) is software system which stores, manipulates, and visualizes spatial data. This information system is useful in analyzing data in various forms in terms of data format, storage etc. This software system helps in decision support, forecast and post analysis in disease management. GIS in epidemiology renders much useful functionalities such as disease mapping, risk assessment and outbreak analysis of disease. This section explores use of GIS in epidemiology.

Epidemiology Hotspot Analysis

Hotspot analysis is a spatial analysis process. This process can be performed using Point spatial data. The density of point data can be visually analyzed using Heatmap. The outcome of hotspot analysis is heatmap. The density of point spatial data describing disease spread, crime, accidents, incidents etc. could be analyzed using hotspot analysis. The Figure 2 shows heatmap describing tuberculosis in UK in 2017. Kernel density estimation function is being used to find spatial regions severely affected by tuberculosis. When the same kernel density function is applied to sparse data describing hospitals in New York State there is no significant clusters describing dense location of hospitals as shown in Figure 3. Hence, the Figure 3 which is not a heatmap shows the presence of hospitals and not the density of hospitals within a proximity distance.

Case Study 1

A survey is made on microbial survival in a flooded pit. This survey has following details: Identity of Site, Depth of pit, Sample name and different classes of bacteria. The result of hotspot analysis process is reported using heatmap generation. Statistical tools and packages have made ease the generation of heatmap. Further, three-dimensional data can be visualized in two-dimensions. The three dimensions taken for hotspot analysis for the data in this case study are *X- (i) Identity of sites and (ii) Depth of the pit in meters; Y- Class of Bacteria survival and Z- Severity.*

Figure 2. Heatmap of tuberculosis in U.K 2017

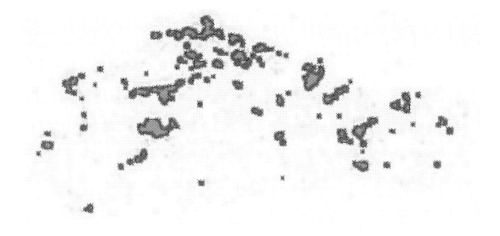

Figure 3. Point diversity which is not a heatmap

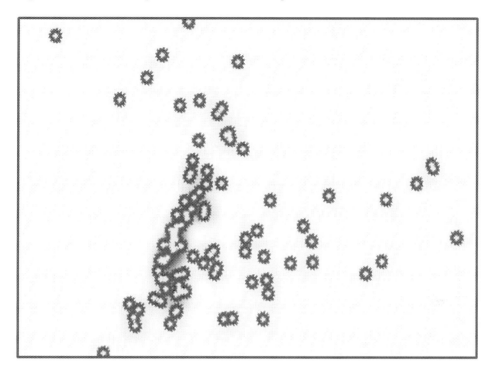

Heatmap describing survival of bacteria in flooded pit is shown in Figure 4. Survey on bacterial survival in each of three sites at different depth (in meters) is considered along the X – axis. The class of bacteria identified at each of site is along the Y-axis. The Z- axis denotes the severity of the class of bacteria surviving in a site at various depth represented using color gradient. Gradient value 0 denotes white color which is representing low number of bacteria while dark green and its variants from 100 to 400 represents high number of bacteria surviving in the pit.

Spatial Analysis: Spatial Join Operation

Joins are operations performed using attributes of vector data of a geo-spatial region. Spatial epidemiological data in vector forms are the source of input to perform join operations. Spatial join helps in identifying spatial relationships between two layers. Join is operation performed between two datasets that satisfy the condition involving attributes common to both the vector datasets. Vector datasets are visualized as layers in GIS as shown in Figure 5. Spatial Join operation is performed using geometric predicates. Spatial relationship between two vector layers is computed using geometric predicates. The geometric predicates are "intersects", "contains",

Figure 4. Heatmap of microbial survivals

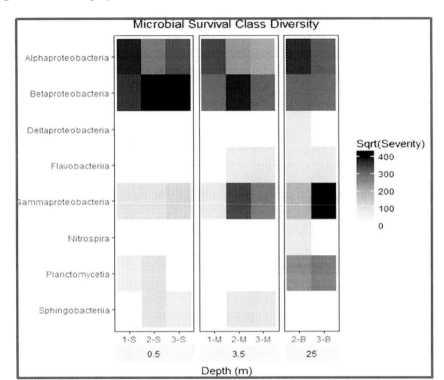

Figure 5. Vector dataset showing administrative boundaries of New York (state)

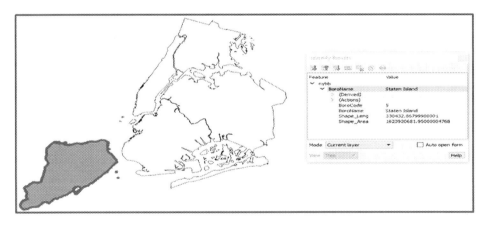

"crosses", "touches", "overlaps", and "within." The spatial join operations can be explained with example. Considering the health care centers located in New York state, the borough boundaries are shown in Figure 6. Spatial join operation using tools in GIS helps in estimating health center capacity for each administrative boundary.

These data sets are available for use of public in NYC Open Data portal. The borough boundaries and location of health centers in New York State are displayed as vector layers in GIS before spatial join operation as shown in Figure 3. The spatial relationship helps in estimating the total health centers in each borough. Hence, join attribute by location is required. The location of each health centers is the common attribute to both the vector layers. Thus, spatial join is performed on location attribute using geometric predicates. The result of spatial join is made known by selecting a feature on the borough layer as shown in Figure 7.

Epidemiology Data Analysis

Epidemiology data describes factors influencing the infection, symptoms of disease and distribution of disease in terms of frequency in a given population. Analyzing such facts helps in diverse applications like (1) Time of exposure and onset of food poisoning outbreak (2) Factors influencing sleepiness disorder (3) The impact of age and education level in marriage (3) The impact of smoke in causing death (4) The impact of age factor in Schizophrenia. The significance of epidemiology data analysis is explored in this section. The distributions of epidemiology considering various factors are illustrated using different case studies. Data analysis is reported using epicalc package in R-3.1.3.

Figure 6. Layers showing healthcare centers located in New York City

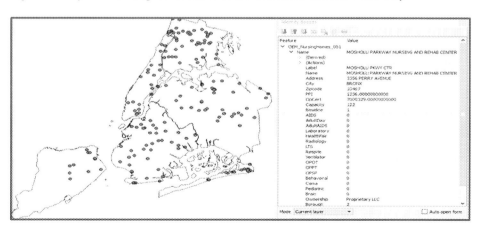

41

Figure 7. Spatial join of healthcare centers in New York City

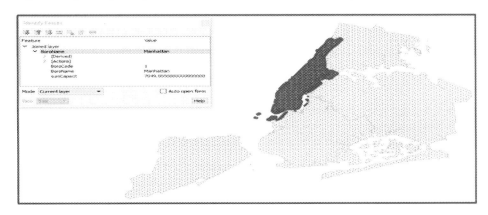

Figure 8. Distribution of food poisoning on sports day

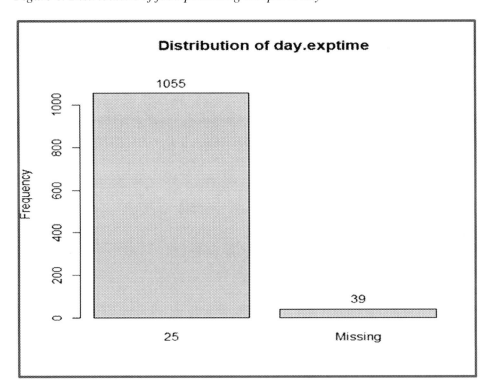

Case Study 2: Temporal Outbreak Analysis

Outbreak of a disease is defined by case definitions. The symptoms like vomiting, diarrhea and other gastrointestinal infections in case definition are recorded to investigate exposure and onset times of food poisoning on sports day meet. The graphs Figure 9 through Figure 13 explain this. The data recorded on the sport day meet for outbreak analysis are id (numeric), sex (numeric), age (numeric), beefcurry (numeric), saltegg (numeric), éclair (numeric), water (numeric), nausea (numeric), vomiting (numeric), abdpain (numeric), diarrhea (numeric). Out of 1094 observations 39 missing values were found as shown in Figure 8. On ignoring the 39 missing values the time of exposure in hours was found to be the maximum at 18 hours of the sports day as shown in Figure 9. The time of exposure to food poisoning is found to be between 6 o'clock and 7 o'clock while it is less during middle of the day 12 noon as shown in Figure 10. It is possible to analyze onset time of food poisoning on the sports day. The onset time is estimated using only case definitions. From the

Figure 9. Distribution of food poisoning in hour

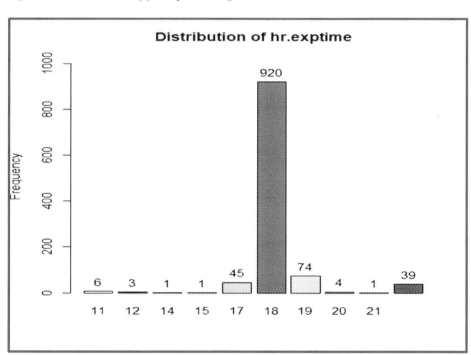

Figure 10. Time of exposure to food poisoning

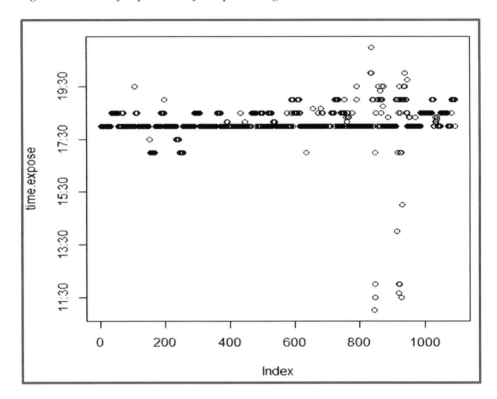

observations it is found that 429 had the symptoms onset on the same day of 25th August, while remaining 33 had on next day. On the 26th August and 632 had no symptoms reported as shown in Figure 11.

The onset time of food poisoning in sport day meet started at 3pm on 25th August and most of case definition shows onset towards end of the day. Few cases were reported on the next day morning as shown in Figure 12. The incubation period of food poisoning is calculated as the difference between onset time and exposure time. It is observed from Figure 13 that incubation period was found to be the maximum at 3.5 hours and skews on right.

Case Study 3: Sleepiness Disorder Analysis

The observations made regarding sleepiness disorder are gender, date of birth, weight (in kg), Height (in cm) and survey on sleepiness during lecture, group work etc. The observation was recorded on 4 males and 11 females as shown in Figure 14. It

Figure 11. Observation on onset of food poisoning

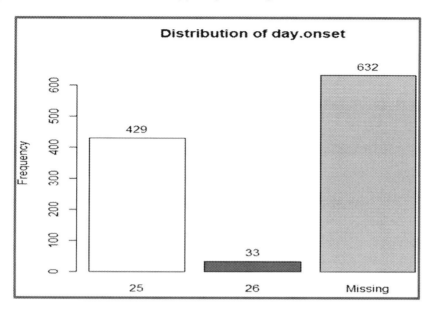

Figure 12. Onset time of food poisoning

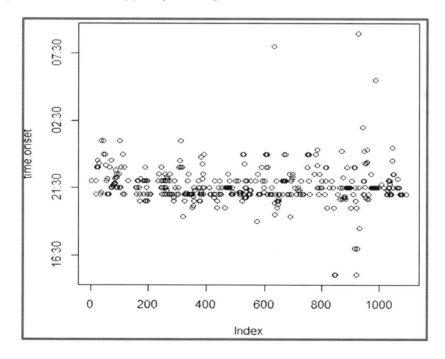

Figure 13. Incubation period of food poisoning

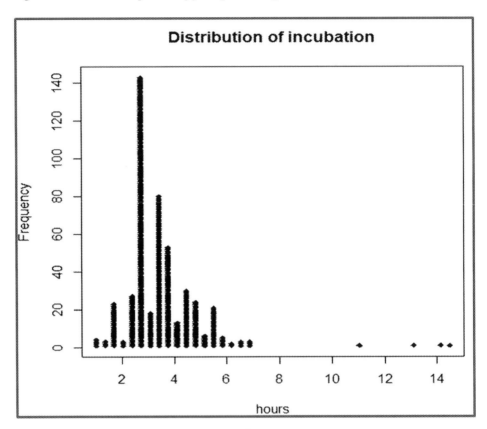

was found that a total of 12 people both male and female together were found to be sleepy in workshop as shown in Figure 15 while 1 was not sleeping during lecture as shown in Figure 16. The distribution of height and weight is shown in Figure 17 and Figure 18 respectively.

Case Study 4: Age and Education in Marriage

The impact of age and education in marriage is analyzed using 27 observations containing the details (1) gender (2) date of birth (3) level of education and (4) marital status. In a given population of 27, 13 observations were reported at bachelor level and 14 observations were reported above bachelor level as shown in Figure 19. The education of females was above bachelor level compared to males as shown in Figure 20.

Figure 14. Observation on gender in sleepiness disorder

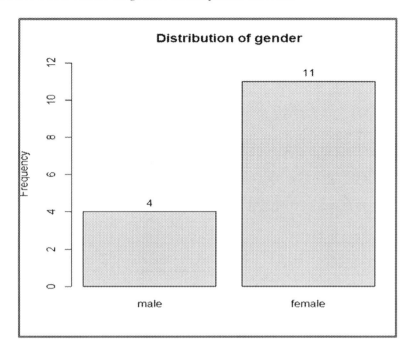

Figure 15. Observation on sleepiness at workshop

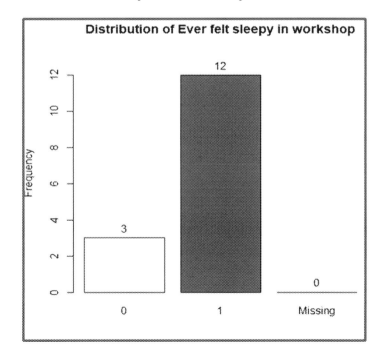

Figure 16. Observation on sleepiness at workshop

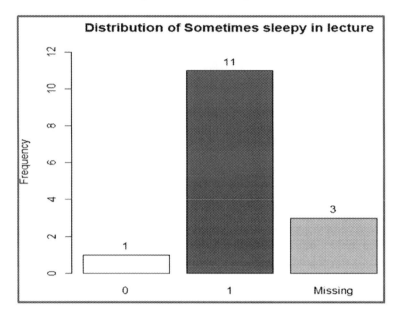

Figure 17. Observation of height in sleepiness

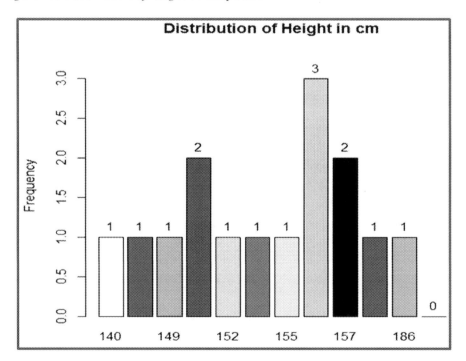

Figure 18. Observation on weight in sleepiness

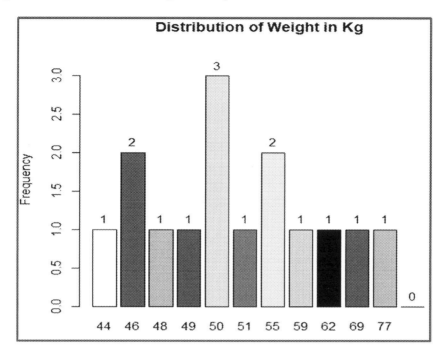

Figure 19. Observation on level of education

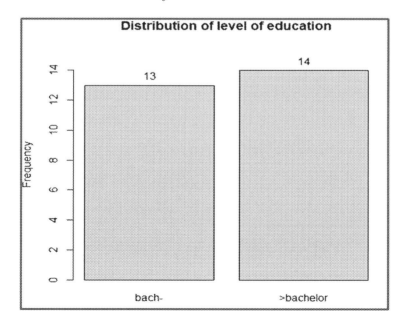

Figure 20. Comparison of level of education among gender

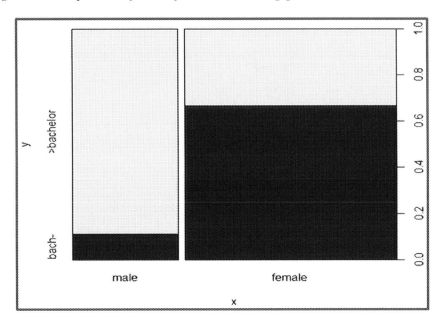

Case Study 5: Air Pollution Causing Death in UK

Air pollution causing death in UK is observed for 15 days. The frequency of death is shown in Figure 21. It is found that death rate highly varies between 200 and 300 compared to death rate between 100 and 200.

Case Study 6: Age Factor in Risk of Schizophrenia

The observation of Schizophrenia was recorded among population consisting of 251 cases. The details are age and gender. The distribution of age in total population among 151 male and 101 female population affected by Schizophrenia is shown in Figure 22. Figure 22 shows that it is commonly found in age between 15 and 30 in both genders.

SPATIO: TEMPORAL ANALYSIS TECHNIQUES

Spatial Autocorrelation

The measure of a phenomenon correlated to itself in geographic space is spatial autocorrelation. This measure was introduced by Cliff and Ord 1973. Spatial

Figure 21. Air pollution causing death

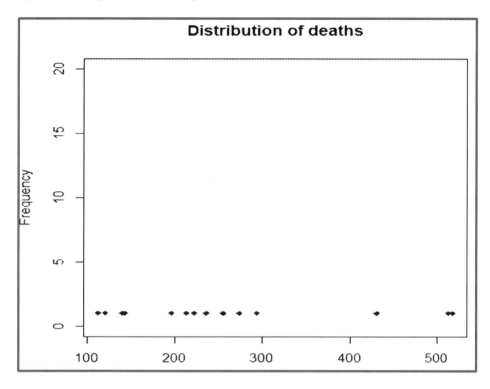

autocorrelation measure helps in examining the dependency of a phenomenon in a spatial region with its neighboring regions.

$$Moran's\_coefficient = \frac{n}{\sum_{i=1}^{n}\sum_{j=1}^{n} w_{ij}} \frac{\sum_{i=1}^{n}\sum_{j=1}^{n} w_{ij}(x_i - x')}{\sum_{i=1}^{n}(x_i - x')^2} \quad (1)$$

Where x_i is quantity measured at i^{th} observation. x' is the sample mean. W_{ij} is spatial weight of relationship between i and j.

Temporal Autocorrelation

Temporal autocorrelation is required to measure relationship between variables indexed by time by correlating variable with itself, say at some lag or delay. Correlation

Figure 22. Age factor in Schizophrenia

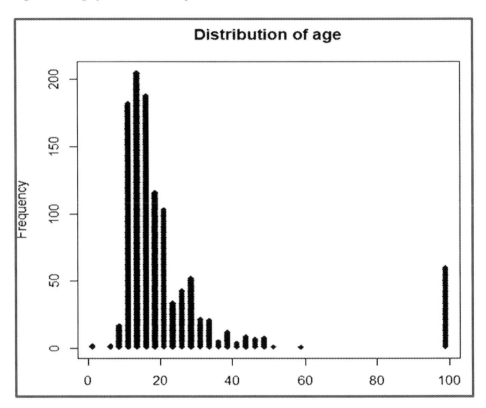

coefficient is used to measure temporal autocorrelation. Pearson Coefficient is given by ρ given in equation 2.

$$\rho = \frac{n\left(\Sigma xy\right) - \left(\Sigma x\right)\left(\Sigma y\right)}{\sqrt{\left[n\left(\Sigma x^2\right) - \left(\Sigma x\right)^2\right]\left[n\Sigma y^2 - \left(\Sigma y\right)^2\right]}} \tag{2}$$

Modeling Spatio-Temporal Epidemic Process

We have proposed modeling of spatial and temporal data using spatio-temporal graph. The advantage of this modeling is that it enables inference of new knowledge from existing data. For instance, if a location A is considered to have disease D and location C which is not spatially connected to location A also has the same disease D. Then there is a possibility that location B which is spatially connected to A and C may have the prevalence of disease as well. This can be inferred by the spatial relations and logical reasoning of these relations (Jayanthi and Uma, 2017). Similarly, if at time t_1, location A is found to have the disease and at time t_2 location B is infected with the same disease then by logical inference it can be found that at a later time instance t_3, people at location C which is spatially connected to B may be infected with the disease. With the knowledge about the time instances and their relationships it is possible to find the order in which the locations got infected with the disease. This inference process will help the health-care administrators to plan ahead so that they can provide better health services to the people so that they may be protected from the disease.

From the above discussion it is found that by modeling the spatial and temporal aspects of the locations and diseases, better inference can be made. For this purpose, the time and point relation proposed by Allen 1983 and 1994 is used. The RCC spatial relations (Randell, 1992) are used in modeling the spatial relations. Spatial-temporal analyzing of epidemic diseases is made possible by modeling spatio-temporal graph $G = (V_s, E_t)$, where V_s is set of vertices representing geographic locations, E_t is the set of edges of the graph describing the spatial relationship between two spatial regions.

Spatio-temporal graph model is shown in Figure 23. The graph can be represented as two dimensional matrix based on adjacency between two spatial locations. The adjacency between two spatial locations A and B is defined by e_1 in the figure where the presence of edge denotes the presence of any of the spatial relation listed in Table 1. Figure 24 shows adjacency matrix of G in Figure 23.

The occurrence of diseases at various locations is stored using the time points or interval relations listed in Table 2a and 2b respectively. If location A is infected with a particular contagious disease at time instance t_1 or over an interval of time t_1 to t_2 then there is a possibility that location B which is spatially connected may be infected with the disease at a later time t_3. The above relation can be represented using after relation. By knowing the temporal order (relations) that exist between

Figure 23. Spatio-temporal graph g

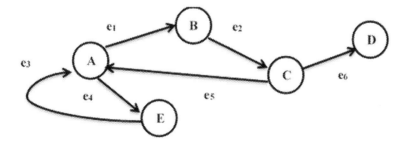

Figure 24. Adjacency matrix of G

	A	B	C	D	E
A	0	e_1	0	0	e_4
B	0	0	e_2	0	0
C	$e5$	0	0	e_6	0
D	0	0	0	0	0
E	$e3$	0	0	0	0

Table 1. Spatial logic relations

Topological Relation	Syntactic Representations
Connected (C_{xy}) "x", "y" are spatial regions	$\forall xy[\ C_{xy} \rightarrow C_{yx}]$
Disconnected (DC_{xy})	$\neg\ C_{xy}$
Part (P_{xy})	$\forall z\ [C_{zx} \rightarrow C_{zy}]$
Proper Part (PP_{xy})	$P_{xy} \wedge \neg P_{xy}$
Overlaps (O_{xy})	$\exists z[P_{zx} \wedge P_{zy}]$
Partial Overlap (PO_{xy})	$O_{xy} \wedge \neg P_{xy} \wedge \neg P_{yx}$
Discrete (DR_{xy})	$\neg O_{xy}$
Externally Connected (EC_{xy})	$\neg O_{xy} \wedge C_{xy}$
Tangential Proper Part (TPP_{xy})	$\exists z[EC_{zy} \wedge EC_{zx}] \wedge PP_{xy}$
Non-Tangential Proper part ($NTPP_{xy}$)	$\neg\exists z[EC_{zy} \wedge EC_{zx}] \wedge PP_{xy}$
Non-Tangential Proper Part Inverse ($NTPP^{-1}_{xy}$)	$NTPP_{yx}$
Tangential Proper part Inverse (TPP^{-1}_{xy})	TPP_{yx}
Proper Part Inverse (PP^{-1}_{xy})	PP_{yx}
Part Inverse (P^{-1}_{xy})	P_{yx}

various time points or intervals, the health-care professionals can know the disease outbreak sequence with respect to locations. The edges can be attributed with the time relations so that inference may be done based on temporal facts.

The diffusion of disease can be inferred using point relation, interval relations, and spatial logic relations shown in Table 2, Table 3, and Table 1 respectively. The diffusion of disease can be logically inferred using properties defined as follows.

1. Spatial logic relation at region A is symmetric to spatial logic relation at region E as A→ E and E→A, where A and E are different spatial regions.
2. Spatial logic relation at region A is transitive to spatial logic relation at region C as A → B, B → C ⇒ A→C, where A B and C are different spatial regions.

Table 2. Point Relations of Temporal Logic

Syntactic Relations	Logical Definition
before (α, β)	$\alpha < \beta$
after (α, β)	$\alpha > \beta$
equal(α, β)	$\alpha = \beta$

α and β are time points

Table 3. Interval Relations of Temporal logic

Syntactic Relations	Logical Definition
before(λ_1, λ_2)	$\lambda_1.End < \lambda_2.Start$
overlaps(λ_1, λ_2)	$\lambda_1.Start < \lambda_2.Start \wedge \lambda_1.End < \lambda_2.End$
starts(λ_1, λ_2)	$\lambda_1.End < \lambda_2.End \wedge \lambda_1.Start = \lambda_2.Start$
during(λ_1, λ_2)	$\lambda_2.Start < \lambda_1.Start \wedge \lambda_1.End < \lambda_2.End$
meets(λ_1, λ_2)	$\lambda_1.End = \lambda_2.Start$ at point P
finishes(λ_1, λ_2)	$\lambda_2.Start < \lambda_1.Start \wedge \lambda_1.End = \lambda_2.End$
equal(λ_1, λ_2)	λ_1, λ_2 occurs in same interval such that $\lambda_1.Start = \lambda_2.Start \wedge \lambda_1.End = \lambda_2.End$

λ_1 and λ_2 are events defined in an Interval

Spatial logic relation at region C is anti-symmetric to spatial logic relation at region D as D $\rightarrow$ C is not defined.

The next section explains the software packages that are used widely in implementing spatial analysis.

FREE OPEN SOURCE SOFTWARE PACKAGE FOR GIS

GIS technology integrates database query operations, geographic analysis, statistical analysis and visualization. There are nearly 100 geospatial software packages available. GIS software tools can be classified as Open source GIS, Web GIS, desktop GIS, CAD GIS, Mobile GIS and general-purpose GIS. Some widely used open source software tools are

1.   QGIS (Quantum GIS)
2.   WHO Health Mapper
3.   GRASS GIS (Geographic Resources Analysis Support system)
4.   GeoDa

5.   R
6.   Python

This section will explain the above software packages and tools briefly.

QGIS (Quantum GIS)

ArcGIS is the widely used proprietary software for spatial analysis. QGIS, a stand-alone GIS application was developed to compete with ArcGIS. The latest version is QGIS 3.2. QGIS API allows integration of plugins in a very easy way. QGIS provides improved geometry editing, searches, projections and layering. It is supported by all common operating systems. It has a user-friendly Graphical user interface (GUI). QGIS supports all common data formats like Excel, CSV and PostgreSQL. Most of the spatial data formats like PostGIS, ESRI shapefiles are supported. Cartographical operations can be performed using QGIS. This can be integrated with other open source GIS platforms. Base maps can be generated easily. Statistical analysis like generation of graphs and charts is not fully supported. QGIS python modules enable us to develop stand-alone applications.

Health Mapper

Health Mapper, an analytical tool is a WHO initiative. It is an information and mapping application related to public health. It supports easy visualization of disease and health information in order to support decision making and advocacy. It provides spatial analysis facility based on clustering technique.

GRASS (Geographic Resources Analysis Support System) GIS

GRASS GIS, a stand-alone GIS application is also available for multiple operating systems. The GUI is not as user friendly as QGIS. This also supports all major data and spatial formats. Manipulating the geometry can be done easily. Spatial Analysis routines are available in GRASS GIS. Base map generation facility is not available. Scripting functionality is not available.

GeoDa

GeoDa, an analytic tool with GIS capabilities is supported by the common operating systems. It has a user-friendly GUI. It provides spatial analysis facility. Cartographic operations are partially supported. It provides querying and scripting functionality and hence can be integrated with programming languages like Python.

R

R is a statistical package which is being supported by major operating systems. It can perform spatial and statistical analysis of spatial data. It provides scripting functionality. It gives support to restricted data formats only. The spatial packages of R include epicalc, gstat, ggmap, rgdal, rgeos, etc. With the support provided by R for various statistical and spatial analyses, it is integrated with tools like QGIS for visualization of the results.

Python

Python has some spatial analysis packages. PySAL is an open source library of spatial analysis functions written in Python. GeoPandas enable spatial operations. Spatial geometries like polygon and lines can be easily manipulated using the spatial libraries. Other analysis libraries are shapely, numpy, scipy, scikit-learn, etc.

CONCLUSION AND FUTURE RESEARCH DIRECTIONS

This chapter discussed about how GIS with respect to public health can help in identifying the distribution of diseases, analyzing their trends so that planning can be done to provide health services to needy people. Recent advancements in geo-spatial data acquisition have made information processing of geo-spatial data simple. This chapter also discussed data visualization in different dimension and types thus showing the easiness with which Geographical Information systems can contribute to health-related analysis. In view of volume of data and diversity in its type, many techniques have been adopted in hotspot, coldspot cluster analysis. Hence, with today's information systems analyzing spatio-temporal facts in epidemiological studies is much sophisticated as many open source software Quantum GIS (QGIS) and packages with libraries like epicalc, maptools in R have emerged. Some of the GIS tools were discussed in this chapter.

The chapter thus provides an in-depth idea about the application of GIS in epidemiology, its advantages and tools used. The future research direction in this field is applying machine learning techniques for prediction of disease outbreak. Machine learning techniques are now applied to raster and vector operations for better information extraction and exploration. These algorithms have strong mathematical computational structures and hence can be employed to devise solution in prediction, risk assessment and monitoring etc. in epidemiological studies.

REFERENCES

Allen, J. F. (1981). An interval-based representation of temporal knowledge. *In International Conference of Artificial Intelligence*. Morgan Kaufmann.

Allen, J. F. (1983). Maintaining knowledge about temporal intervals. *Communications of the ACM*, *26*(11), 832–843. doi:10.1145/182.358434

Allen, J. F. (1984). Towards a general theory of action and time. *Artificial Intelligence*, *23*(2), 123–154. doi:10.1016/0004-3702(84)90008-0

Allen, J. F., & Ferguson, G. (1994). Actions and events in interval temporal logic. *Journal of Logic and Computation*, *4*(5), 531–579. doi:10.1093/logcom/4.5.531

Bhunia, G. Kesari, S., Chatterjee, N., & Kumar, V, Das. P. (2013). Spatial and temporal variation and hotspot detection of kala-azar disease in Vaishali district (Bihar), India. *BMC infectious diseases*, *13*(1), 64. doi:. doi:10.1186/1471-2334-13-64

Cockburn, M., Mills, P., Zhang, X., Zadnick, J., Goldberg, D., & Ritz, B. (2011). Prostate cancer and ambient pesticide exposure in agriculturally intensive areas in California. *American Journal of Epidemiology*, *173*(11), 1280–1288.

Esteva, A., Kuprel, B., Novoa, R. A., Ko, J., Swetter, S. M., Blau, H. M., & Thrun, S. (2017). Dermatologist-level classification of skin cancer with deep neural networks. *Nature*, *542*(7639), 115–118. doi:10.1038/nature21056 PMID:28117445

Giorgi, E., Diggle, P., Snow, R., & Noor, A. (2018). Geostatistical methods for disease mapping and visualization using data from spatio-temporally referenced prevalence surveys. *International Statistical Review*, *86*(3), 571–597. doi:10.1111/insr.12268

Ikeda, E., Stewart, T., Garrett, N., Egli, V., Mandic, S., Hosking, J., ... & Moore, A. (2018). Built environment associates of active school travel in New Zealand children and youth: A systematic meta-analysis using individual participant data. Journal of Transport & Health. doi:10.1016/j.jth.2018.04.007

Jayanthi, G., & Uma, V. (2018). Modeling Spatial Evolution: Review of Methods and Its Significance. In C. Pshenichny, P. Diviacco, & D. Mouromtsev (Eds.), *Dynamic Knowledge Representation in Scientific Domains* (pp. 235–259). Hershey, PA: IGI Global. doi:10.4018/978-1-5225-5261-1.ch010

Kirby, R. S., Delmelle, E., & Eberth, J. M. (2017). Advances in spatial epidemiology and geographic information systems. *Annals of Epidemiology*, *27*(1), 1–9. doi:10.1016/j.annepidem.2016.12.001 PMID:28081893

Meliker, J. R., & Sloan, C. D. (2011). Spatio-temporal epidemiology: Principles and opportunities. *Spatial and Spatio-temporal Epidemiology*, *2*(1), 1–9. doi:10.1016/j.sste.2010.10.001 PMID:22749546

Mutheneni, S. R., Mopuri, R., Naish, S., Gunti, D., & Upadhyayula, S. M. (2018). Spatial distribution and cluster analysis of dengue using self-organizing maps in Andhra Pradesh, India, 2011–2013. *Parasite Epidemiology and Control*, *3*(1), 52–61. doi:10.1016/j.parepi.2016.11.001 PMID:29774299

Randell, D. A., Cui, Z., & Cohn, A. G. (1992). A spatial logic based on regions and connection. *KR*, *92*, 165–176.

Seligman, B., Tuljapurkar, S., & Rehkopf, D. (2018). Machine learning approaches to the social determinants of health in the health and retirement study. *Social Science and Medicine Population Health.*, *4*, 95–99. doi:10.1016/j.ssmph.2017.11.008 PMID:29349278

Yu, G., Yang, R., Wei, Y., Yu, D., Zhai, W., Cai, J., & Qin, J. (2018). Spatial, temporal, and spatiotemporal analysis of mumps in Guangxi Province, China, 2005–2016. *BMC Infectious Diseases*, *18*(1), 360. doi:10.118612879-018-3240-4 PMID:30068308

ADDITIONAL READING

Allen, J. F. (1981). An interval-based representation of temporal knowledge. In *International Conference of Artificial Intelligence*. Morgan Kaufmann.

Allen, J. F. (1983). Maintaining knowledge about temporal intervals. *Communications of the ACM*, *26*(11), 832–843. doi:10.1145/182.358434

Box, P., Jenkins, G., Reinsel, G., & Ljung, G. M. (2012). *Time Series Analysis Forecasting and Control*. Wiley.

Clarke, B. L. (1981). A calculus of individuals based on connection. *Notre Dame Journal of Formal Logic*, *22*(3), 204–218. doi:10.1305/ndjfl/1093883455

Dan, W. (1995). *Patterson, Introduction to Artificial Intelligence and Expert Systems*. Pearson.

McCarthy, J., & Hayes, P. J. (1969). Some philosophical problems from the standpoint of artificial intelligence. In *Readings in Nonmonotonic Reasoning* (pp. 26–45). Morgan Kaufmann Publishers Inc.

Pani, A. K., & Bhattacharjee, G. P. (2001). Temporal representation and reasoning in artificial intelligence: A review. *Mathematical and Computer Modelling, 34*(1–2), 55–80. doi:10.1016/S0895-7177(01)00049-8

Randell, D. A., Cui, Z., & Cohn, A. G. (1992). *A spatial logic based on regions and connection.* Proceedings Knowledge Representation and Reasoning.

Rich, E. (2017). *Kevin Knight and Shiva Shankar Nair, Artificial Intelligence* (3rd ed.). Mc Graw Hill India.

KEY TERMS AND DEFINITIONS

A-Spatial Data: Data that do not represent a geographic location such as color, shape, size, type etc., are a-spatial data.

Attribute Table-Database: Database that contains information about the geographic features.

Autocorrelation: The correlation between observation as a function of time delay or lag between the observations.

Base Map: The map that provides the fundamental information upon which other maps can be built.

Buffer: Polygon surrounding a geographic feature in selection is buffer space which is used for proximity analysis.

Cartesian Co-Ordinate: Point coordinate on real axis.

Cartography: It is study of map making techniques.

Cluster Analysis: Grouping of candidate dataset without prior knowledge of its identity.

Communicable Disease: Diseases transmitted from person to person, one organism to another etc.

Connectivity: Two linear features A, B are said to be connected when there is path to traverse from A to B and B to A.

Control Point: The point coordinate on real world that references the geographic features on map.

Determinant: Factors influencing disease spread.

Data Base Management System (DBMS): The collection of software program that organizes, manipulates data in database.

Data Model: The way of organizing and representing data is data model.

Database Schema: The representation of entity and attribute in a database is schema.

Diffusion Modeling (Disease Spreading/Transmission): The estimation of disease spread using scientific formulations.

Distribution: The pattern describing the propagation of disease.

Elevation: The height of a geographic location is represented using contour lines.

Endemic: Infectious disease is said to be endemic when infection does not propagate extremely rather it is maintained at some baseline.

Entity: Physical object in real world is an entity in database.

Epidemic: Infectious disease rapidly spread within short duration or time period.

Etiology: The study on origin of disease and its causes.

Features: Set of attributes that describes the spatial object.

Feature Classes: Represent homogenous collection of spatial features in terms of point, line and polygon. For example area of land cover region is represented as polygon feature.

Frequency: The count of number of disease in various categories.

Geocoding: It is the process of transforming physical identity of an object to location in point coordinates form.

Geographic Information System GIS -: The software that integrates storage, analysis, mapping and visualization of both spatial and a-spatial data of a geographic area.

Geo-Database: It is organized collection of spatial data in raster and vector format.

Geo-Epidemiology: Study of etiology of diseases.

Geometry: Points on plane connected to form different shapes.

Geo-Referencing: It is mapping raster image by associating it with real co-ordinate system.

Heatmap: Density of data points representing geographic feature is analysed using heatmap.

Hotspot Analysis: Spatial locations identified based on statistical significance measure.

Incidence: The rate of occurrence of an undesirable medical condition.

Infectious Disease: The disorders due to living organism.

Interpolation: Numerical analysis in which new data points are estimated from known set of discrete data points.

Latitude: The angle ranges from $0°$ at the equator to $90°$ at the poles.

Layer: Geographic dataset is represented using symbols and labels.

Line: The path connecting two spatial points is line.

Longitude: The angle ranges from $0°$ at Prime meridian to $+180°$ East and $-180°$ West.

Map Algebra: Mathematical set theory based algebraic operations used for analysis and manipulation of geographic data.

Map Clusters: The identification of hotspot, outlier, spatial similarity based on geographic features that are statistically significant. They can be visualized as layers in GIS.

Map Projection: Transformation in which a point coordinate on earth is projected on a plane.

Metadata: Data that provides description of existing data.

Mortality Rate: Death rate of particular community.

Nearest Neighbor: It is proximity analysis in which nearest neighbor is computed based on distance.

Network: Collection of nodes interconnected via communication link.

Node: In network, node is a point that either initiates or terminates communication.

Overlay: Map overlay is operation performed for relating different geographic features by superimposing more than one dataset with different themes.

Point: Point is a geographic location represented in Latitude and Longitude.

Polygon: The closed path of finite length forms polygon.

Prevalence: The phenomenon by which a medical condition found to exists or found to be common.

Prognosis: Outcome of disease that could be predicated or likely to occur as expected.

Raster Data: The spatial data stored as picture element (pixel) with row and columns in matrix form. Each pixel contains spatial information. Example: image in .tiff, .png

Spatial Autocorrelation: The measure of a phenomenon correlated to itself in geographic space.

Spatial Data: Geographic location of an existing physical object or constructed structures represented using co-ordinate system is spatial data.

Spatial Epidemiology: The study of disease spread considering risk factors in behavioral, genetics, environmental etc., in various geographic locations of interest.

Spatial Statistics/Spatial Analysis: Formal mathematical techniques applied to study properties of spatial features.

Temporal Autocorrelation: The measure of relationship between variable indexed by time by correlating variable with itself at some delay.

Temporal Data: Data representing quantity recorded at different time intervals or points.

Thematic Map: A Layer describing geographic features in a dataset represented using specific theme.

Topography: The mapping of earth surface that comprises of hilly terrains, land cover, natural and man-made structures etc.

Topology: Physical structures represented as point, line, and polygon describing connectivity, adjacency and continuity.

Vector Data: The spatial data stored in the form of point, line and polygon constitute vector data format. Example: shapefiles

Zonal Operation: Zone in raster data is area of interest in which raster spatial analysis is performed using the cells present in the zone.

Chapter 3
Digital Professionalism:
Challenges and Opportunities to Healthcare Professions

Joana Vale Guerra

https://orcid.org/0000-0001-7426-5579
University of Coimbra, Portugal

ABSTRACT

The widespread use of digital technology allows for a number of transformations in the organization of work which renders the importance of professional and expert knowledge more open to challenges. The digital age is impacting and changing many aspects of professional development, therefore must be examined in its effects on reshaping healthcare professions and its implications on professional autonomy and discretionary judgment. To achieve this goal, advantages and disadvantages will be highlighted about the usage of electronic health record software to the healthcare professional's autonomy and discretionary power. The increased use of digital technologies is deeply affecting most professional occupations, transforming their identities, structures, and practices. In recognizing the challenges and opportunities to professional work of the digital transformation is underlined the importance of trying to understand how to remain professional in different digital environments and how to work in contexts with ambient surveillance.

DOI: 10.4018/978-1-5225-8470-4.ch003

INTRODUCTION

Currently, we are witnessing a life time that enjoys the extraordinary development of new technologies, the multiplication of channels of communication and information, the superabundant consumption of the image and where the cyber world has become global and universal (Vago, 2004; Lipovetsky, 2013; Innerarity, 2010).

The digital revolution has been very pervasive to people, enterprises and even to structures as solid as governments and public administration. The digitization of just about everything is one of the most important phenomena of recent years (Brynjolfsson, 2016). The digital age can be defined as a historical period marked by the widespread use of digital technologies in different aspects of human activity, including the economy, politics and most forms of human interaction (Eurofund, 2018). The term digital describes generating, storing and processing data in a way that is considerably faster and more efficient than any previous means at society's disposal (OECD, 2017). The increased use of digital technologies enables meaningful and useful information to be generated and shared, potentially creating much utility and value (idem).

The widespread use of digital technology allows for a number of transformations in the organization of work which renders the importance of professional and expert knowledge more open to challenges (Parton, 2000, 2008; Lorenz 2006; Carvalho, 2015). Several authors agree digitization enables immense amounts of information to be compressed on small storage devices that can be easily preserved, transported and also quickens data transmission speeds (Schafer, 2003). Since the mid-twentieth century digital technology has created new fields of potential professional work though undermined others. Commonly, the most mention changes are: the appearance of new professions and the extinction of others; the opening of virtual organizational contexts for work accomplishment; frontiers between public, private sectors and civil society are becoming blurred (emerging new forms of collaboration, e.g. public/ private partnerships); new forms of competition, quality, trust and transparency requirements; new mechanisms of regulation, auditing and evaluation. Adding this, under the same technological leverage, consumer's expectations have become more knowledgeable and thereafter more demanding (given the abundance of information associated with a hyper consumer profile).

The author assumes that digital age is impacting and changing many aspects of professional development, therefore must be examined in its effects on reshaping healthcare professions and its implications on professional autonomy and discretionary judgement. It has been well-established in Andrew Abbott's Systems of Professions (1988) that the forces that impinge on professions reshaping arose within the professions and others are exogenous forces. From a wide field of possibilities to study, the main goal reflecting on the effect of digitalization on professionalism, emphasizes the interest in analyzing digitization as a source, an instrument and an outcome of professional changes and control at macro, mezzo and micro social levels (Ellaway, 2015; Evetts, 2014). To achieve this goal, advantages and disadvantages will be highlighted about the usage of electronic health record software to healthcare professional's autonomy and discretionary power.

Digital professionalism discourse or its benefits are strongly supported by managers, governments and transnational political organizations, as stated on Recommendations on Digital Government Strategies: today's technology is not only a strategic driver for improving public sector efficiency, but can also support effectiveness of policies and create more open, transparent, innovative, participatory and trustworthy governments (OECD, 2014). But as far as it can be seen, this emerging form of professionalism is debatable since there are elements of change which encroach professional jurisdictions, causing disturbances such as: control of work by practitioners; collegial authority; occupational identities; discretion and decision-making; trust and confidence between professional/client; and codes of ethics provided by professional associations (Freidson, 2004; Rodrigues, 2012).

The increased use of digital technologies leads to different changes within organizations and organizational principles, strategies and methods are deeply affecting most professional occupations, transforming their identities, structures and practices (Crotty, 2011; Ellaway, 2015; Penã-Casas, 2018). The main concern is to understand if the discourse of digital professionalism is a way of occupational control to promote efficient management of the organization or an opportunity to reshape practical knowledge and improving professional status. Probably both.

Although no perspective exhausts it completely it poses new challenges that need to be known and overcome so that people and societies reap the benefits of the transformations that are operating worldwide. The new digital environment offers opportunities to express professional work with a powerful discourse based on transparency, real-time data, smarter use of information, accountability and accessibility for all (notwithstanding the need to discuss the new digital discrimination or virtual inequality). Health care providers and professionals must take advantage of a digital transformation strategy in order to adapt their professional communication to meet the expectations and needs of consumers.

This chapter draws on the work of sociology of professions to address the concept of professionalism as an occupational value and the concept of digital professionalism as the result of social development changes supported by the perspective of organizational professionalism. To trace this linkage, the chapter introduces an overview of the changes to professional work and highlighted some professional implications trying to figure out what is the reality of the digital age for healthcare professionals.

BACKGROUND

The study of professions has a long path during the second half of the 20th century. However, it seems that the digital revolution is been remarkable reframing the understanding of how the processes of professionalization and professionalism evolve or recast in organizational settings and its implications to expert knowledge (Guerra, 2017; Brock, 2016). Currently, a managerially oriented theory discuss developments on professionalism requiring its reconceptualization considering two prominent factors: 1) professional practice guided by management and administration models centered on rationality and economic efficiency; and 2) the use of the discourse of professionalism outside the internal dynamics of professional groups; for example, managers requiring and providing mechanisms of work control imposing limits on the autonomy and discretionary power of professionals judgment and decision-making (Evetts, 2014; Brock, 2016; Guerra, 2017). For a better understanding about the potential conflict between professionalism as an occupational value and as a discourse used by managers in work organizations it is important, firstly, to present the well-known definition of professionalism by Elliott Freidson (2004). Considering his work, professionalism is established in the endorsed belief that the knowledge and skills of a particular specialization follow underpinning abstract concepts, formal education, training, and experience. He has defended professionalism as a desirable way of providing complex, discretionary services to the public and firmly, argues that organizational control of work based on managerial models impoverish and standardize the quality of service to consumers and demotivates practitioners. More recently, sociologist Julia Evetts (2012a; 2012b; 2104) described the organizational professionalism laying emphasis on the replacement of professional values for organizational demands and market endeavor. The following examples stand out this new direction, it became more common to praise bureaucratic, hierarchical and managerial controls rather than collegial relations; to pursue managerial and organizational resolutions rather than professional expertise; to bring off budgetary restrictions and financial rationalizations rather than customer needs; to standardize work practices rather than professional discretion; to achieve targets and accountability based on political control rather than professional autonomy based on expert knowledge. Intuitively, it is easy to predict that digital technology enhances some of the requirements of organizational professionalism allowing managerial tools to control professional's work. Here is the thing, increasing use of software programs in daily work can be seen as an adjustment to organizational demands with consequences to professional discretion or it can also be seen as an opportunity to strengthen customers trust and provide confidence for professional practice. Standardization is often presented as a way to reduce uncertainty and unpredictability for professionals and clients, since standardized tools offer predictability, uniformity and transparency (Ponnert, 2016). In a way or other, in the light of digital and standardized tools, professionals will need to debate if digital work is enhancing or reducing professionalism.

The interpretation of professionalism can evolve a double meaning aspect driven in opposite directions. Summarizing, it is possible to say that professional discourse market-based managements have brought the values and techniques which claim economic efficiency, transparency, self-responsibility, center-citizen approach, positive organizational image to customers, measurable goals and a competitive environment. And the professional discourse based on professional values involves different features, as the following: abstract knowledge; work, tasks and procedures control; discretionary power; professional autonomy; licensing and training in universities; advocacy and supportive with the customers interests; strong sense of identity; sense of purpose and trusted by employers and clients. But are these two logics completely appositive? Or there will be mix logics in contemporary professional and organizational developments?

Removing opposing scenarios of complete compatibility or incompatibility between two discourses – professional values versus organizational values – Evetts (2012a, 2012b, 2014) introduced the possibility of a new form of professionalism. There are little doubts that organization logics have an attractive dimension to professions because some of their principles and methods are quite interesting to improve professional development regarding public's trust. The organizational discourse centered on good values for public, employers and professionals as quality, innovation and transparency became stilly accepted and embodied in professions' legacy. On the other side, organizations success benefit a lot from work and specialized knowledge of professionals to ensure its existence and development.

This combination of perspectives on professionalism with steady and conflicting points can create opportunities for debate, but can also generate a new form of professionalism. Recently, many authors from the background of the sociology of professions provide many different studies to identify the elements of occupational professionalism that still remain in the nature of the work and those that have been changed. It is significant to gain insight and dimension on the transformations that emerge from the point that professionalism was a synonym of trust or social closure to a discourse of organizational marketing (Freidson, 2004; Burton, 2009; Rodrigues, 2012; Evetts, 2014; Brock, 2016;)

This opportunity to mix logics found good reception in the New Public Management framework and the dissemination of good governance principles interfered in organization, structuring, functioning and coordination of professional work (Pollitt, 2011, 2013; Ponnert, 2016). At the same time, an interesting phenomenon started to appear, the occupation of management positions by professionals, notwithstanding their professional expertise, assumed a managerial-oriented practice defending bureaucratic procedures, cost-effectiveness and measurement of performance and standardized practices. It became very common for professionals, regardless their academic background, to study for a graduate degree in business management and qualify for a management position (Noordegraaf, 2006, 2007; Brock, 2016; Guerra, 2017). Another driving force to combine professional and organizational logics is the increasing dissemination of collaborative work between public and private sector organizations to address issues and problems that can only be solved in partnership, with a multiplicity of stakeholders and professional from diverse backgrounds (Keating, 2002).

Those are just a few boosters which contribute to understanding hinging mechanisms between professions and organizations. It is important to look for potential tensions and at the same time consensual emerging spaces in professional environments. Within this theoretical framework, it is possible to appreciate an increasing number of empirical studies depicting this new approach to the process of professionalism. In Portugal, Carvalho and Santiago's (2015) developed research focusing the impact of public health reforms on nurses' performance in hospital settings and the impact of higher education reforms on teachers. The researchers argue that the new government rationality and the introduction of economic and managerial norms and values exposed professional groups to a strong scrutiny that confronts professionals with unprecedented challenges. Portuguese government has open up a new digital environment to actively shape political priorities, to collaborate in the design of public services and to participate in their delivery, and to provide integrated solutions to complex challenges. The state can be very demanding on professional jurisdictions. However, it is possible to theoretically present two opposite views of the relationships between states and professions, each one corresponding to a specific political and institutional environment. Liberal states play a passive role in the professionalization process, restricting their intervention to the granting of legally-based privileges. Even if public authorities gave the initial impulsion by employing a great number of professionals, gradually, they should emancipate from state control. In Continental countries, the state has a high impact on and within professions leaving little room to professionalism resist the logic of bureaucratic organizations, particularly when depending functionally and institutionally from the state's legal authority (Noordegraaf, 2007, Evetts, 2014). For this reason, the literature bases its theoretical and empirical production on the two models of explanation of professional power: the continental and the liberal model. The state's role is limited to the provision of a certain type of political and institutional environment which sometimes favor professionalism (in liberal states), and sometimes hampers it (in highly centralized states) (Bianic, 2003).

However, the development of the welfare state and, more recently, the reconfiguration of the State under the neoliberal currents and the implementation of the New Public Management in the Public Administration display a scenario of convergence in the analysis of professional power that tends to overcome the divergences imposed by the two models. As Evetts (2014) points out continental or liberal states are increasingly similar and the convergence between bureaucratization and professionalization can be seen as two mutually reinforcing phenomena (a recovered idea from Neoweberians).

In this perspective, the most recent theoretical studies, of Evetts (2014), Noordegraaf (2007) and Brock and Saks (2016), for example, appeal for greater flexibility in defining the concept of professionalism. Given a scenario in which work is changing and being changed by organizations, empirical trends demonstrate that the analysis of the compatibility between organizational professionalism and occupational professionalism propose what Evetts (2012a, 2012b) called "new professionalism", or what Faulconbridge and Muzio (2008) and Noordegraaf (2007) referred to as "hybrid professionalism".

Additionally, professional work is changing and has been changed, increasingly finding and exploring information and communication technologies that provide new abilities to an old form of social organization (Castells, 2005, 2012; Cappellin, 2009). However, technology does not determine society, but incorporates it. Neither society determines technological innovation, but uses it (Rodrigues, 2005). It is possible to produce the same analogy with the world of professions. Technology does not determine professions or the reverse, but through a dialectical relationship they transform each other.

Branching out from organizational professionalism, Rachel Ellaway and colleagues (2015) described digital professionalism around concepts of proficiency, reputation, and responsibility and highlighted the following question: how professions are preparing the workplace and practice in an increasingly digitally mediated world? The use of digital media has accelerated the speed and scale of our actions. Unprecedented quantities of information can be retrieved instantly wherever a network connection can be accessed, allowing us to communicate and collaborate with others spatially or timely free. Digital technologies refer to information and communication technologies (ICT), including the Internet, mobile technologies and devices, as well as data analytics used to improve the generation, collection, exchange, aggregation, combination, analysis, access, search ability and presentation of digital content, including for the development of services and apps (OECD, 2014; Brynjolfsson, 2016; Eurofund, 2018).

To intertwine digital technologies and health settings suggests identifying what kind of digital tools healthcare professionals are dealing with, and not only tools for health authorities and professionals, but also personalized health systems for users, such as the electronic record of patient's data, telemedicine, and a whole set of technology-based instruments designed for prevention, diagnosis, treatment, monitoring and management of the patient's health. These are some examples of formal and technological systems used in an organizational context in health settings, for health care purposes or for administrative or management purposes. These digital tools can be found in public and private hospitals, clinics, pharmacies, service providers related to additional diagnostic tests, nursing services and therapies to support treatments (Collste, 2006; Couch, 2015; Gholami-Kordkheili, 2013). Citizens and patients may or may not be users of such systems, however the number of users is growing and widespread to all population (Portuguese Ministry of Health, National Health Plan, 2015). A disseminated example which is interesting to point out is the Electronic Prescription that allows the dematerialization of medical prescription. It is based on an efficient and secure process of emission / prescription control and medical dispensing, requiring an authenticated electronic access, through a qualified digital certificate in the case of professionals, and citizen card for users (idem). Adding examples of technological devices or procedures used by professionals, it is possible to point out all kinds of digital platforms to support professional work: enabling a faster and clear measurement of professional activities, writing final reports, production of monthly statistical data, evaluation based on previously defined quantifiable goals and "better" organization of the service.

It is undeniable that the human creativity and innovations with "positive" technologies can embrace or reach new solutions to human problems (Gaggioli, 2017). What potentiality has the virtual world to people, professionals, organizations and governments when adopting "positive" technologies?

MAIN FOCUS OF THE CHAPTER

Regarding digital transformation, significant changes in healthcare settings pawned the traditional work model and introduced a debate about new organizational principles and its influence in professional values and skills. As put in before, how are professions preparing practice in an increasingly digitally mediated world? What are the jurisdictional consequences? Outlining options of response, we can anticipate three scenarios: a) professionals transfer and adopt new configurations to professional practice; according to this, professionals accept and put into action without questioning the required changes; or b) they analyze new configurations and their context of action and adjust their objectives to new experiences and information. In this sense professionals analyze, discuss roles and procedures, and adapt, creating a good combination of both worlds; or c) professionals maintain pre-established patterns of action creating a dependency of the professional path, and resisting to the loss of its main features. Perhaps this kind of reaction can dictate profession's extinction over time.

To reflect about these three possibilities in this chapter we analyze how an electronic health register can influence or change professional practice. The starting point is the National Network of Long-Term Integrated Care (RNCCI)[1] – a Portuguese health public policy based on multilevel and multidisciplinary work and executed through a digital platform to deliver healthcare services to patients with hospital discharge but clinically disabled to go home. This program, based on horizontal and vertical governance, has an organizational model created by the Ministries of Labor, Social Welfare and Health and is formed by clusters of public and private institutions that provide long-term healthcare and social support at local level. The main goal is to provide integrated healthcare and social support to people who, regardless of age, have a temporary or permanent disability caused by a disease. Long-term care is intended to the overall recovery of the person, promoting their autonomy and improving their functionality, considering people's disability, needs and potential of rehabilitation. As follow, the values are: continuous care promoted between different levels of differentiation; equity access and mobility between services; provision of healthcare services close to patient's residential place, empowering community services; multidisciplinary work; systematic evaluation of patients' needs to determine a rehabilitation plan; supportive to continuous recovery or maintenance of functionality and autonomy; involvement of patient and families, or legal representative, in the preparation of the individual intervention plan and care delivery; efficiency and quality of care delivery (PMH, 2016).

In order to gain a sense of Network's size and dynamics, the Portuguese ministry of health (2016) reported that there are 7837 vacancies to receive patients admitted in the National Health Service's hospitals or from the community (home, private hospital or other places of residence). When patients are at the hospital, the Discharge Management Team aims to prepare and manage hospital discharge in coordination with community services, for patients who require follow-up of their health and social problems. The evaluation of patient's need for integrated continuous care is preferably performed at the beginning of the hospital admission, because it is necessary to prepare, in time, the stage following clinical discharge. When patients are at home, the proposal to join the RNCCI is presented to the Local Coordinating Team by a multidisciplinary team composed by one doctor, one nurse and one social worker from the health center.

Network coordination is carried out at national level, without prejudice to regional and local coordination. The coordination at regional and local levels aims to accomplish its operationalization at two territorial levels, guaranteeing flexibility and sequentially use of the units and teams that compose it. At regional level, coordination of the

Network is ensured by five teams involving representatives of the regional health administrations (North, Center, Lisbon and Vale do Tejo, Alentejo and Algarve) and the district social security centers in a multidisciplinary strategy, as defined in Joint Order No. 19040/2006, of the Ministries of Labor, Social Welfare and Health of Portugal. The regional coordinating team (RCT) is dimensioned according to the population's needs and existing resources and work with professionals with knowledge and experience in the areas of planning, management and evaluation. At local level, coordination is ensured by teams of municipal scope. The local coordinating teams are multidisciplinary and are composed by representatives of the Regional Health and Social Security Administration. They must include at least one doctor, one nurse, one social worker and, where necessary, a representative of the local authority designated by the respective mayor of the city.

After this brief description of the RNCCI, which pretend to demonstrate the importance of expert knowledge in the fields of health, social support and management, it will be presented the main features of the electronic health informational systems that support work at national, regional and local levels. Patient information is stored in a cloud-based electronic health recording solution designed for hospitals, primary care facilities, and long term/post-acute care. The software enables multi-provider, multi-location practices by coupling real-time data captured with custom practice management tools. Having a virtual tool, professionals and managers can respond in real time to the demands of all levels of the Network (High Management Teams, Health Centers, Local Coordination Teams, Regional Coordination Teams, Providers - Units and Teams), by accessing to the information needed to produce high health gains to RNCCI users.

An Electronic Health Record is an evolving concept defined as a systematic collection of electronic health information about individual patients or populations. It is a record in digital format that is capable of being shared across different health care settings and includes a range of data like demographics, medical history, medication and allergies, immunization status, laboratory test results, radiology images, vital signs monitoring, personal statistics like age and weight, and more. In many cases this data sharing can occur by network-connected enterprise-wide information systems and by other internal information networks (Couch, 2015; Evans, 2016).

About this program, it is important to highlight that there are more than 1,300 entities in Portugal that use the digital platform with connection between the Ministry of Health and health care providers of the National Health Service. Since 2007, more than 167,000 users have been registered. In addition to the monitoring of the RNCCI workflow circuit, the platform integrates three key evaluating modules, associated to patient's episodes in healthcare facilities of RNCCI, namely, medical, nursing, and social work evaluations. Each dimension registers the following topics: integrated assessment tool (biopsychosocial); risk and assessment of pressure ulcers, and diabetes; diagnostic tests; bandage registration; registration of drugs; adverse drug reactions; infection registration; medical benefits calculation; other reviews like pain evaluation; risk of falls; palliative care evaluation; Edmonton symptom assessment; registration of diaper consumption; identification of the need for social support; registration of care at home; complications / reservation of vacancy; discharge note, among others.

Using digital platforms professionals respond to a mechanical form of work where actions are prescribed in a pre-packed form, rather than judged according to the specific situation at the moment. Freidson (2004) referred to these kinds of tools as expressions of mechanical specialization.

Challenges and Opportunities to Healthcare Professions

The challenges and opportunities to professional work can be found in the organizational professionalism, but to what extend typical features of the traditional professionalism will be blurred? Considering all aspects that are possible to analyze is quite difficult to separate challenges from opportunities, so in this sense we present some of the topics that can provide advantages to the world of professions in healthcare settings.

As follow, it is important to retain that the discourse of managers in public administration defends a national governmental project generating a sense of professional belonging to a complex organization and with good value for all population, like hospitals. It is a discourse that raises the idea of efficiency, citizen empowerment, innovation, public interest and promises autonomy and decision-making power to professionals. It provides also: visibility of the work within the institution and to managers and supervisors, and to the public audience; shared responsibility because all programs are standardized by rules and guidelines and platforms can offer greater and faster contact with hierarchical superiors; control over work at distance. The individual performance is linked to the success of the organization and the definition of measurable objectives and competencies transform the intervention process into quantitative tasks. The principles of good governance integrate codes of ethics and a sense of mission defined by the organizational managers, as well as procedures and solutions defined by the organization. These solutions are based on budgetary constraints, which can justify all changes in procedures and professional roles, and more proximity with the language of management and with managers or administrators. In the same way, they generate: ability to discuss organizational and professional logics; ability to argue and negotiate with the hierarchical superiors for the protection of citizens; ability to mediate and interact with different types of actors in the search for solutions; multidisciplinary work training, and management as a career opportunity (Harding, 2000; Falconbridge, 2008; Hartfouche, 2008; Evetts, 2014; Brock, 2016).

The creation of a positive and modern image and a greater visibility of professional work are reasons that influence the acceptance of the use of digital platforms. Working speedy and efficiently can be increased by the use of technology: meetings taking place in a virtual environment; updating notes on the same document in real time; email inboxes and word processors; easy communication across national and international territories; track procedures steps and standardized procedures, etc. (Evetts, 2014; Guerra, 2017).

The ease that professionals have in using new technologies allows them to adapt to communication and information systems, such as the use of electronic mail that guarantees the timely communication of information relevant to the service. However, there are also hospitals that, through their own virtual information systems, guarantee communication between professionals. Increasingly, the use of new technologies is not a barrier; on the contrary, their absence is considered a problem. However, the urgency of using the computing devices is directly related to the statistical commitments and with all the tools to promote the visibility of professional work.

The purpose of this chapter is to reflect on the impact of new systems related to a range of new information and communication technologies and the shift from a narrative based on traditional knowledge to digital work. It is important to deepen the question: Is the use of digital media a way of organizational control by managers or a path to maximize professional know-how? In order to discuss the benefits of digital professionalism, what has changed and what still remains in the world of professions. The redefinition of professionalism and its connection to digitization grants opportunities to reflect about professional work and about the processes in which professions can evolve, maintain or be dismantled.

SOLUTIONS AND RECOMMENDATIONS

In recent years, there has been an increasing of hospital's production, despite the reduction in the number of hospitals beds in the context of the Portuguese National Health Service. Healthcare benchmarking analysis in all types of intervention (emergency, appointments, hospitalization and surgeries) translates unparalleled progress in science and technology in the healthcare field. However, the scenarios of healthcare services performance and production have become more evident due to the reforms in the health sector in Portugal. Hospital's privatization, the creation of hospitals-corporation, created the imperative to monitor and evaluate the production and performance of each healthcare unit. The notion of performance has become a key element in the modernization process of the National Health Service in Portugal (Simões, 2004). The changes in the management model of healthcare system interfere in the processes of professionalization of all professional groups directly related to healthcare institutions.

Taking the example of Portugal, hospital units provide computer platforms to monitor daily work and professionals are well adapted to the use of computer tools. Using virtual platforms to access services is a common practice. In this chapter we present an example of integrating patients into the National Network of Long-Term Integrated Care.

The level of sophistication of equipment and software varies from hospital to hospital. It is still possible to notice that there are professionals executing paper record-keeping due to lack of equipment. On the other hand, there are hospital units able to reduce the use of paper to the minimum, since they are equipped with technological resources to face the whole dynamics of work through virtual environments (Guerra, 2017).

The adoption of principles of marked-based management with emphasis on measurable production, creation of new management structures, incentive to competition and the creation of performance indicators have generate the bases for the transformation of the healthcare services management model with reflexes in the different health professional groups. The New Public Management presented itself as an alternative to the traditional bureaucratic model of directing public management. This model argues that government should only intervene in activities that cannot be privatized or managed by private and employ means that would allow the presentation of several options to citizens. It also suggests a specific role for managers, requiring improvements in terms of economic efficiency and productivity, through management by objectives and results (Hartfouche, 2008). Understanding health policy reforms and strategies that professionals have assumed in adapting to the new organizational environment that has been created is quite important and interesting. It is about considering new forms of professionalism which result from coalescing organizational and professional discourse in work's organization. The main analytical points pretend to reflect on professional action limited by new forms of control and management that emphasize the defined economic rationalization, not by professional decision but mainly by the organizational goals of management.

According to the Neoweberian theoretical framework it will always be possible to establish a threefold hypothetical scenario on the reaction of the professions to the new management guidelines. One possibility indicates that there is no compatibility between the two logics: the professions consider themselves threatened by organizations, losing their autonomy of judgment and decision-making, favoring administrative and managerial authority and, in this sense, they struggle to maintain their own path and keeping apart of organizational/managerial demands. A second possibility accepts that professional groups resist to organizational changes and are able to protect and preserve their jurisdictions and privileges. Yet, in this case, their defense strategies cannot come only from their cautious or conservative point of view, but from their ability to adapt to new demands, to combine opportunities, and to create an orientation well-matched with organizational principles. The third hypothesis, which is less damaging to the organizational system, considers the possibility of non-existing tensions and a compatible agenda, through the existence of a joint system between professions and organizations, abolishing potential pressures.

FUTURE RESEARCH DIRECTIONS

By recognizing the challenges and opportunities to professional work framed by digital transformation is underlined the importance of trying to understand how to remain professional in different digital environments and how to work in contexts with virtual surveillance. It would be interesting to explore changes at three different levels.

At macro level, the diffusion and adoption of new technologies is giving rise to new forms of public engagement increasing relationships that combine public, private and social spheres. To what extend new digital governance contexts reshape professions and state relationships? Are all stakeholders ready to a cultural shift towards modernization within the public sector?

At mezzo level, how practitioners are learning technological skills in order to maintain their jobs and perform their duties and grant employability over the long term. What efforts have been taken by employers to translate the opportunities of the digital transformation into productivity gains?

And at micro level how citizens benefit from digital professionalism? The shift to use technology should be closely linked to improve people lives. Are professionals improving their expert knowledge to accomplish citizens' expectations of problem-solving? New forms of public governance inspired by digital transformation are improving digital technologies' effectiveness for delivering public value and strengthening citizen trust? This chapter pretends to highlight the connection between professions and digital transformation in changing societal expectations and look up for this promising field of research.

CONCLUSION

The world is undergoing an important shift, which can be called transition to an economy of intensive knowledge. A new model of creation, diffusion and use of knowledge is becoming consistent resulting from three main factors: the acceleration due to information and communication technologies; the increasingly sophisticated process of coding, learning and knowledge management and its social perception as a strategic asset of companies, nations and populations (Rodrigues, 2005). Digitization, globalization, mercantilism, hyperconsumption and individualism have become the framework of all domains of human life with clear connection to the world of professions (Innerarity, 2010, Lipovetsky, 2013, Evetts, 2014). For all of these transformations, the world of work is also transforming and being transformed (Evetts, 2010, 2014; Lorenz, 2006; Freidson, 2004). Each profession is bound to a set of tasks by ties of jurisdiction and none of these connections are absolute or permanent because they change continually (Rodrigues, 2012).

REFERENCES

Abbott, A. (1988). *The System of Professions. An essay on the division of expert labor*. Chicago: The University of Chicago Press. doi:10.7208/chicago/9780226189666.001.0001

Bianic, T. (2003). Bringing the State back in the study of professions. Some peculiarities of the French model of professionalization. In the *6th ESA Conference, Research Network Sociology of Professions*, University of de Murcia. Retrieved from https://www.um.es/ESA/papers/Rn15_28.pdf

Brock, D. M., & Saks, M. (2016). Professions and organizations: A European perspective. *European Management Journal, 34*(1), 1–6. doi:10.1016/j.emj.2015.11.003

Brynjolfsson, E., & McAfee, A. (2016). *The second machine age: work, progress, and prosperity in a time of brilliant technologies*. New York: W.W. Norton & Company.

Burton, J., & Broek, D. (2009). Accountable and Countable: Information Management Systems and the Bureaucratization of Social Work. *British Journal of Social Work, 39*(7), 1326–1342. doi:10.1093/bjsw/bcn027

Cappellin, R., & Wink, R. (2009). *International Knowledge and Innovation Networks: Knowledge Creation and Innovation in Medium-technology Clusters*. Cheltenham, UK: Edward Elgar Publishing Limited. doi:10.4337/9781848449084

Carvalho, T., & Santiago, R. (Eds.). (2015). *Professionalism, Managerialism and Reform in Higher Education and the Health Services. The european welfare state and the rise of the knowledge society*. Londres: Palgrave Macmillan.

Castells, M. (2012). *Era da Informação II: Economia, Sociedade e Cultura* (4th ed.). Lisboa, Portugal: Fundação Calouste Gulbenkian.

Castells, M., & Cardoso, G. (Eds.). (2005). *The Network Society: From Knowledge to Policy*. Washington, DC: Johns Hopkins Center for Transatlantic Relations.

Collste, G., Duquenoy, P., George, C., Hedström, K., Kimppa, K., & Mordini, E. (2006). *ICT in Medicine and Health Care: Assessing Social, Ethical and Legal Issues*. Retrieved from https://www.researchgate.net/publication/31597715

Couch, D., Han, G. S., Robinson, P., & Komesaroff, P. (2015). Public health surveillance and the media: A dyad of panoptic and synoptic social control. *Health Psychology and Behavioral Medicine*, *3*(1), 128–141. doi:10.1080/21642850.2015.1049539

Crotty, B., & Mostaghimi, A. (2011). Professionalism in the Digital Age. *Annals of Internal Medicine*, *154*(8), 560–562. doi:10.7326/0003-4819-154-8-201104190-00008 PMID:21502653

Ellaway, R. H. (2014). Panoptic, synoptic, and omnoptic surveillance. *Medical Teacher*, *36*(6), 547–549. doi:10.3109/0142159X.2014.914680 PMID:24873680

Ellaway, R. H., Coral, J., Topps, D., & Topps, M. (2015). Exploring digital professionalism. *Medical Teacher*, *37*(9), 844–849. doi:10.3109/0142159X.2015.1044956 PMID:26030375

Eurofound. (2018). *Automation, digitalisation and platforms: Implications for work and employment*. Luxembourg: Publications Office of the European Union. Retrieved from http://eurofound.link/ef18002

Evans, R. S. (2016). Electronic Health Records: Then, Now, and in the Future. *Yearbook of medical informatics*, *25*(S 01), S48-S61. doi:10.15265/IYS-2016-s006

Evetts, J. (2012a), Professionalism in turbulent times: changes, challenges and opportunities. *Sociologia, Problemas e Práticas, 88,* 43-59. Retrieved from https://revistas.rcaap.pt/sociologiapp/article/view/14797

Evetts, J. (2012b). Sociological Analysis of the New Professionalism: Knowledge and Expertise in Organizations. In T. Carvalho, R. Santiago, & T. Caria (Eds.), *Grupos Profissionais, Profissionalismo e Sociedade do Conhecimento* (pp. 13–27). Porto: Edições Afrontamento.

Evetts, J. (2014). The Concept of Professionalism: Professional Work, Professional Practice and Learning. In S. Billett, C. Harteis, & H. Gruber (Eds.), *International Handbook of Research in Professional and Practice-based Learning* (pp. 29–56). Dordrecht, Sweden: Springer. doi:10.1007/978-94-017-8902-8_2

Faulconbridge, J. R., & Muzio, D. (2008). Organizational professionalism in globalizing law firms. *Work, Employment and Society*, *22*(1), 7–25. doi:10.1177/0950017007087413

Freidson, E. (2004). *Professionalism: The Third Logic*. Cambridge, UK: Polity Press.

Gholami-Kordkheili, F., Wild, V., & Strech, D. (2013). The Impact of Social Media on Medical Professionalism: A Systematic Qualitative Review of Challenges and Opportunities. *Journal of Medical Internet Research*, *15*(8), 1-8. Retrieved from https://www.jmir.org/2013/8/e184/

Griffin, D. (2012). *Hospitals: What They Are and How They Work*. Burlington: Jones & Bartlett Learning.

Guerra, J. (2017). *Serviço Social, Profissão e Professionalismo no Contexto do Estado-Providência em Portugal. Os assistentes sociais nos hospitais do Serviço Nacional de Saúde*. Unpublished doctoral dissertation, Catholic University of Portugal, Lisbon, Portugal.

Harding, A., & Preker, A. S. (2000). *Understanding organizational reforms: the corporatization of public hospitals*. Retrieved from http://siteresources.worldbank.org/HEALTHNUTRITIONANDPOPULATION/Resources/281627-1095698140167/Harding-UnderstandingOrganizational-whole.pdf

Harfouche, A. P. (2008). *Hospitais Transformados em Empresas. Análise do impacto na eficiência: estudo comparativo*. Lisboa, Portugal: Instituto Superior de Ciências Sociais e Políticas da Universidade Técnica de Lisboa.

Hill, A., & Shaw, I. (2011). *Social Work and ICT*. London, UK: Sage Publication.

Innerarity, D. (2010). *O Novo Espaço Público*. Lisboa, Portugal: Teorema.

Keating, M. (2002), Working Together – Integrated Governance. *United Nations*. Retrieved from http://unpan1.un.org/intradoc/groups/public/documents/apcity/unpan007118.pdf

Lapão, L. V. (2016). The Future Impact of Healthcare Services Digitalization on Health Workforce: The Increasing Role of Medical Informatics. *Studies in Health Technology and Informatics*, *228*, 675–679. PMID:27577470

Lipovetsky, G., & Serroy, J. (2011). *Cultura-Mundo. A cultura-mundo, respostas a uma sociedade desorientada*. São Paulo, Brazil: Companhia das Letras.

Lorenz, W. (2006). *Perspectives on European Social Work: From the Birth of the Nation State to the Impact of Globalisation*. Opladen: Barbara Budrich Publishers.

Noordegraaf, M. (2006). Professional Management of Professionals: Hybrid Organizations and Professional Management in Care and Welfare. In J. W. Duyvendak, T. Knijn, & M. Kremer (Eds.), *Policy, People and the New Professional: De-professionalisation and Re-professionalisation in Care and Welfare* (pp. 181–193). Amsterdam, The Netherlands: Amsterdam University Press.

Noordegraaf, M. (2007). From "Pure" to "Hybrid" Professionalism: Present-Day Professionalism in Ambiguous Public Domains. *Administration & Society*, *39*(6), 761–785. doi:10.1177/0095399707304434

OECD. (2014). *Recommendation of the Council on Digital Government Strategies*. Retrieved from http://www.oecd.org/gov/digital-government/Recommendation-digital-government-strategies.pdf

OECD. (2017). *New Health Technologies: Managing Access, Value and Sustainability*. doi:10.1787/9789264266438-

Parton, N. (2000). *Social Theory, Social Change and Social Work (The State of Welfare)*. London, UK: Routledge.

Parton, N. (2008). Changes in the Form of Knowledge in Social Work: From the 'Social' to the 'Informational'? *British Journal of Social Work*, *38*(2), 253–269. doi:10.1093/bjsw/bcl337

Peña-Casas, R., Ghailani, D., & Coster, S. (2018). Digital transition in the European Union: what impacts on job quality? In B. Vanhercke, D. Ghailani & S. Sabato (Eds.), *Social policy in the European Union: state of play 2018*, Brussels, European Trade Union Institute (ETUI) and European Social Observatory (OSE). Retrieved from http://www.ose.be/EN/team/ose/ghailani.htm

Pollitt, C. (2013, January). What do we know about public management reform? Concepts, models and some approximate guidelines. *Paper presented at the Workshop Towards a comprehensive reform of public governance*, Lisboa, Portugal. Retrieved from https://www.bportugal.pt/pt-pt/obancoeoeurosistema/eventos/documents/pollitt_paper.pdf

Pollitt, C., & Bouckaert, G. (2011). *Public Management Reform. A comparative analysis - New Public Management, Governance, and the Neo-Weberian State.* New York: Oxford University Press.

Ponnert, L., & Svensson, K. (2016). Standardisation – the end of professional discretion? *European Journal of Social Work, 19*(3-4), 586–599. doi:10.1080/136 91457.2015.1074551

Portuguese Ministry of Health (PMH). (2015). National Health Plan (PNS) 2012-2016. Retrieved from https://www.dgs.pt/em-destaque/plano-nacional-de-saude-revisao-e-extensao-a-2020-aprovada-pelo-governo.aspx

Portuguese Ministry of Health (PMH). (2016). *Plano de Desenvolvimento da RNCCI 2016-2019.* Lisboa: Ministérios do Trabalho e da Solidariedade Social e da Saúde. Retrieved from https://www.sns.gov.pt/wp-content/uploads/2016/02/Plano-de-desenvolvimento-da-RNCCI.pdf

Gaggioli, A., Riva, G., Peters, D., & Calvo, R. A. (2017). Positive Technology, Computing, and Design: Shaping a Future in Which Technology Promotes Psychological Well-Being. In M. Jeon (Ed.), Emotions and Affect in Human Factors and Human-Computer Interaction (pp. 477–502). Academic Press; doi:10.1016/B978-0-12-801851-4.00018-5

Ragnedda, M., & Muschert, G. W. (2013). *The Digital Divide: The internet and social inequality in international perspective.* Abingdon: Routledge. doi:10.4324/9780203069769

Rodrigues, M. J. (2005). The European Way to a Knowledge-Intensive Economy—The Lisbon Strategy. In M. Castells & G. Cardoso (Eds.), *The Network Society: From Knowledge to Policy* (pp. 405–424). Washington, DC: Johns Hopkins Center for Transatlantic Relations.

Rodrigues, M. L. (2012). *Profissões. Lições e Ensaios.* Coimbra: Almedina.

Schafer, E. (2003). *Digital Technology.* Retrieved from http://www.encyclopedia.com/doc/1G2-3401801216.html

Simões, J. (2004). *Retrato Político da Saúde. Dependência do percurso e inovação em saúde: da ideologia ao desempenho.* Coimbra: Almedina.

Vago, S. (2004). *Social Change* (5th ed.). New Jersey: Pearson Education, Inc.

ADDITIONAL READING

Friedewals, M., & Pohoryles, R. J. (Eds.). (2016). *Privacy and Security in the Digital Age: Privacy in the Age of Super-Technologies*. Abingdon: Routledge. doi:10.4324/9781315766645

Gagnon, K., & Sabus, C. (2015). Professionalism in a Digital Age: Opportunities and Considerations for Using Social Media in Health Care. *Physical Therapy, 95*(3), 406–414. doi:10.2522/ptj.20130227 PMID:24903111

Heidkamp, B., & Kergel, D. (Eds.). (2017). *Precarity within the Digital Age: Media Change and Social Insecurity*. Wiesbaden: Springer. doi:10.1007/978-3-658-17678-5

Mather, C., Douglas, T., & O'Brien, J. (2017). Identifying Opportunities to Integrate Digital Professionalism into Curriculum: A Comparison of Social Media Use by Health Profession Students at an Australian University in 2013 and 2016. *Informatics, 4*(2), 1-14. Retrieved from https://www.mdpi.com/2227-9709/4/2/10

Qudrat-Ullah, H., & Tsasis, P. (Eds.). (2017). *Innovative Healthcare Systems for 21st Century*. Cham, Switzerland: Springer. doi:10.1007/978-3-319-55774-8

Shachak, A., Borycki, E. M., & Reis, S. P. (Eds.). (2017). Health Professionals' Education in the Age of Clinical Information Systems, Mobile Computing and Social Networks. Cambridge, UK: Academic Press inc Elsevier.

Skurka, M. A. (Ed.). (2017). *Health Information Management: Principles and Organization Health Information Services* (6th ed.). San Francisco, CA: Jossey-Bass.

Vanacker, B., & Heider, D. (Eds.). (2018). *Ethics for a Digital Age* (Vol. 2). New York: Peter Lang Publishing. doi:10.3726/b14177

KEY TERMS AND DEFINITIONS

Digital Health: Is representing a shift paradigm on healthcare and it is creating a different model of healthcare professional versus patient relationship. Software will be able to detail guidance about specific nutrition, supplements, exercise, medication and treatment for individuals. Consumer devices helping to monitor many aspects of life such as weight, vital signs, physical activity, sleep, skin resistance, perspiration and location.

Digital Professionalism: Is the competence or values expected of a professional when engaged in social and digital communication

Health Information Systems: Provide new information through its four main functions: data collection, processing, analysis and dissemination in order to enable decision-makers at multi-levels of the health system to identify problems and needs, make evidence-based decisions on health policy and allocate scarce resources on the most favorable way.

Interoperability: Is a way to communicate and data sharing through software to exchange and make use of information by different organizations, it allows to work in conjunction with each other.

Jurisdiction: Is based on abstract knowledge, express the capability of a profession to solve problems, find solutions for the good of people.

Positive Technology: Technology designed to improve the quality of life representing a potential way to increase accessibility, affordability, and effectiveness of positive interventions in many areas of society, including health (e.g. Electronic Health Records, Mobile Health Apps, Telemedicine, electronic prescribing).

Professional Autonomy: The right or possibility to determine professional work, procedures, and tasks, because of the expert knowledge achieved in universities or practice.

Standardization: Is a framework of agreements to which professionals in an organization must accept to ensure that all processes associated with the creation of a product or service are performed within set guidelines, achieving uniformity to certain practices or operations within the selected environment. It can be seen as a professional strategy to strengthen professional trust and provide a sense of certainty for professionals or it can be interpreted as a way to lose professionalization and as an adjustment to organizational demands.

ENDNOTE

[1]   In Portuguese: Rede Nacional de Cuidados Continuados Integrados.

Chapter 4

The Matrix of Complexity Associated With the Process of Social Intervention With Chronic Kidney Disease Patients

Marta Freitas Olim
iD https://orcid.org/0000-0001-5151-9425
Diaverum, Portugal

Sónia Guadalupe
iD https://orcid.org/0000-0003-4898-3942
University Coimbra, Portugal

Fernanda da Conceição Bento Daniel
iD https://orcid.org/0000-0002-2202-1123
University Coimbra, Portugal

Joana Pimenta
iD https://orcid.org/0000-0002-7617-7270
Diaverum, Portugal

Luís Carrasco
iD https://orcid.org/0000-0002-7835-5296
Diaverum, Portugal

Alexandre Gomes da Silva
iD https://orcid.org/0000-0001-5163-9670
University of Coimbra, Portugal

DOI: 10.4018/978-1-5225-8470-4.ch004

ABSTRACT

This chapter discusses the standardization of instruments and typologies in social work assessment and introduces, from a multidimensional perspective, a new standardized instrument evaluating the level of complexity associated with the social intervention process in a sample of chronic kidney disease (CKD) patients. The authors evaluated the matrix's metric properties by internal consistency and defined a rating index through the best cutoff points, using receiver operator curve and Youden Index. Matrix construction and validation used focus groups of experts in blinded classification of 100 CKD patients and indicator weighting. The matrix shows good internal consistency and reliability (Cronbach's alpha = .742). Cutoff points indicate three levels of complexity classification. The matrix is a good instrument to identify the complexity associated with the social intervention process in the area of Nephrology, and is a relevant contribution to the social information management of social workers, the health teams and the administration of health units.

INTRODUCTION

The computerization of social assessment in the context of health organizations poses enormous challenges. The complexity of patients' social situations rarely emerges from linear and fragmented statistics derived from records based on isolated variables. Understanding Social Work's intervention process, the actions it entails and the time involved are often difficult to justify to management departments because they arise from a complex set of interlocking factors that are difficult to quantify. In close complementarity with the clinical diagnosis and prognosis, the social diagnosis must be expressed through methods that recognize this complexity.

In a society dominated by technology, the pressure to record social information related to the processes of study, diagnosis, planning and social intervention has increased sharply to quantify this information, as well as the evaluation of professionals' workloads. Scientificity, instrumental rationality and technicality cannot, however, overshadow the values of the profession and its humanistic realm, under penalty of realizing the risks of de-professionalization associated with fragmentation and over-bureaucratization emphasized by managerialism and social technology (Amaro, 2014). Despite of the McDonaldization of the social care and care management in Social Work, the "adherence to professional values, supported by professional registration, and an awareness of power, both instrumental and normative, can promote good practice" (Dustin, 2007, p. 164). Opting for a scientific-humanist profile, Amaro (2012) mentions that the instruments are defined and mobilized based on the analysis of a given situation, requiring a reflexive and critical position about them. Bureaucratic and standardized procedures should integrate professional reflexivity and emerge not as ends in themselves, but as methodological strategies to achieve professional goals. These can be evidence of the relevance of a particular social problem, and support intervention programs or institutional policy measures, or even, social policy favoring the well-being of a given population, for example.

Although standardization and categorization emerge as serious trends in the health field, Social Work has been resisting this tendency in his social evaluation procedures, avoiding reductionist and linear evaluations. However, the challenges of computerizing social information require innovation and overcoming such gaps with the construction of standardized multidimensional instruments that could support non-linear social diagnostics and guide intervention plans.

In this chapter the authors debate the controversial approaches to standardization and the potentialities and risks of the use of classificatory typologies in social diagnosis, presenting an innovative assessment tool, in the field of nephrological Social Work, that overcomes some of the identified risks.

Thus, this chapter shows the development and validation of a new standardized instrument that evaluates the level of complexity associated with the social intervention process in a sample of chronic kidney disease (CKD) patients. The matrix presented (MCAPIS_DRC[1]) aims to identify and classify the complexity associated with the social intervention process with CKD patients, in three levels of complexity, making a relevant contribution to the work of social workers in this intervention area, as well as to the management of health services. This study intends to show the process of constructing an index to be used by social workers in professional evaluation and research in the specific scope of work with a population with a clinical diagnosis of chronic kidney disease and patients undergoing hemodialysis.

BACKGROUND

The Standardization in the Social Diagnosis Under Debate[2]

The use of standardized instruments in Social Work is not widespread and it is controversial. We do not recognize nosological and typological systems for social diagnosis. However, we find commonly used concepts that may be unassigned typologies (Guadalupe, 2016), which may give rise to a blurred conceptual field, poorly reflected and inexpertly grounded in theory and purpose and professional values. The evaluation based on standardized instruments can contain reducing realms but can also enhance the construction of knowledge, provided it can systematize the complexity of the situations.

The social diagnosis has evaded the rule regarding other disciplinary areas of the social and human sciences regarding the etymology of social problems, the adoption of typologies and the definition of nosological entities and taxonomies. Greenwood (1955) affirmed the need to construct diagnostic and intervention typologies ("treatment") in Social Work, arguing that a well-developed practice would be associated with a descriptive and prescriptive diagnostic typology of social problems, intensively analyzed in the context of Social Sciences.

The classification scheme in categories or types of "problem-definition" and "problem-solution" would be a constellation of factors and would base a set of generalizable and comparable propositions without leaving aside singularities, so Greenwood (1955) claims to require a high level of professional specialization. The author stresses that "the descriptions of the of diagnostic and treatment typologies, in all their ramifications, implications and rationalizations, are the principles of practice and constitute the unique body of knowledge of the discipline" (Greenwood, 1955, p. 26), which he calls "practice theory". Along the same lines, Hamilton (1958, p. 266) stated that "it would be useful to have some sentences for which problems could be expressed, but such classification has not yet had practical results as diagnostic statements", adding that "it was trendy (…) to criticize the diagnostic classification, while it is really indicative of a certain amount of professional knowledge" (Hamilton, 1958, p. 277). While such ideas integrate works published in the 1950s, it would not be a complete anachronism to think of them in the scope of contemporary Social Work.

The lack of a categorization of social problems, needs and social resources in the context of social diagnosis has a facet of non-generalization, with which we tend to agree as a principle, but which has simultaneously emerged as a conditional gap in the development of a language of its own, in the appropriation of constructs, or in the construction of objects and perspectives unequivocally associated with the disciplinary area.

However, we understand that Social Work does not escape classificatory systems. Although systematic classifications are unknown, they tend to proliferate in the professional daily life disconnectedly, mainly driven by the need to record social information. Thus, classifying concepts and constructs are commonly used without there being explained, scrutinized and validated criteria and descriptors that favor their use in Social Work education and their unequivocal operation by the professional category. The same seems to occur with the social information registration instruments, lacking theoretical grounds as well as validity and methodological trustworthiness (Guadalupe, 2016), requiring to be gauged through the discussion and further development of the meta-theoretical presuppositions that traverse them, explaining and understanding the paradigms, models and their underlying ontological, gnosiological and epistemological principles.

Reflexivity has to find space, not letting drop the record and the professional action in a bureaucratic-administrative exercise (Amaro, 2012; Howe, 1992; Portes & Portes, 2009; Sousa, 2008). Thus, Restrepo (2003) warns that the critical use of categorical action-orienting systems prevents the practice from falling into empiricism or unreflective self-regulation, or methodological finalism (Amaro, 2012, 2014), and it is fundamental that the technical-operational realm is appropriated critically (Silva, 2013).

However, we must be aware that daily pressure tends to restrict the complex professional action to provide mechanized and superficial responses (Lacerda, 2014), and can also negatively favor a homogenization of the unique situations through managerialist instruments, not allowing to equate the movement between the singular and universal vis-à-vis the elements underlying the professional exercise and their interconnections with social dynamics.

This work recognizes such critical realms that traverse the standardized instruments and is a contribution to the field of social evaluation in the area of health care.

Typologies and Classifications in Social Diagnosis: Potentialities and Risks

Any diagnosis contains potentialities and risks. Potentialities concern the assessment of the problem-situation and the possibilities it provides for planning and evaluating the intervention. On the other hand, risks are associated with their potential for labeling, stigmatization, linearity, reductionism, superficiality, mechanicism, emphasizing the negative realm of the situations evaluated, crystallizing a perspective from other possible perspectives and concealing the dynamism and complexity of situations.

In a discussion from the systemic epistemology, Elkaïm (1985) states peremptorily that it does not authorize the definition of explanatory etiological systems, warning that the regularities in systems should not hide their singularities. In this line of questioning, Rey and Prieur (1991, p. 61) strongly criticize clinical diagnosis and argue that "the system is itself the best explanation", indicating that this postulate will avoid the conceptual trap of "deplorable construction of 'realities' (...) through the use of apparently scientific diagnostic terms". In contrast, Ausloos (1996, p. 58) counteracts and points out that "it is said that typologies are not systemic", but he deconstructs the idea by arguing that they will be so if they integrate the interaction in the systems and are not focused on the individual realm. These are some arguments that encompass the context of psychopathology but that we can also extrapolate to other areas.

Expressing complex realities, dynamics and singularities through digital (written or spoken) language, which involves syntax but not semantic, avoiding extensive and tangled descriptions, will be an unworkable exercise. Thus, the use of typologies allows the expression of perspectives on consensual realities through a reference construct that allows us to outline the contours of a given situation without an extensive descriptive exercise. The use of professional jargon cannot pretend to exhaust the confronted realities and does not always facilitate the construction of a narrative that corresponds to its "multiversus" (multiple universes).

These ideas refer to the controversial concept of reality. From a constructivist perspective, it is understood that the systems we observe are not 'the reality.' In parallelism with the famous sentence of Alfred Korzybski, "the map is not the territory", it is a risk to confuse what reality is and how we organize reality to get to know it (Castelucci, Fruggeri, & Marzari, 1984, as cited in Campanini & Luppi, 1996). Watzlawick (1991, p. 7) asserts that it is dangerous to presume the existence of a single reality and is convinced that what exists are multiple and unique perspectives of reality, constructed by each and their "lenses", references, experiences, as well as their academic and professional education. So, the constructivists opt for the plural concept of realities. The idea assumes polysemy senses as a premise but does not rule out the existence of common and coincident constructions, although the vertexes we clarify and underscore when reading these realities may differ. This is an interesting idea to think about the social diagnosis, "because regardless of the technical scrutiny to which it is submitted, it is still the construction of a given social worker about the reality of a given situation in a given moment" (Guadalupe, 2016, p. 58). The German pioneer of the profession, Alice Salomon, believed that the diagnosis is not established by the compilation of data, but involves evaluation, comparison and interpretation, resulting in a general picture that is not obtained by the accumulation of details (Salomon, 1926, as cited in Lorenz, 2004). Thus, the author appeals to the idea of totality, so special to the systemic perspective, in the construction of readings on the realities.

Typologies, taxonomies and classifications function as reference and analytical resources for the reading of realities, in their plurality and singularity, equated as theoretical models and ideal types, in the Weberian conception.

We agree with Fook (2002, p. 124) when she states that "the process of making meaning of a situation is interactive and reflective". Albuquerque (2011, p. 110), discussing the processes of legitimization and recognition of social work practices, states that they are part of "retroactive dynamics between the singularity of a situation, the set of experiences and resources accumulated and reinterpreted by the agent, the constituent elements of the contexts and the set of perspectives of the various actors, in the construction and weighting of a given situation". However, the author positions herself unfavorably vis-à-vis the categorization in the process of translating and publicizing the construction of the situation in the public domain, advocating for the path of "de-singularization", which would safeguard the idiosyncrasy of the situations described, stating that "the use of categories and typologies to fit populations and search translates a discourse of rationalization and homogenization" (Albuquerque, 2011, p. 110). Regarding favoring the recognition of the production of knowledge in the area, the author considers the diagnostic elements as one of its argumentative linkages. The professional production on diagnostic elements involves a process of identification, interpretation and connection of data, assuming suitability for the screening of relevant elements, release against contingency and circumstantiality, as well as the capacity to produce complex and pluralistic records and readings, and the sharing of social diagnoses requires the definition and clarification of a conceptual and operational field of action capable of reviving and appropriating composite concepts (Albuquerque, 2011).

The construction of typologies in Social Work is exceptionally found. Hollis (1970), an author associated with casework, proposed a typology constructed on the basis of an investigation that analyzed the content of social processes, noting the potential risks of careless labeling and the stereotyped categorization of people in a given category, recognizing, however, that its proper use would add value to the diagnostic understanding and intervention. Also, in the same period, Ogren, Norris-Shortle and Showalter (1979) present two typologies within the scope of clinical social work also based on the review of social processes, a multidimensional family-centered classification and a prescriptive typology, warning that these should be seen as tools rather than stereotypes for social work practice. Such warnings in the use of categorizations also appear in contemporary works. For example, in Spain, a manual of indicators for social diagnosis adopted by the General Council of Social Work (Muñoz, Barandalla, & Aldalur, 1996), which shows five categories based on a classification of needs and social indicators, aiming to achieve greater operability in the diagnosis, although choosing to sacrifice the singular nuances that involve the different social situations. The definition of diagnostic indicators should be theoretically supported (Prizzon, 2006) and accurate terminology should be used in the evaluation (Campanini, 2006).

Digital age represents several ethical challenges in assessment, data registration and in the intervention process, namely using diverse digital, online or electronic tools (Reamer, 2013), thus, any innovation has to be strongly based on ethical principles and the reflexivity of the professionals.

Despite the possible risks or limitations, we understand that the use of standardized instruments and typologies in the Social Work's diagnosis can contribute to the development of the profession and the scientific area. In order to overcome any linearity or reductionism, the instruments must be multidimensional and integrate complex approaches, mirroring the complexity of people's realities in situations monitored by Social Work, in an area traversed by enormous complexity and mutation, and by ethical determinations.

Multidimensional Assessment of Chronic Kidney Disease in Health Social Work

The multidimensionality of chronic kidney disease (CKD) and its implications has been reaffirmed (Pilotto et al., 2012; Rascanu & Radu, 2014). Health and disease express a complex and dynamic reality based on a whole set of bio-psyco-ecological-cultural-social factors.

Although the informatization of health and social care is a key element of the modernization in Social Work methodologies, the dilemmas and opportunities presented by different paths to informatizing social data have to be central also (Hardey & Loader, 2009).

Analytically, in the approach to health and disease, we can identify subjective dimensions (related to meanings of well-being and malaise) and objective dimensions (related to somatic functioning and functionality) (Ribeiro, 1994), where realms such as emotional, social, relational, intellectual, spiritual and physical health (O'Donnel, 1986, as cited in Ribeiro, 1994) can be independent, and the latter realm is only one of several, in interaction, which underlines the relevance of its holistic conception. While they are two opposing social processes, we cannot delimit health and disease, equating their relationship in a continuum with different and mixed degrees and expressions (González et al., 1988).

The quality of life and well-being of CKD patients depends on a favorable combination of different domains that enhances adjustment and adaptation to the demands of the disease and its treatments (Lopes, et al. 2014). The chronicity of the disease, described as "the great crossing" by Rolland (2000, p. 78), has implications in all areas of the patient's life, whether on a personal, emotional, relational, family, professional level or another level (Guadeloupe, 2012). If the impact of the disease on society is remarkable (Jha, Wang, & Wang, 2012), due to its costs to health systems and productive years lost (Schieppati & Remuzzi, 2005; Turchetti et al., 2017), the impact on the personal and family sphere is undeniable and plural. The literature has shown the socioeconomic impact (Jha, Wang, & Wang, 2012), as well as the impact on mental health (Goh & Griva, 2018, Shirazian et al., 2017) on declining autonomy and functionality (Bowling, Sawyer, Campbell, Ahmed, & Allman, 2011) and, in general, on the quality of life (Brown, et al., 2017, Lopes et al., 2014), where the clinical, economic and humanistic burden of the CKD is highlighted (Braun, Sood, Hogue, Lieberman, & Copley-Merriman, 2012). The family´s role has been referred to as central in the adjustment to the disease (Guadalupe, 2012; Rascanu & Radu, 2014).

This multidimensionality of impacts is associated with a wide range of social needs whose adequate response is intended to compensate for the vulnerability that these patients often evidence. In Social Work, professionals daily address complex and cross-cutting social issues, involving multidimensional relationships expressed in a particular way in each context (Serafim & Santo, 2012). In the context of health, the relationship between the social worker, the patient (with his/her health-disease process) and the family is extremely complicated and interferes in the intervention process in the face of the various social problems, the dynamics of the organization of health and social policies, among other dimensions (Serafim & Santo, 2012). Therefore, Vourlekis and Rivera-Mizzoni (1997) identify three interrelated components that inform social assessment: 1) the body of knowledge about the characteristic significance and impact of the psychosocial factors of the disease; 2) a general model of the evaluation process; 3) a detailed understanding of the psychosocial circumstances and the specific and changing clinical conditions of each patient.

With chronic disease, we see the emergence of a dynamic systemic puzzle that takes into account different impacts and interferences on a personal and interpersonal (emotional, relational, professional, life plans) and family level (taking into account the age of the patient and his/her role in the family, family structure diversity, personal and sociocultural meanings, the life cycle stage, previous experiences of disease in the family, living and economic conditions, reconciliation of professional life with care, family support and social support network) (Guadalupe, 2012). The puzzle also contains the idiosyncrasies of CKD, its evolution, the care plan, the demands of treatments, the associated limitations, the prognosis and eventual disability. Completing the puzzle are: the organizational system, which includes the health system; the rights and access to health care and social policies; the specific health unit, and the relationship with other social services (Guadalupe, 2012).

Working with patients with CKD, understood as a complex and debilitating condition (Braun et al., 2012), requires an in-depth knowledge of the various vectors in interaction, and of all the intersecting analytic, comprehending and intervening spheres (Guadalupe, 2012; Vourlekis & Rivera-Mizzoni, 1997). Thus, Social Work must be provided with instruments that respond to this complexity in the intervention in order to facilitate the systematization of information.

However, few specific instruments developed by the Social Work for use with the population concerned are found in the literature. The ECB Renal Patient Questionnaire is an exception. This was developed by Calder and Banning (2000) to screen patients for Social Work's priority intervention, taking into account the number of requests registered in the framework of the Medicare subsystem (USA) that provides the monitoring of Social Work to all patients. This self-administered questionnaire (in the context of a psychosocial interview) produces the Social Work Assessment Index that classifies the need for intervention in: 1) no intervention required; 2) monitoring; 3) immediate intervention. From the analysis of its underlying 30 items, it emphasizes its multidimensionality, inscribing itself in the psychosocial evaluation.

Thus, the challenge of developing multidimensional tools and the scarcity of specific instruments give particular relevance to the contribution of this chapter.

MATERIAL AND METHODS

MCAPIS_DRC is a hetero-administered matrix. It is intended to be classified by social workers or other members of the multidisciplinary team with specific training to do so.

The initial version of MCAPIS_DRC was developed based on the literature and contains the adaptation and transformation of 5 items that underpin the Scale of Complexity of Social Intervention with Adults in the Hospital Context (ECISACH) (Serafim & Santo, 2012). A first version was modified after the focus group with social workers' experts in the intervention with chronic kidney patients. For its validation, 100 chronic kidney patients were followed up by 25 private clinics in Portugal in 2017 by a group of 5 experts based on the data in patients' social processes. No sociodemographic or other data were collected to identify the participants, and the evaluation was blind. The experts are social workers with work experience with CKD patients.

A univariate analysis of the data was carried out initially using central tendency and dispersion measures, and the internal consistency of the items was also evaluated. Data were analyzed using the statistical software SPSS® - Statistical Package for Social Sciences version 24.0 for Windows®.

We requested experts to classify 100 chronic patients through MCAPIS_DRC, with the experts quoting each item of the matrix in three levels of complexity (low, moderate, high) to validate the cutoff points. Experts further classified each "case" in general, with the same scale of levels of complexity.

The metric properties of the matrix were evaluated through the sensitivity and specificity of the scale for several possible cutoff points, through pairs of sensitivity and specificity for each cutoff point. A Receiver Operating Characteristic (ROC) curve was used to define the best cutoff point, evaluating the efficiency of MCAPIS_DRC through the Area Under the ROC Curve (AUC), accuracy (ACC) and the Youden Index with a confidence interval of 95%. The AUC has a range between 0.5 to 1.0, with higher values indicating greater adjustment. Youden's index (J) is equal to sensitivity plus specificity minus one. The "J" has a variation between 0 and 1, with values close to 1 indicating the perfect precision and the 0 value precision obtained by mere chance (Schisterman, Perkins, Liu, & Bondell, 2005). We requested the weighting discussed by nine experts to evaluate the need to distinguish between matrix item weights for the complexity index.

RESULTS

Internal Consistency

The Cronbach's alpha value reveals good internal consistency (.74), indicating reliability of the measure. Variations in Cronbach's alpha value when the item is eliminated (between .70 and .75) indicate that there is no advantage in eliminating any item.

Index of Complexity Associated With the Process of Social Intervention With Chronic Kidney Disease Patients

We asked nine experts to weigh and write down the weighting for each item to evaluate the need to distinguish between matrix item weights for the complexity index. Scores were weighted on a decimal basis. Our analysis defined a syntax to calculate the complexity index that results from the matrix.

Table 1. Internal consistency evaluated by Cronbach's Alpha

N.º of items	15
N	100
Cronbach' s Alpha	.74

Table 2. Item-total statistic for the scale if the item is deleted

Item	Scale Mean if Item Deleted	Scale Variance if Item Deleted	Corrected Item-Total Correlation	Squared Multiple Correlation	Cronbach's Alpha if Item Deleted
1	22.48	19.02	.35	.54	.73
2	22.31	18.10	.31	.54	.73
3	22.12	18.27	.31	.43	.73
4	21.25	18.25	.2	.33	.75
5	22.23	18.87	.23	.21	.74
6	22.47	19.79	.5	.18	.75
7	21.54	16.90	.48	.43	.71
8	22.25	18.43	.31	.29	.73
9	22.13	17.39	.38	.32	.72
10	21.60	16.44	.54	.5	.71
11	21.68	16.12	.58	.58	.71
12	21.98	17.70	.38	.34	.73
13	21.81	18.14	.33	.45	.73
14	22.25	18.98	.16	.23	.75
15	22.02	17.05	.54	.48	.71

Table 3. Weightings of items by experts

Items of the MCAPIS_DRC	Classification by the Nine Experts									Weightings	
1	1	1	0	0	0	1	1	1	0	5	1.56
2	0	0	1	0	0	1	0	1	1	4	1.44
3	1	1	0	1	0	0	1	0	0	4	1.44
4	0	1	0	0	0	1	0	1	0	3	1.33
5	0	1	0	1	1	1	1	1	1	7	1.78
6	0	1	0	0	1	1	0	1	0	4	1.44
7	1	0	0	0	0	0	0	0	0	1	1.11
8	0	0	0	0	0	0	0	0	0	0	1,00
9	1	1	1	1	1	1	1	1	0	8	1.89
10	1	0	1	0	1	0	1	0	1	5	1.56
11	0	0	0	0	0	0	0	0	0	0	1,00
12	0	1	1	1	0	1	1	1	0	6	1.67
13	1	1	0	1	0	1	1	1	0	6	1.67
14	0	0	0	0	0	0	0	0	0	0	1,00
15	1	0	0	0	0	0	0	0	0	1	1.11

From this procedure, the Complexity Index Associated with the Social Intervention Process with Chronic Kidney Disease Patients (ICAPIS_DRC) resulted with the following syntax:

ICAPIS_DRC = (1x1.56) + (2x1.44) + (3x1.44) + (4x1.33) + (5x1.78) + (6x1.44) + (7x1.11) + (8x1.00) + (9x1.89) + (10x1.56) + (11x1,00) + (12x1.67) + (13x1.67) + (14x1,00) + (15x1.11).

Cutoff Points

The best cutoff point with the highest sensitivity (75.0%) is 38.56 with a specificity value of .08% and a value below the ROC curve of .85 (95% CI = .72-.98) (Figure 1). The best cutoff point with the highest sensitivity (91.5%) is 31.22 with a specificity value of 30.2% and a value below the ROC curve of .89 (95% CI = .82-.95) (Figure 2).

Table 4. Correlation between weightings and the associated level of complexity (Evaluated by Experts)

		Weighting	Level of Associated Complexity
	Pearson Correlation	1	.70**
Weighting	Sig. (2-tailed)		< .001
	N	100	100
Level of associated complexity	Pearson Correlation	.70**	1
	Sig. (2-tailed)	< .001	
	N	100	100

**Correlation is significant at the 0.01 level.

Table 5. Areas under the ROC curves

	Area	Standard Error [a]	Asymptotic Sig. [b]	Asymptotic 95% Confidence Interval	
				Lower Limit	Upper Limit
Cutoff point 1 (38.56)	.85	.07	< .001	.72	.98
Cutoff point 2 (31.22)	.89	.03	< .001	.82	.96

Captions: ROC Curve, Sensitivity, Specificity, Diagonal segments are reproduced by ties.

Figure 1. ROC Curve cutoff point 1

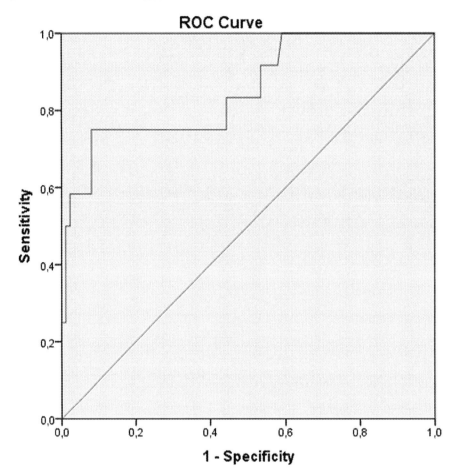

Diagonal segments are produced by ties.

From the analysis performed, we conclude that the cutoff points for the Complexity Index Associated with the Social Intervention Process with Chronic Kidney Patients (ICAPIS_DRC) are as follows:

1. ICAPIS_DRC Low <= 31.22;
2. ICAPIS_DRC Medium 31.23 – 38.56;
3. ICAPIS_DRC High >= 38.56.

Figure 2. ROC Curve cutoff point 2

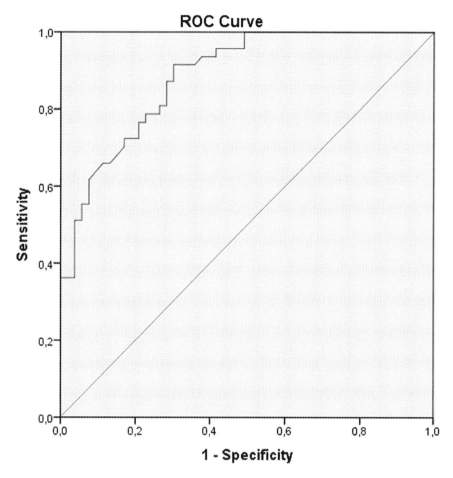

Diagonal segments are produced by ties.

Description of the Matrix: Dimensions, Indicators and Descriptors of the Matrix

MCAPIS_DRC includes two dimensions:

1. Determinants of health-related intervention complexity;
2. Determinants of intervention complexity related to the psychosocial situation.

Table 6. Descriptive statistics for the Cutoff Points

Cutoff Points	n	%
<= 31.22	41	41.0
31.23 – 38.56	43	43.0
38.57+	16	16.0
Total	100	100

The first dimension includes seven indicators: Guidance, Mental Health, Autonomy (AVD), Implications of clinical diagnosis/prognosis, Individual's adaptation to the disease and treatment, Family's adaptation to the disease and treatment and Health literacy level.

The second dimension includes eight indicators: Life context (residential); Family relationships (dominant); Attitude in activating resources to satisfy needs; Competencies to activate rights and medical-social guarantees (own or the support network); Support in monitoring and provision of care (formal and informal); Monthly household's income; Housing conditions; Signaling for evaluation due to psychosocial problems.

Each indicator is classified in a 3-point Likert scale that stipulates the level of complexity associated with the social intervention process as Low (1), Medium (2) and High (3), where the classification of zero is considered when it "does not apply" (0) to the actual situation, or it is not possible to evaluate the indicator.

DISCUSSION

The advantages of the systematic use of standardized instruments in assessing social and psychosocial health problems, particularly at CKD level, are referred to by Vourlekis and Rivera-Mizzoni (1997) because they allow the identification of priority intervention realms, as well as monitoring and documenting changes and results in the follow-up process of Social Work. The use of computerized technology to record the clinical and social information of patients in the dialysis units is widespread in the contemporary world, fostering a comprehensive interdisciplinary approach to the care plan (Browne, Peace, & Perry, 2014). Thus, this scale constitutes a contribution to innovation in the health field, articulating the holistic principles with the linearity of the informatics register that tends to proliferate.

Table 7. Dimensions, indicators and descriptors of evaluation

DIMENSION 1. DETERMINANTS OF HEALTH-RELATED INTERVENTION COMPLEXITY	
INDICATORS	**DESCRIPTORS OF EVALUATION**
1. Guidance*	1. Individual oriented in time, space and person 2. Individual with periods of disorientation 3. Non-oriented individual
2. Mental Health**	1. No indication of mental health problems 2. With indication of mental health problems (without clinical diagnosis) 3. With clinical diagnosis of mental illness
3. Autonomy (AVD)*	1. Total independence 2. Modified independence (a) 2. Moderate dependence (b) 3. Total dependence (c)
4. Implications of clinical diagnosis/ prognosis*	1. Chronic kidney disease without comorbidities 2. Chronic kidney disease with one comorbidity 3. Chronic kidney disease with multiple comorbidities
5. Individual's adaptation to the disease and treatment	1. With adaptation strategies 2. With difficulties of adaptation 3. Rejection
6. Family's adaptation to the disease and treatment	0. Not applicable (non-existent family) 1. With adaptation strategies 2. With difficulties of adaptation 3. Rejection
7. Health literacy level	[Ability to make informed health decisions] 1. High 2. Medium 3. Low
DIMENSION 2. DETERMINANTS OF INTERVENTION COMPLEXITY RELATED TO THE PSYCHOSOCIAL SITUATION	
INDICATORS	**DESCRIPTORS OF EVALUATION**
8. Life context (residential)	1. Cohabiting with family 1. Institutionalized 2. Living alone, close to the family/social network 3. Cohabiting with dependent people 3. Living alone and isolated
9. Family relationships (dominant)	1. Close relationships 2. Distant relationships 3. Interrupted relationships / no known family relationship 3. Conflicting relationships
10. Attitude in activating resources to satisfy needs	1. Proactive, diligent 2. Collaborative, not very proactive 3. Passive, apathetic
11. Competencies to activate rights and medical-social guarantees (own or the support network);	1. With competencies, knowing their rights 2. Competent but unaware of their rights 3. Without competencies and unaware of their rights

continued on following page

101

Table 7. Continued

12. Support in monitoring and provision of care (formal and informal)*	[The support network follows and cares for the patient. It provides care and supports patient's special needs.] 1. A lot of support 2. Moderate support 3. No support [no network] / Low support
13. Monthly household's income	1. Ensures without any problem coverage of monthly expenses 2. Only ensures coverage of monthly expenses 3. Does not ensure coverage of monthly expenses
14. Housing conditions	1. Suited to the needs 2. Unfit for household size or architectural barriers *** 3. In a poor state of conservation or without conditions of habitability (healthiness and comfort)
15. Signaling for evaluation due to psychosocial problems	1. Without signaling 2. With signaling due to psychosocial problem (s) of average complexity **** 3. With signaling due to psychosocial problem (s) of high complexity *****

Notes:

(a) performs the activities with auxiliary resources, requiring more time, but does so autonomously and safely

(b) requires supervision/support in performing some ADLs

(c) requires full support in all ADLs

* Information collected in the clinical process

** Self-indication or indication by relatives

*** (WC with bathtub, w/elevator, with steps in access; without accessibility)

**** Transient psychosocial problems or medium complexity intervention.

***** Chronic psychosocial problems, of prolonged development or high interventional complexity.

Source: own elaboration.

The MCAPIS_DRC reveals good internal consistency (Cronbach's alpha = .74), indicating the reliability of the assessment instrument. The cutoff points were at scores 38 and 31, showing a value below the ROC curve of .85 and .89, respectively, indicating that it is an excellent instrument to identify and classify the complexity associated with the social intervention process.

With few instruments to compare, considering their characteristics and structure, we note that regarding the Scale of Complexity of Social Intervention with Adults in the Hospital Context (ECISACH) (Serafim & Santo, 2012), where this matrix was based on the initial phase of its development, characteristics of internal consistency and correlation between items and dimensions were also mentioned. This is an original scale with three subscales (socio-familial context, clinical situation and hospital social work), and the last one is dedicated to the classification of the social intervention process as to its complexity, so, considered of great utility for use by social workers working in hospitals (Serafim & Santo, 2012). Another multidimensional instrument is the scale of social evaluation of elderly people' conditions, (González et al., 1999), known as the Socio-familiar Scale of Gijón (Alarcón & Montalvo, 1998). This scale is specifically constructed for the detection of risk situations or social problems in the elderly population, and referred as being useful in the hospitals (Alarcón & Montalvo, 1998). However, it is a scale with less dimensions (five: family situation, economic situation, housing, relationships and social support), and with less internal consistency (González et al., 1999), not covering the levels of complexity that MCAPIS_DRC includes.

SOLUTIONS AND RECOMMENDATIONS

In the health care area, but outside the field of Social Work, we found a reference to an instrument of classification of care complexity of home care patients (Bôas, Shimizu, & Sanches, 2016), also using cutoff points based on a methodology similar to the one we followed, which allows a validated classification. This instrument was useful, showed evidence of validity and reproducibility, advantages in the use of multi-professional teams were mentioned, allowing improved organization of services, the transition between care, care plan and quality of care (Bôas et al., 2016).

The 15 different indicators that integrate MCAPIS_DRC ensure its multidimensionality. The indicators were carefully selected and meet the proposals for psychosocial assessment by the Council of Nephrology Social Workers of the National Kidney Foundation (USA) (Browne, Peace & Perry, 2014). This multidimensional characteristic allows an approximation to the complexity of situations that result from the impact of the disease on the life of a person and a family. Most scales refer to non-multidimensional constructs. Tools that evaluate the perception of the quality of life are one of the exceptions. Its multidimensionality justifies their frequent use by social workers in the area of nephrology (Manavalan, Majumdar, Kumar, & Priyamvada, 2017; Vourlekis & Rivera-Mizzoni, 1997). In future studies, it will be interesting to study the correlation between the results of the MCAPIS_DRC and quality of life assessment scales.

As mentioned before, the ECB Renal Patient Questionnaire (Calder & Banning, 2000) is one of the few Social work instruments in this area. Vourlekis and Rivera-Mizzoni (1997) acknowledge its usefulness as a screening tool but consider that it cannot replace interview in social assessment. It should be noted that standardized evaluation tools, although valid and reliable, may be less flexible than the social and personal realities require. Therefore, it may be recommended that they be complemented with eminently qualitative techniques (Berkman et al., 2003).

However, the instruments cannot be understood as static, and they can be created and recreated according to the goals and requirements of professional action (Azevedo, 2013; Berkman et al., 2003).

We tend to agree with these recommendations, since the instrument proposed in this paper involves evaluation and follow-up interviews, and is completed by the social worker, thus not constituting a self-administered instrument. The use of instruments and procedures should allow for the apprehension of reality beyond immediacy (Guerra, 2012), preventing the professional from falling prey to instrumental reason (Guerra, 2000).

FUTURE RESEARCH DIRECTIONS

The extraction of an index is one of the characteristics shared by the MCAPIS_DRC and ECB instrument and is classified into three levels of intervention priority, possibly aligned with the complexity level of the situations. Therefore, it will be interesting to use simultaneously these two instruments in future studies for co-validation.

Thus, we agree with Streeter and Franklin (1992), when they consider that social workers should strive to improve the evaluation instruments, favoring their suitability and usefulness. The authors draw attention to evaluation measures with valid and reliable psychometric properties, as well as to the need for standardized procedures to favor the development of comparative empirical studies. The use of standardized tools is part of a transition in professionalism, surpassing unsystematic or unsatisfactory documentation practices, but these structuring demands must achieve a balance between standards and flexible fields, that demand forums for collegial reflection, favoring the use of the tools in context to contributing for the improvement of professional practice for social workers (Skillmark & Oscarsson, 2018).

We believe that the use of MCAPIS_DRC will not only be useful for Social Work, but for the whole multi-professional health team. The precise identification of levels of complexity associated with the intervention process contributes to the definition or reorientation of clinical and treatment protocols. The team may benefit from information about signaling of disease-related and psychosocial dimensions that interfere with the disease process of each patient more or less intensely (Vourlekis & Rivera-Mizzoni, 1997). Such information, which is systematized in a classification index, favors the decision-making of teams and administrations, since social (initial) evaluation and systematic or periodic social re-evaluation not only provide information about individual situations but also about a given population. On the one hand, social information systematized in an instrument of this nature, allows the social worker to support the team with condensed information that identifies competencies and vulnerabilities in patients' social situations, so that it makes the most appropriate options in the care plan, for example (Browne et al., 2014). On the other hand, it is possible to provide answers to concrete problem situations, but also to define broader programs. In fact, the instruments and techniques do not achieve results or ensure the effectiveness of the action by themselves (Azevedo, 2013). They depend on the planning and the purposes of the action in the concrete situations, and are not, therefore, detached from the professional commitment and the theoretical-methodological and ethical-political competencies of the social worker (Azevedo, 2013; Pires, 2007; Santos, 2012).

In Social Work there is the need to "think about techniques and instruments from the context in which professional practice takes place, and, therefore, it is fundamental to think of them from the analysis, by reading the reality, within the values and from what needs to be mobilized" (Santos, Filho, & Backx, 2012, p. 28). The instruments and techniques are mediations that enhance the theoretical-political intentions of professional action (Sarmento, 2012). MCAPIS_DRC arose precisely from the need for a team of social workers to give systematic visibility to the scattered data they collected. In this regard, Sheppard (1995) considers that the methods used by researchers are often refinements of the methodologies daily-used by social workers as practical qualitative researchers, implying a critical awareness in the construction of good evaluative practices. In fact, the use of instruments and techniques can be useful to obtain and systematize empirical data, but this must be submitted to the ontological reason. Uncritical instrumental rationality in Social Work is not acceptable (Silva, 2013). Therefore, the matrix presented must be understood as an open instrumental means that must be improved in this dialectic.

MCAPIS_DRC can be also interesting to the assessment in other areas, especially in the intervention with chronic diseases, but further studies of scale validation will be required to identify if the matrix needs adaptation or specificity.

Transforming the instruments used in daily professional life into instruments with scientific validity and replicable in similar contexts is an essential challenge for affirmation in the professional and scientific fields. At this level, Pires (2007) also notes that the selection of techniques requires intellectual competence to establish nexus between the concreteness of the action and the theoretical-methodological contribution, as well as competencies in its use brought by training and professional experience, since, in each professional act knowledge, know-how and practices are mobilized (Martinelli, 2007).

CONCLUSION

MCAPIS_DRC is a relevant contribution to social evaluation in Social Work in the health field, particularly in the context of CKD. This matrix, as well as the resulting index, is an instrumental means to give visibility to the complex impact of the disease on the life of people with CKD, both at the level of the teams of the services that follow them, and at the level of the administrations of the health care units, or even policymakers.

Specifically, the tool allows social workers to synthesize and systematize social diagnosis, prioritize social risk situations, outline sociographic profiles, define problems and geographic areas of priority intervention, define specific intervention programs, and produce knowledge from the information collected. At the team level, it favors care planning and informed decision making due to the complexity of the patient's social situation. At the level of health services management and administration, it helps to allocate human resources (defining workforce and workloads), financial and material resources to respond to the different levels of complexity of the situations.

Thus, the ensuing systematized knowledge enhances a more apprehensible understanding of the multidimensionality of the impacts of the disease and the complexity and demand of the intervention of social workers with this population, as well as evidences differentiated care needs.

Funding

This research received no specific grant from any funding agency in the public, commercial, or not-for-profit sectors.

REFERENCES

Alarcón, T. A., & Montalvo, J. I. G. (1998). La Escala Socio-Familiar de Gijón, instrumento útil en el hospital general. *Revista Espanola de Geriatria y Gerontologia, 33*(3), 127–192. Retrieved from http://www.elsevier.es/es-revista-revista-espanola-geriatria-gerontologia-124-articulo-la-escala-socio-familiar-gijon-instrumento-13006000

Albuquerque, C. P. (2011). Legitimidade e reconhecimento da prática de serviço social. *Serviço Social Em Revista, 13*(2), 104–118. doi:10.5433/1679-4842.2011v13n2p104

Amaro, M. I. (2012). *Urgências e emergências do serviço social.* Lisboa: Universidade Católica Editora.

Amaro, M. I. (2014). Um admirável mundo novo? Tecnologia e intervenção na contemporaneidade. In M. I. Carvalho & C. Pinto (Eds.), *Serviço social: Teorias e práticas* (pp. 97–111). Lisboa: Pactor.

Ausloos, G. (1996). *A Competência das Famílias – Tempo, caos e processo*. Lisboa: Climepsi Editores.

Azevedo, I. S. (2013). A relação teoria/método/instrumentais: uma leitura a partir da concepção de profissão. *Textos & Contextos, 12*(2), 325–333. Retrieved from http://revistaseletronicas.pucrs.br/fass/ojs/index.php/fass/article/view/15323

Berkman, L. F., Blumenthal, J., Burg, M., Carney, R. M., Catellier, D., Cowan, M. J., & Schneiderman, N. (2003). Effects of Treating Depression and Low Perceived Social Support on Clinical Events After Myocardial Infarction. *Journal of the American Medical Association, 289*(23), 3106. doi:10.1001/jama.289.23.3106 PMID:12813116

Bôas, M. L. C. V., Shimizu, H. E., & Sanchez, M. N. (2016). Creation of complexity assessment tool for patients receiving home care. *Revista Da Escola de Enfermagem, 50*(3), 433–439. doi:10.1590/S0080-623420160000400009 PMID:27556714

Bowling, C. B., Sawyer, P., Campbell, R. C., Ahmed, A., & Allman, R. M. (2011). Impact of chronic kidney disease on activities of daily living in community-dwelling older adults. *Journals of Gerontology - Series A Biological Sciences and Medical Sciences, 66*(6), 689–694. doi:10.1093/gerona/glr043

Braun, L. A., Sood, V., Hogue, S., Lieberman, B., & Copley-Merriman, C. (2012). High burden and unmet patient needs in chronic kidney disease. *International Journal of Nephrology and Renovascular Disease, 5*, 151–163. doi:10.2147/IJNRD. S37766 PMID:23293534

Brown, S. A., Tyrer, F. C., Clarke, A. L., Lloyd-Davies, L. H., Stein, A. G., Tarrant, C., ... Smith, A. C. (2017). Symptom burden in patients with chronic kidney disease not requiring renal replacement therapy. *Clinical Kidney Journal, 10*(6), 788–796. doi:10.1093/ckjfx057 PMID:29225808

Browne, T., Peace, L., & Perry, D. (2014). *Standards of practice for nephrology social work* (6th ed.). Council of Nephrology Social Workers, National Kidney Foundation, Inc. Retrieved from http://www2.kidney.org/members/source/Custom/ CNSW/pdf/CNSW-SOP_6thEd-FINAL_July2014.pdf

Calder, A., & Banning, J. (2000). The ECB renal patient questionnaire: An assessment tool to determine renal patients' needs for immediate social work. *Advances in Renal Replacement Therapy, 7*(2), 184–191. doi:10.1053/rr.2000.5274 PMID:10782737

Campanini, A. (2006). *La valutazione nel servizio sociale: Proposte e strumenti per la qualità dell'intervento professionale*. Roma: Carocci Faber.

Dustin, D. (2007). *The McDonaldization of social work*. Hampshire: Ashgate Publishing Limited.

Elkaïm, M. (1985). From general laws to singularities. *Family Process*, 24(2), 151–164. doi:10.1111/j.1545-5300.1985.00151.x PMID:4018238

Fook, J. (2002). *Social Work: Critical theory and practice*. London: Sage.

Goh, Z. S., & Griva, K. (2018). Anxiety and depression in patients with end-stage renal disease: Impact and management challenges - a narrative review. *International Journal of Nephrology and Renovascular Disease*, 11, 93–102. doi:10.2147/IJNRD.S126615 PMID:29559806

González, A. M., Fuentes, F. C., & García, M. M. (1988). *Psicologia comunitaria*. Madrid: Visor.

González, J., Palacios, E., García, A., González, D., Calcoya, A., & Sanchez, A. (1999). Evaluación de la fiabilidad y validez de una escala de valoración social en el anciano. *Atencion Primaria*, 23(7), 434–440. Retrieved from http://www.elsevier.es/es-revista-atencion-primaria-27-articulo-evaluacion-fiabilidad-validez-una-escala-14810 PMID:10363397

Greenwood, E. (1955). Social science and social work: A theory of their relationship. *The Social Service Review*, 29(1), 20–33. doi:10.1086/639761

Guadalupe, S. (2012). A intervenção do serviço social na saúde com famílias e em redes de suporte social. In *M. I. Carvalho (coord.), Serviço Social na Saúde* (pp. 183–217). Lisboa: Pactor.

Guadalupe, S. (2016). *Intervenção em rede: Serviço social, sistémica e redes de suporte social* (2nd ed.). Coimbra: Imprensa da Universidade de Coimbra. doi:10.14195/978-989-26-0866-2

Guadalupe, S. (2017). *As redes de suporte social informal em Serviço Social: as redes sociais pessoais de idosos portugueses nos processos de avaliação diagnóstica em respostas sociais*. Unpublished doctoral dissertation, ISCTE – Instituto Universitário de Lisboa, Escola de Sociologia e Políticas Públicas e CIES, Centro de Investigação e Estudos de Sociologia, Lisboa, Portugal. Retrieved from http://hdl.handle.net/10071/16706

Guerra, Y. (2000). Instrumentalidade do processo de trabalho do serviço social. *Serviço Social & Sociedade, 62*(XX), 5–34.

Guerra, Y. (2012). A Dimensão técnico-operativa do exercício profissional. In C. M. dos Santos, S. Backx, & Y. Guerra (Eds.), *A dimensão técnico-operativa no Serviço Social: desafios contemporâneos* (pp. 39–68). Juiz de Fora: UFRJE.

Hamilton, G. (1958). *Teoria e prática do serviço social de casos.* Rio de Janeiro, Brazil: Agir.

Hardey, M., & Loader, B. (2009). The Informatization of Welfare: Older People and the Role of Digital Services. *British Journal of Social Work, 39*(4), 657–669. doi:10.1093/bjsw/bcp024

Hollis, F. (1970). The psychosocial approach to casework practice. In R. W. Roberts & R. H. Nee (Eds.), *Theories of Social Casework* (pp. 33–46). Chicago, IL: University of Chicago Press.

Howe, D. (1992). Child abuse and the bureaucratisation of social work. *The Sociological Review, 40*(3), 491–508. doi:10.1111/j.1467-954X.1992.tb00399.x

Jha, V., Wang, A. Y. M., & Wang, H. (2012). The impact of CKD identification in large countries: The burden of illness. *Nephrology, Dialysis, Transplantation, 27*(Suppl. 3), 32–38. doi:10.1093/ndt/gfs113 PMID:23115140

Lacerda, L. E. (2014). Exercício profissional do assistente social: Da imediaticidade às possibilidades históricas. *Serviço Social & Sociedade, 117*(117), 22–44. doi:10.1590/S0101-66282014000100003

Lopes, J. M., Fukushima, R. L. M., Inouye, K., Pavarini, S. C. I., Orlandi, F. de S., Lopes, J. M., & Orlandi, F. de S. (2014). Quality of life related to the health of chronic renal failure patients on dialysis. *Acta Paulista de Enfermagem, 27*(3), 230–236. doi:10.1590/1982-0194201400039

Lorenz, W. (2004). Towards a European paradigm of social work - Studies in the history of modes of social work and social policy in Europe. Retrieved from http://webdoc.sub.gwdg.de/ebook/dissts/Dresden/Lorenz2005.pdf

Luppi, F., & Campanini, A. (1991). *Servicio Social y modelo sistemico: una nueva perspectiva para la practica cotidiana.* Barcelona, Spain: Paidós Ibérica.

Manavalan, M., Majumdar, A., Harichandra Kumar, K., & Priyamvada, P. (2017). Assessment of health-related quality of life and its determinants in patients with chronic kidney disease. *Indian Journal of Nephrology, 27*(1), 37. doi:10.4103/0971-4065.179205 PMID:28182041

Martinelli, M. L. (2007). O exercício profissional do assistente social na área da saúde: algumas reflexões éticas. *Serviço Social & Saúde, 6*(6), 21–34. Retrieved from www.bibliotecadigital.unicamp.br/document/?down=46133%5Cn

Muñoz, M. M., Barandalla, M. F. M., & Aldalur, A. V. (1996). *Manual indicadores para el diagnóstico social*. Bilbao: Colegios Oficiales de Diplomados en Trabajo Social y Asistentes Sociales de la Comunidad Autónoma Vasca. Retrieved from https://www.cgtrabajosocial.es/files/51786ad45be4d/Manual_de_indicadores_para_el_diagnstico_social.pdf

Ogren, E. H., Norris-Shortle, C., & Showalter, A. (1979). Typologies in social work practice. *Social Work in Health Care, 4*(3), 319–330. doi:10.1300/J010v04n03_07 PMID:472982

Pilotto, A., Panza, F., Sancarlo, D., Paroni, G., Maggi, S., & Ferrucci, L. (2012). Usefulness of the multidimensional prognostic index (MPI) in the management of older patients with chronic kidney disease. *Journal of Nephrology, 25*(Suppl. 19), 79–84. doi:10.5301/jn.5000162 PMID:22641578

Pires, S. R. A. (2007). O Instrumental Técnico na Trajetória Histórica do Serviço Social Pós-Movimento de Reconceituação. *Serviço Social Em Revista, 9*(2), 15–25. Retrieved from http://www.uel.br/revistas/ssrevista/c-v9n2_sandra.htm

Portes, L. F., & Portes, M. F. (2009). A observação e a abordagem no exercício profissional: revisitanto a dimensão técnico-operativa no serviço social. *Cadernos Da Escola de Educação e Humanidades, 1*(4), 28–35. Retrieved from http://revistas.unibrasil.com.br/cadernoseducacao/index.php/educacao/article/view/35

Prizzon, C. (2006). Assessment e qualità dell'azione professionale dell'assistent sociale. In A. Campanini (Ed.), *La valutazione nel servizio sociale* (pp. 115–144). Roma: Carocci Faber.

Rascanu, R., & Radu, S. M. (2014). Psycho-social assessment of patients with chronic renal diseases undergoing dialysis. *Procedia: Social and Behavioral Sciences, 127*, 379–385. doi:10.1016/j.sbspro.2014.03.275

Reamer, F. G. (2013). Social Work in a Digital Age: Ethical and Risk Management Challenges. *Social Work, 58*(2), 163–172. doi:10.1093wwt003 PMID:23724579

Restrepo, O. L. V. (2003). *Reconfigurando el trabajo social – Perspetivas y tendencias contemporâneas*. Buenos Aires: Espacio.

Rey, Y., & Prieur, B. (1991). Systèmes, éthique, perspectives en thérapie familiale. Paris: EME Editions Sociales Françaises (ESF).

Ribeiro, J. L. (1994). A importância da qualidade de vida para a psicologia da saúde. *Análise Psicológica, XII*(2–3), 179–191. doi:10.1177/1089253207311685

Rolland, J. S. (2000). *Famílias, enfermedad y discapacidad – Una propuesta desde la terapia sistémica*. Barcelona: Gedisa.

Santos, C. M. (2012). *Na prática a teoria e outra? Mitos e dilemas na relação entre teoria, pratica, instrumentos e técnicas no serviço social*. Rio de Janeiro: Lumen Juris.

Santos, C. M., Filho, R. S., & Backx, S. (2012). Dimensão técnico-operativa no Serviço Social. In C. M. dos Santos, S. Backx, & Y. Guerra (Eds.), *Dimensão técnico-operativa no Serviço Social: desafios contemporâneos* (pp. 15–38). Juiz de Fora: Editora UFJF.

Sarmento, H. B. de M. (2012). Instrumental técnico e o Serviço Social. In C. M. dos Santos, S. Backx, & Y. Guerra (Eds.), *Dimensão técnico-operativa no Serviço Social: desafios contemporâneos* (pp. 103–121). Juiz de Fora: Editora UFJF.

Schieppati, A., & Remuzzi, G. (2005). Chronic renal diseases as a public health problem: Epidemiology, social, and economic implications. *Kidney International. Supplement, 68*(98), 7–10. doi:10.1111/j.1523-1755.2005.09801.x PMID:16108976

Serafim, M. do R., & Santo, M. I. E. (2012). Criação e validação de uma escala de complexidade da intervenção social com adultos em contexto hospitalar (ECISACH). *Intervenção Social, 39*, 45–87. Retrieved from http://revistas.lis.ulusiada.pt/index.php/is/article/viewFile/1186/1297

Sheppard, M. (1995). Social work, social science and practice wisdom. *British Journal of Social Work, 25*(3), 265–293. doi:10.1093/oxfordjournals.bjsw.a056180

Shirazian, S., Aina, O., Park, Y., Chowdhury, N., Leger, K., Hou, L., & Mathur, V. S. (2017). Chronic kidney disease-associated pruritus: Impact on quality of life and current management challenges. *International Journal of Nephrology and Renovascular Disease, 10*, 11–26. doi:10.2147/IJNRD.S108045 PMID:28176969

Silva, J. F. S. (2013). Serviço Social: Razão ontológica ou instrumental? *Katalysis, 16*(1), 72–81. doi:10.1590/S1414-49802013000100008

Skillmark, M., & Oscarsson, L. (2018). Applying standardisation tools in social work practice from the perspectives of social workers, managers, and politicians: A Swedish case study. *European Journal of Social Work*, 1–12. doi:10.1080/1369 1457.2018.1540409

Sousa, C. T. (2008). A prática do assistente social: Conhecimento, instrumentalidade e intervenção profissional. *Emancipação*, *8*(1), 119–132. doi:10.5212/Emancipacao.v.8i1.119132

Streeter, C. L., & Franklin, C. (1992). Defining and measuring social support: Guidelines for social work practitioners. *Research on Social Work Practice*, *2*(1), 81–98. doi:10.1177/104973159200200107

Taylor, A. (2017). Social work and digitalisation: Bridging the knowledge gaps. *Social Work Education*, *36*(8), 869–879. doi:10.1080/02615479.2017.1361924

Turchetti, G., Bellelli, S., Amato, M., Bianchi, S., Conti, P., Cupisti, A., & Scatena, A. (2017). The social cost of chronic kidney disease in Italy. *The European Journal of Health Economics*, *18*(7), 847–858. doi:10.100710198-016-0830-1 PMID:27699568

Vourlekis, B. S., & Rivera-Mizzoni, R. A. (1997). Psychosocial problem assessment and end-stage renal disease patient outcomes. *Advances in Renal Replacement Therapy*, *4*(2), 136–144. Retrieved from http://www.ncbi.nlm.nih.gov/pubmed/9113229. doi:10.1016/S1073-4449(97)70040-2 PMID:9113229

Watzlawick, P. (1991). *A Realidade é Real?* Lisboa: Relógio D'Água.

ADDITIONAL READING

Brunsson, N., & Jacobsson, B. (2000). *A World of Standards*. Oxford: Oxford University Press. doi:10.1093/acprof:oso/9780199256952.001.0001

Callahan, M. B. (2011). The role of the nephrology social worker in optimizing treatment outcomes for end stage renal disease patients. *Dialysis & Transplantation*, *40*(10), 444–450. doi:10.1002/dat.20618

Cowles, L. A. F. (2003). *Social Work in the health field – A care perspective* (2nd ed.). New York: The Haworth Press.

Gray, M., Plath, D., & Webb, S. A. (2009). *Evidence-Based Social Work - A critical stance*. New York: Routledge. doi:10.4324/9780203876626

Matos, M. C. (2013). *Serviço Social, ética e saúde – Reflexões para o exercício professional*. São Paulo: Cortez.

Olim, M. F., Guadalupe, S., Mota, F., Fragoso, P., & Ribeiro, S. (2018). Sociographic profile of hemodialysis patients in Portugal. *The Journal of Nephrology Social Work / the Council of Nephrology Social Workers, National Kidney Foundation, 42*(1), 9–20. Retrieved from https://www.kidney.org/sites/default/files/v42a_a1.pdf

Ponnert, L., & Svensson, K. (2016). Standardisation. The end of professional discretion? *European Journal of Social Work, 19*(3-4), 586–599. doi:10.1080/136 91457.2015.1074551

White, S., Fook, J., & Gardner, F. (2006). *Critical reflection in health and social care*. Maidenhead: Open University Press.

KEY TERMS AND DEFINITIONS

Complexity: A property of systems that emerges from the interaction between its parts or dimensions. The more dimensions and more intersystemic interactions, the greater the complexity.

Multidimensional Assessment: It is a type of evaluation that articulates different dimensions or different constructs with theoretical coherence.

Nephrology Social Work: Field of the Social Work profession focused on the specificity of psychosocial characteristics and social rights of the population with chronic kidney disease, working with patients and families in the different disease stages and life cycle.

Social Evaluation: Phase of the social intervention process that implies the study, analysis and synthesis of information of a given problem-situation in context, which aims to determine the nature and magnitude of social needs, strengths and problems. Methodologically, this is a continuous and reflexive applied research that supports the intervention plan. It is a cornerstone of the Social Work profession, designating also for social assessment and social diagnosis.

Standardized Instrument: An evaluation or measurement instrument that is valid and reliable, replicable, without changes or adaptations in its structure and content, in different populations with similar characteristics.

Systemic Puzzle of Disease: Refers to the dynamic interaction between the different impacts and interferences on a personal, interpersonal and family level, such as the idiosyncrasies of disease, the diagnosis, the prognosis, its evolution, the care plan, the demands of the treatments, the associated limitations or eventual disability that occur, as well as the relationship with the health care system and other social services, the rights and access to health care, and the social policies.

Typologies in Social Diagnosis: Concepts and constructs that constitute references and analytical resources to typify and classify the synthesis of social evaluation. They must be built based on the theory, evidence, values and reflection, through the debate in the profession as a collective.

ENDNOTES

[1] The acronym refers to the original Portuguese designation: Matriz de Complexidade Associada ao Processo de Intervenção Social com Doentes Renais Crónicos.

[2] This section was adapted from the PhD Thesis in Social Work of one of the authors (Guadalupe, 2017).

Section 2
Innovation, Privacy, and Inclusion:
Critical Approaches and Recommendations

Chapter 5
The Emerging Concept of an Inclusive mHealth Ecosystem in India

Pradeep Nair
Central University of Himachal Pradesh, India

ABSTRACT

The reason for considering ICT-based communication platforms, especially mobile phones, as the most efficacious media tool to interconnect health care providers, practitioners and other stakeholders to a substantially large number of consumers in the healthcare system is that the mobile phone subscribers in India has reached to 1,013.23 million in the third quarter of 2018. The prices of smartphones have also come down by 11 percent with a demand for 4G devices capturing 6 percent of smartphone unit demand in India. Hence, it is an appropriate time to understand that the future of healthcare business in India lies with mobile based healthcare services. This chapter explores some of the significant innovations taking place in mobile healthcare business in India and examines the emerging approach of integrated health care ecosystems to provide quality health services to everyone where and when it is required.

INTRODUCTION

India has the highest population growth rate in the world. The WHO, in its ranking of health-care systems of the world, placed India at a dismal 112th position out of 190 countries it studied. This is corroborated by the fact that India spends just 4.2 percent of its GDP on health care, of which public health spending is mere 1.2

DOI: 10.4018/978-1-5225-8470-4.ch005

percent, compared to 3 per cent in China and 8.3 per cent in the United States. India needs to add 1.7 million beds, double its medical manpower and increase its para-medical manpower three-fold to match the WHO standards. Therefore, it becomes imperative to create an environment conducive to facilitate infrastructure creation and increase investments across the health-care ecosystem. Although the Indian government has accorded priority in its Union Budget 2018, by allocating INR 3,073 crore to create a digital economy with emerging technologies like Artificial Intelligence (AI), the Internet of Things (IOT), blockchain and 3D printing, which are necessary for building a modern technology landscape in health care delivery. The budget announced positive steps to encourage start-ups and other schemes for establishing biotech clusters to develop innovative healthcare applications and services based on mobile and other wireless technologies. The budget also emphasized on converting 1.5 lakh sub centers in Indian villages to health and wellness centers by integrating ICT based health technologies to bridge the rural-urban divide. The Niti Ayog, policy think tank of the Government of India, also suggested the government to work with health care organizations, to provide intuitive and interactive modes of communication, treatment, data transmission and retrieval to doctors, hospitals and patients using mobile based applications (BCC & PwC, 2018). The objective of the chapter is to explore the canvas of Indian healthcare delivery and the scope for an integrated and inclusive mHealth based healthcare ecosystem in India to fulfil the dream of universal healthcare for all.

HEALTHCARE BUSINESS IN INDIA

With increased digital adoption in last one decade, the Indian health care market, which is worth around US $ 100 billion, will likely to grow at a CAGR of 23 per cent to US $ 280 billion by 2020. The Indian health care market has a possibility to increase three-fold to US $ 372 billion by 2022 (Shetty, 2018). Although, India ranks 112th on the World Health Organization's (WHO) ranking of the world's health system, and the doctor-to-patient ratio for rural India, as per the Health Ministry statistics stands at 1:30,000, much below than the WHO's recommended 1:1,000. The overall healthcare spending (public and private) accounts for a mere 4 per cent of India's GDP, far below than the average of 9.5 per cent across Organisation for Economic Co-operation and Development (OECD) countries. Even in this, the private healthcare sector accounts for more than 70 per cent of this spend; while the public healthcare spends only 1.4 per cent. In term of the total health expenditure per capita, India spends about 1 per cent of its GDP on public health, compared to

3 per cent in China and 8.3 per cent in the United States. In 2018, the Union budget has allocated 52,800 crore INR for the healthcare sector but still the allocation is much less than other BRIC nations.

With the rising middle-class population, the average real household disposable income is doubled from 2010 to 2018 leading to an increased expenditure on healthcare. It is estimated that, by the end of 2020 the country will require an additional 1.8 million new beds to fulfil the targeted 2 beds per thousand people. The emerging challenges will be the infrastructural requirement for primary and community health centres, nursing homes, clinics, hospitals; and the skill gap - shortage of doctors and trained para-medical staff. The solution is the deployment of wireless mobile communication technology and its linkages to rural areas to bridge the gap between the increasing healthcare demands and the services need to provide (Blaya, Fraser & Holt, 2010).

Healthcare Ecosystem

The healthcare ecosystem is basically known as an ecosystem of interconnected stakeholders, where each one takes initiatives to improve the quality of care while lowering the cost. With an objective to provide people quality health care services in a healthcare ecosystem, the stakeholders build new relationships both inside and outside the four walls of healthcare institutions. The healthcare service provider and the patient who are the key payers now have a collaboration which is at the centre of the new consumer-centric business models of healthcare. In this collaboration, both the healthcare service provider and the payer really concern each other, and the services are designed on the basis of the actual needs (Carroll, Kennedy & Richardson, 2016).

In this ecosystem, the pharmacists are direct partners in patient care rather than just executors of the orders of the service providers. The pharmacist can not only encourage the patient to adhere the prescription given by the doctor, but can also help the patients in minimizing his clinical visits by adjusting dosage and prescription when needed. Since, the ecosystem shares data about prescription and information about patient care between the service providers and pharmacists; it helps the medical practitioner to understand the patients more and also helps to integrate pharmacists into the web of care and thus saves money and resources and improves patient satisfaction (Carroll, Kennedy & Richardson, 2016).

Across healthcare, investment in preventive care is on the rise. People are using biomarker trackers and monitors to manage the disease they already have. Shifting these devices to a more feature-oriented utility requires the expertise of medical practitioners as well the design wisdom of device manufacturers (Copeland, 2018). The healthcare ecosystem provides an opportunity for the clinicians to work closely with the device manufacturers to devise analytical applications for the patients by incorporating evidence-based data about wearable medical devices, optimum lifestyle decisions, preventions and care methods. This helps to improve the usefulness of the monitoring and tracking devices by bringing the communication from the healthcare service providers and manufacturers on the front lines (Coyle & Meier, 2009).

Presently, the cost structure of managed healthcare has changed as the payers/consumers moved from a business-to-business model to a business-to-consumer model (Okpala, 2018). The consumers are more aware about the cost of their healthcare and are more dependable on their health insurance providers to act in their best interests. So, it is very important for the healthcare service providers to educate their patients/consumers about the overall cost of their treatment so that they can understand the new cost structure of healthcare (Ivatury, Moore and Bloch, 2009).

As healthcare consumers become more aligned and integrated with healthcare management, data will be the key to build trust and intelligence in healthcare business. Both the service providers and consumers of healthcare have ample scope to capitalize on new appetite for information thus harnessing the self-interest and autonomy of the information providers and consumers. In this new healthcare ecosystem, innovative tools can be easily designed for self-monitoring which can further provide the patients/consumers to have more access to information and resources to make health changes and choices. Thus it has the potential to provide the healthcare service providers, consumers and other stake-holders new power and new prominence (Marjanovic et al., 2018).

Integrated Healthcare

Integrated healthcare is an approach that is being used widely these days. This is not about structures or common ownership or bearing insurance risk, but about networks and connections, often between separate organizations, that focus the continuum of healthcare delivery around patients and populations. The objective of integrated healthcare is to ensure providing quality health care to everyone where and when it is needed. The approach is to share information on quality, costs and outcomes across healthcare delivery- the core of connected health (Ray, 2017).

The present approach to integrated healthcare services in India leverages the systematic application of healthcare information technology to facilitate the accessing and sharing of information, as well as to allow subsequent analysis of health data across systems. The aim of connected health is to connect all parts of a healthcare delivery system, seamlessly, through interoperable health information processes and technologies so that critical health information shall be made available whenever and wherever require (Kaplan, 2006). By structuring and exchanging healthcare information to facilitate health care delivery to patients even in remote places, the connected health facilities can improve care coordination, diseases management and the use of clinical practice guidance to help reduce errors and improve quality care.

Digital Hospitals

Digital hospital is an ICT-based hospital that connects all of its digital medical equipment with a standardized program to increase the efficiency of the hospital operations, diagnosis and treatment. It is a cost-efficient hospital that provides an enhanced quality of medical service and is paper-less, slip-less, chart-less and film-less, allowing for greater number of treatments per hour with minimized costs for each patient. Digital hospital is a hospital that offers continuous after-care through remote-assistance, bi-directional communication between medical staff and patients, and efficient management of information (Giles, 2012).

The concept of digital hospital is to improve care both inside and outside of the four wall of a hospital, integrating health and social care for a 'virtual health community', ensuring that patients should be well and remain at home, out of the hospital. Digital hospital is a transformation of the conventional 'doctor's clinic' into an efficient, interconnected, patient-centric health environment for the 21st century. Health experts are also visioning it as a fully integrated element of a health and wellness system within the community. Digital health is an extension and integration of information and communication technologies that can drive the vision of virtual health management in India by focusing on wellness, prevention, treatment, recovery, and rehabilitation outside the hospital. It provides the patients an opportunity to have control on their health and medical details, ensuring that they should be assessed by the right people, at right time, at the right point of care well administered and delivered (Duffy & Holland, 2009).

Digital hospitals ensure a 360-degree view of patient health and social service care by integrating multiple levels of care delivery – home care, primary, secondary, ambulatory, emergency, and long-term recovery care and leverages innovative technology to orchestrate care coordination, improve operational efficiency, and improve patient outcomes. It provides a real-time health information integration environment that enables optimized care coordination, more efficient hospital operation and administration, and improves patient care quality. It further comprises a completely automated and deeply integrated set of health information services that fulfil clinical, financial, and administrative requirements. Core technologies in a digital hospital includes –

- **Physician Documentation**: Electronic medical records, computerized physician order entry, evidence-based medicine.
- **Smart Technology**: Stretchers, nurse call, patient cards, phones.
- **Point of Care Technology:** Bar coding, infrared, voice recognition, handheld devices.
- **Digital Imaging**: Radiology, cardiology, multi-modality, advanced imaging.
- **Device Integration**: Medical equipment and medications.

The concept of digital hospitals relies on information and communication technology as an integral part of its operational strategy. Technology is used at every level to integrate people, process, equipments, and socio-cultural elements. The technology deployed in a digital hospital is more advanced than the modern clinical systems and have a greater integration of information and communication technologies and medical technologies thus including both input and output instruments (Singh, 2016). That is why the concept of digital hospital represents a rallying point and architectural goal for deploying and linking health information

Figure 1. The essential components of a digital hospital

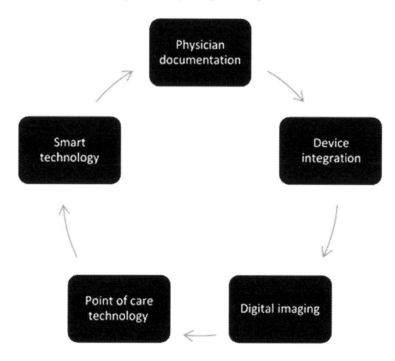

systems and medical devices. Using these systems and devices with an ICT roadmap and framework helps the health experts and policy makers to reshape how people think about hospitals and their services, and the roles and responsibilities of all the stakeholders in a healthcare ecosystem – care providers, patients, administrators and policy makers.

Thus, digital hospitals have the potential to deliver high quality healthcare in efficient and affordable ways. They entail a broader array of health information technologies than conventional hospital settings and the technologies are implemented in more integrated manner. When a hospital or a healthcare centre aspires to become digital, it needs to encompass all information processing, tracking and workflow management functions. The services are designed in such a manner that it should reduce development and maintenance costs to make the whole concept cost-effective (Schulz et al., 2018).

mHealth Initiatives in India

Today, mobility is one of the most promising innovations and is expected to transform the way healthcare services reach the patient. India has witnessed significant activity in the mobile health space with the launch of several different services; however, the majority of initiatives are focused on spreading prevention and awareness messages. Entrepreneurship in mobility for health has now entered in Indian market as lot of ICT-enabled health solution providers like Rockefeller Foundation, United Nations Foundation, Vodafone Foundation, GSM Association, PEPFAR (President's Emergency Plan for AIDS Relief) and Health 3.0 have made their presence in India.

Mobile technologies include mobile phones, personal digital assistants (PDA) and smartphones like blackberry, palm pilot, iPhone, enterprise digital assistants (EDA), and handheld and ultra-portable computers such as tablet PC, iPad and smartbooks. These devices have a range of functions and applications like photos and video (MMS), telephone and World Wide Web access and software application support. Technological advances and improved computer processing power has made the smart phones and iPads capable of high lever performance in many of these functions. The features of mobile technologies that make them particularly appropriate for improving healthcare service delivery processes relate to their popularity, mobility, and technological capabilities (Curioso & Michael, 2010). The popularity of mobile technologies has led to high and increasing ownership of these technologies to deliver interventions to large numbers of people. The mobility of mobile technologies means that many people carry their mobile phones with them wherever they go. This allows the temporal synchronization of the intervention delivery and allows intervention to claim people's attention when it is most relevant (Gatner Report, 2016). For example, healthcare consumers can be sent appointment reminders that arrive the day before or morning of their appointment. Real-time (synchronous) communication also allows interventions to be accessed or delivered within the relevant context, i.e. the intervention can be delivered and accessed at any time and wherever it is needed. For example, at the time healthcare service providers see a patient; they can access management support system providing information and protocols for management decisions to whoever requires them. This is relevant for providing clinical management support in settings where there is no senior or specialist health care provider support or where there is no such support at night or at weekends. As mobile technologies can be transported wherever one goes, interventions are convenient and easy to access (Bhat, 2005).

From a technology perspective, the transformation of Indian healthcare can be seen via online databases, applications, e-hospital applications, mobile apps, platforms and SMSes. All these applications have changed the way healthcare service is perceived, received and consumed in India. Online data bases give patients the ability to check for what drugs are available in which pharmacies thereby saving them the effort to hunt for their medications. Applications enable the service providers to track the patient's medical records and allow them to take multiple opinions from other care providers. With the help of Mobile apps, one can very easily track calorie intake, help manage diets and monitor fitness schedules and provide useful reports on demand. Platforms like MOTECH (Mobile Technology for Community Health) have transformed disease management in rural India by managing sample tracking, treatment registration and adherence, patient tracking, treatment reminders and alerts and reporting. SMS services are widely used to disseminate information on NGO/government led health care campaigns (Atun & Mohan, 2005). New services like Mediphone offer a tele-triage facility for immediate care related to acute minor ailments over the phone. The service allows everyone to get medical advice by an expert team of doctors and qualified para-medical staffs. This service can be used for all the daily medical needs and can provide health advice anywhere a mobile connection is available at an affordable cost (Singh, 2016).

All these services and applications are leveraging healthcare mechanisms to drive efficiency and effectiveness across the country. Lot of efforts are taken by the health industry and policy makers to sustain these applications and services. Policy makers are developing policies and agendas for mHealth. Both government and non-government organizations are committed to encourage the use of mobile enabled services by public healthcare providers, and a lot of healthcare organizations and agencies are providing incentives to private providers to invest in mobile and other wireless health information technologies. The issues of certification, standardization and interoperability are also addressed at various public domains (Nahar et al., 2017).

With increasing penetration and rising transmission capabilities of mobile networks, mobile technology is a robust and sustainable option. A synergy of building up healthcare capabilities, initiatives by policymakers and private businesses to build policies and business models are making this tool effective. Mobile Health is presently INR 3000 crore market in India (Source PwC). M-health (use of mobile phones) and E-health have already made an entry into India's primary health centres (PHCs) and sub-centres as the health ministry in 12th Five Year Plan has decided to go hi-tech. From remote monitoring to disease management, wireless technology is helping to improve healthcare outcomes and address the healthcare worker shortage. In India, chronic disease treatment costs more than USD 1.4 trillion each year, but using mHealth could mean a savings of more than USD 21.1 billion per year. Six years back in 2012, Government of India made some promising announcements. The Health ministry of India announced the citizen health information system (CHIS) – a biometric based health information system which will constantly update health record of every citizen-family. Today, the system incorporates registration of births, deaths and cause of death, maternal and infant death reviews, nutrition surveillance, particularly among under-six children and women. The service delivery in the public health system, hospital information service besides improving access of public to their own health information and medical records are now the primary function of the CHIS. The steering committee constituted for this purpose in year 2011-12 had suggested that disease surveillance should be put on a GIS platform. Disease surveillance based on reporting by providers and clinical laboratories (public and private) to detect and act on disease outbreaks and epidemics would be an integral component of the system (Planning Commission, 2012).

With the advancement of technologies and applications, healthcare agencies are providing mHealth services through voice, SMS, mobile websites as well as apps. The maturing of the mobile environment has led to the service providers offering a bouquet of solutions over the mobile phones that have become ubiquitous in their presence. Starting from basic services like finding a doctor or a specialist nearby to fixing up an appointment with a doctor, there are solutions available that allow the patient to connect to a doctor immediately, irrespective of the location (Khokhar, 2009). mHealth solutions have made it possible for persons seeking a second opinion to get it from specialists. The government too has been actively hitching on the mHealth bandwagon. It has launched 'Dial a Doctor' services in states like Kerala, which connect rural people to doctors in urban areas under its National Health Mission (NHM) scheme. This has proved to be beneficial to the rural people. Some notable innovations in mHealth are:

- **mDhil:** A start-up that provides healthcare information through SMSes, mobile web and apps.
- **Sana:** That enables community health workers on how to screen and diagnose patients and link that data to doctors through Open MRS via open source mobile apps.
- **mPedigree:** A mobile platform to track and check the validity of medicines to combat drug counterfeiting.
- **E-Health Points:** That provide families in rural villages with clean drinking water, medicines, comprehensive diagnostic tools, and advanced tele-medical services.
- **World Health Partners:** A multi-level service delivery network which leverages the latest in telemedicine and point-of-care diagnostic technology to improve access and quality of care.
- **ZMQ Software Systems:** That develop mobile games to combat HIV in India.

All this has helped the health experts and healthcare providers to realize that they can use mHealth as a mean to combat epidemics. Though the mHealth service providers agree that they may not be able to provide treatment in case of a spread, their services are very useful in disseminating information to the people so that they can entertain caution and prevent a sudden outbreak. The currently available mHealth leveraged applications can help in disease surveillance, tracking, monitoring, prevention as well as management. Many experts believe that if a service like mHealth is available to even a small portion of people and they get regular tips, it will make a lot of difference in their understanding and taking of precaution against the disease.

THE CURRENT PRACTICES

Kilkari

In 2015, India recorded 174 per 100, 000 maternal and 6, 00,000 lakh new born and infant deaths because of poor sanitary conditions and stark poverty. Preventable health hazards like pneumonia, jaundice and poor nutrition were the cause of most of these deaths. A project like Kilkari, based on the delivery of health advice through voice messages is a cost-effective health intervention to combat the situation to some extent. The country currently has mobile connections of 1,013.23 million, second largest in the world. This will definitely help the government and public health system to reach to the places where health workers hesitate to visit due to poor geographical locations and lack of transport services.

The project was launched on August 15, 2013 initially in eight states of India. Within 18 months, near about 1,00,000 rural families in Bihar itself have signed up for the voice messages. Other implemented states have also shown over-whelming responses. The project is very similar to the Mobile Midwife project already implemented in Ghana. Pregnant women were encouraged to enrol themselves in the project to receive interactive voice response (IVR) calls in their local languages reminding them of healthy behaviours and encouraging them to follow the schedule of care prescribed by the state and union government for their pregnancy and the first two years of their child's life.

Ananya

Ananya is a constellation of health services delivered over mobile platforms. The project has specific mobile handset application for case management by the front-line health workers (FLWS). Any pregnant women or child less than one year of age can be enrolled as a 'case' in the system. Each case is tracked along the continuum of care (starting from pregnancy till two years of age of the child) with specific protocols devised on birth preparedness, delivery, post-natal period, exclusive breastfeeding, and complementary feeding till two years of age of the child. The protocol is developed by the NGO *CARE,* whereas, the CommCare handset application is developed by *Dimagi*, a non-profit social organization. The system is very well used by the front-line health workers – accredited social health activist and anganwadi workers (ASHAs and AWWs) to facilitate better interactions with pregnant women or mothers during home visits. The application further helps in sharing data among the frontline health workers working in the same catchment area and their supervisors. In its pilot experiments itself, the project has proven its usefulness in improving the co-ordination between the health workers and in establishing an effective supervisory and monitoring mechanism.

The application is very helpful for the health workers to organize and plan their home visit schedules, as the application has an in-built checklist to follow right protocol during the interaction of health workers with women and children. Many multi-media applications were integrated within the system to facilitate the counselling process. In the process, the data is collected through mobile handsets during home visits and is stored in *MOTECH* suite. The client data is synchronized between the handsets of the frontline health workers and their supervisors who serve the same client population and is compiled at one virtual place. The MOTECH suite then integrates the patient/client information and case history with external database like Mother Child Tracking System (MCTS) of the respective state governments where the project is implemented. To make the frontline health workers familiar with this system, regular internet voice response (IVR) based training and certificate programmes were conducted for these health workers.

Dial a Doctor

To strengthen the public health services, the government of Kerala in India, launched a project in March 2014 to enable the public to seek health-related advice over phone round-the-clock from doctors/health specialists by dialing a toll-free number known as *'Dial a Doctor'* programme. Under the programme, any person can dial 1056 and can avail the advice of doctors especially regarding first aid, vaccination and health problems. The service is being made available through the state government's health department's call centre, *Disha*, which can be accessed through the phone number. For this project, a selected panel of 74 doctors from various specialities have been set up to help the health department to deliver the service. At a time, atleast eight doctors were available online at phone. The calls from the patients were handled by 21 trained counsellors who route it further to the concerned doctors/health specialists quickly. The project is managed by the National Health Mission.

mDhil

mDhil is another online health network with 12 channels, 7 channels in English and 5 channels in Hindi language. The network provides a range of information on various topics and issues of health and wellness. The network also has regional channels in Malayalam, Tamil, Telugu and Kannada. The channel can be easily accessed by mobile phone with the help of an application. mDhil tells a lot of well-researched health stories through text, video and photographs to a wide range of audience. The network claims that it has 20 million views in the first year of its implementation.

Mediphone

Mediphone is a cellular health service that allows people to get medical advice by a health expert. The service is provided by Airtel, the largest private mobile communications network in India. The service provides health advice anywhere, anytime to anyone at an affordable price. The service is manned by qualified medical professionals who assess and ensure accuracy in recording and evaluating the clinical symptoms and advice treatment on that basis. Besides offering medical advice, including self-care, consultations and permissible medical advice, the service also provides information about nearest emergency facilities, transfers the calls to nearest ambulance services and hospitals. It also provides information of all health facilities available in a particular location as per the requirement of the customer.

Citizen Health Information System

After the strong recommendation of the Steering Committee on Health for the 12th Five Year Plan, the Government of India has placed a biometric based health information system to constantly update the health record of every citizen of India. The system incorporates registration of births, deaths and cause of death, maternal and infant death reviews, nutrition surveillance, particularly among under-six-year-old children, and women, service delivery in the public health system, hospital information service etc. The system improves the access of personal health information to everyone and helps to identify geographic concentration of disease. It further provides hospital information service to improve the quality of care to patients through electronic medical records. It has cut down the delay in response time in emergency and helps the hospital administration to improve their health-care services. The system compiles and makes available all the essential information to encourage evidence-based health practices and helps the health practitioners to take prompt medical decisions on the basis of the information available with this system.

mPedigree

mPedigree is a free text-messaging service partnered with several pharmaceutical manufacturers to place an authenticity code on product packaging so that patients, providers, distributors and manufacturers can utilize the fee service to confirm the product's authenticity at the point of sale or transfer of medicines/drugs. The network helps the consumer of the drugs to verify that the drugs they are consuming are the genuine version and not counterfeit. A country like India, which face a huge demand for medicine but at the same time also faces counterfeit medicines/drugs, the service is very useful as it helps the government and patients to identify and check counterfeit medicines /drugs which is dangerous and is a major cause for the death of people from various diseases/epidemic. Anyone can check and verify the medicines by checking the code assigned by the system to that medicine through a text message.

THE CONCERNED ISSUES AND PROBLEMS

Today, the patients are connected and linked with the healthcare service providers through the communication technological interventions. The interventions mentioned in the chapter are providing consistent access to health care service providers – doctors, health specialists, pharmacists, and frontline health workers relevant information for diagnosis and treatment of various diseases. The full and secure access to patient information, diagnosis and treatment information, information of medicines and its availability, information to monitor the progress of treatment helps all the stakeholders in a healthcare ecosystem to play their role positively and helps them to have a visibility into patient status and health history to improve the diagnosis and delivery of care (Kobusingye, 2005). All the information can be accessed within minutes which earlier took days. The power of mobile connectivity in health care is empowering the health practitioners with new diagnostic tools. The practitioners can now share imaging and test results with their colleagues and seniors across the globe for able guidance. Patients also have an instant access to their own treatment records and history, which they can send, transmit and carry from one service provider to another for further treatment and advice. A connected health care system reduces errors, redundancies, lost information and the cost of information sharing to an unbelievable extent. The various initiatives at policy, program/project conceptualization and implementation level taken by the government, public and private healthcare providers and technology firms are committed to ensure that the information about diseases, diagnosis, treatment, medical facilities, should be available to all the stakeholders so that optimizing care should be provided to everyone whenever and wherever it is required (Krishna, Boren & Balas, 2009).

The cost of setting and maintaining a conventional healthcare centre in a remote area and making all the necessary arrangements for diagnosis and treatment in developing countries like India is a costly and tedious effort (Shankar et al., 2017). In this case, health mobility seems to be the best alternative solution as it not only provides all the required patient information accurately but also helps to retrieve patient's case history quickly (Lindquist, et al., 2008). This reduces the need for multiple visits to healthcare centres and the drop-rate in readmission cases by providing access to monitory and diagnoses patients from remote and geographically tough terrain. The use of mobile phones in collecting and capturing patient's data has shown remarkable cost-benefit ratios in several pilot initiatives in India (Mechael et al., 2010). The digitization of conventional paper-based record of patient's not only saves the cost of storing the information on paper but also reduces the error causes due to illegible handwriting and drug name confusion. This further helps to detect anomalies and errors in automating alerts (Patnaik, Brunskill & Thies, 2009).

The technological capabilities of mobile technologies are continuing to advance at a high pace. The technologies currently in practice allow low cost interventions. There are potential economies of scale as it is technically easy to deliver interventions to large population – as mobile technology applications can easily be downloaded, and automated systems can deliver text messages to large numbers of people at low cost. The technological features that have been used for health interventions include text messages (SMS), software applications, and multiple media (SMS, photos, audio and video) interventions. The technology allows interventions to be personalized and interactive (Patrick, 2008).

In many developing countries, there has been a shift from wired communication technologies towards wireless communication technologies. A number of low- and middle-income countries have made a technological leap with a 'mobile-first' based approach to communications. The market penetration of mobile phones has reached 80% worldwide. The cost-effective mobile devices provide new and potentially transformative opportunities for all those working to improve health outcomes. The mHealth interventions implemented in last five years in low- and middle-income countries and the specific outcomes are an evidence of this. The expanding mobile network coverage and availability of mobile handsets, especially smartphones, are capitalizing all possible health benefits in developing economies. The mobile technologies have now moved beyond calls, simple short messaging service (SMS) text and voice messaging to incorporate mobile internet browsing, voice over internet protocol services (e.g. Skype), instant messaging services (WhatsApp, Uber), photographic capabilities, and a wide variety of device-based software applications. These various mobile technology functionalities offer a range of opportunities for mHealth interventions – from health promotion via SMS texts and interactive voice response campaigns and content to mobile phone-based imaging having potential diagnostic capabilities (Varshney, 2007).

Low call tariff rates in the county has made mobile communication a feasible choice for implementing health interventions. Near about 35-40 mobile applications dealing with diverse health problems have already been placed on National Health Portal. Mobile health voice calls integrated with translation applications is a good alternative for SMS alerts and thus encourages the young generation which is more mobile application friendly to seek health and medical advice and ensures the participation and inclusion of people needing health care in their native language. Health information can be easily subscribed by paying a nominal subscription fee or by paying on use basis. In many cases like endemic regions or in case of outbreaks, health calls were made toll free. Further, applications like WhatsApp calling allow users to call other WhatsApp users for free. A minute of WhatsApp call costs around 0.15 MB to 0.20 MB of 3G data, which is quite easy to afford.

Without mobile internet plans, the standard data rates for most cellular operators in India are 4 paisa per 10 KB (3G) and 10 paisa per 10 KB (2G). This roughly translates to Rs. 1 per minute of WhatsApp call on 3G and Rs. 2.50 per minute on 2G network. The BSNL 3G data plans are also very affordable as it has Rs. 750 per month charges with unlimited download. Some other cheapest data plans for 3G services are Rs. 197 for 500 MB. Now anyone can have a 3G prepaid connection from most service providers at just Rs. 59. This starter pack comes with U-SIM (3G Sim Card). These cost-effective affordable 3G internet plans had already boost up the consumers and service providers to access and provide health information over mobile phones. The pilot studies of many mHealth interventions have shown that these interventions have not only reduced the cost but have also delivered healthcare information timely and accurately without putting a burden on the public and private health agencies in terms of infrastructure development and manpower requirement (Waldman et al., 2004).

THE SOLUTIONS AND RECOMMENDATIONS

The mHealth ecosystem in India is still at the edge of technical feasibility. A lot of implementation efforts are required at various levels of stakeholders to bring desirable changes. In the absence of mature standards of implementation, the challenges of integrating multiple healthcare systems and technologies remain daunting (Zayyad & Toycan, 2018). Advanced clinical information system is required to take the vision of mHealth ecosystem in India further as the Indian healthcare industry is still struggling in pushing the envelope of healthcare automation. The functional requirement for the automation of clinical healthcare system requires more technological supports to provide and maintain 24 x 7 digital healthcare solutions. Unless the entire healthcare system automates all the processes in a single big-bang strategy, the transformation of diagnostic decisions and treatment is not possible in a time bound manner.

mHealth ecosystem in India needs an incremental automation and interconnectivity of the broader collection of healthcare organizations. It is really a challenge for a developing economy like India to integrate the care processes of the hospitals and clinics with other care agencies (Somvanshi, 2018). But this comprehensive integration can upgrade the healthcare components from a care perspective to a service perspective. This will further help to monitor the progress of patients outside a hospital or healthcare setting, which can help the Indian healthcare system to overcome the patients rush in hospitals.

The other challenge for a mHealth ecosystem in India is to improve patient safety and security while designing mobile based clinical information systems (Rajagopal, 2018). Treatment and care mostly depends on pathological reports. If they will be provided easily on time, most of the medical errors could be eliminated easily. The quality and accuracy of healthcare delivery can be improved if the healthcare system can deliver patient's history, the ongoing medications and the problems of the patient quickly to the care provider (Carman et al., 2010). A mobile based healthcare information system can accomplish this at anytime, anywhere. If we look at the rural healthcare system of India, the problems faced by the primary and community health centres are mostly related to connectivity. There is huge gap between the diagnostic/pathological information and the treatment (Phadke, 2016). In the absence of healthcare data sharing mechanism, the required information for a treatment mostly doesn't reach on time. A national level central and integrated healthcare portal can help the care provider to access the patient data which is mostly pocketed with isolated private clinics and doctors. A mHealth ecosystem can not only deliver an integrated, patient-centric diagnosis, treatment and recovery environment but can also improve the outcomes of public healthcare systems by providing various information tools to provide diagnostic and EMR solutions. Since fifty percent of Indian population still resides in rural areas, without a mHealth ecosystem it will be very difficult to cover rural health in India (Shankar et al., 2017). The reach and scale of mobile technologies can help the Indian healthcare system to serve billions by increasing access to quality healthcare. But the challenge is to formulate a strong National Health Policy to implement mHealth based innovations in a simpler way with supportive infrastructure. Sharing the realistic patient data across various medical facilities and stakeholders through mobile networks can speed up the process of healthcare within the shortest possible time (Levin & Bertschi, 2018).

FUTURE RESEARCH SOLUTIONS

The rapid advancements in mobile communication technology is providing enormous benefits to all the stakeholders in a health care ecosystem by helping them to track the genuineness of medicines, by enhancing patient-care provider communications promptly for updates required for diagnosis and treatment (Nair & Bhaskaran, 2015). It helps to monitor the improvements in the treatment through real time data. The information which was distinct at one time and is placed at different places – hospitals, clinics, laboratories, pathologies are now possible to store at one place accessible by the patients and the service providers from anywhere at any platform – web, mobile, desktop, iPad, tablet. All this is happening not only because of the technology especially the wireless mobile technology but also because of the shift taking place in the mindset and behaviour of the patients, healthcare providers, pharmacists, para-medical staff, and the technology vendors. Thus, the impact on the quality of health care is now clearly visible to some extent.

The requirement is to collaborate across the healthcare industry to integrate technology systems, applications and workflows to unleash the power of health mobility to facilitate safe and secure exchange of accurate and timely information to increase the efficiency of healthcare service providers. It could further drive value and improve quality in healthcare ecosystem. When the authentication of medication is possible to done electronically before the patient leaves the care centres, the benefits goes far beyond improved patient care. Electronic information of critical health care on finger tips means saving of time wasted on wired phone, or fax machine, or physical travel assuring that the patients gets immediate and right treatment quickly as soon as the problem is diagnosed.

For making all this possible to a larger number, it is an appropriate time to utilize and connect the country's all available information highways, networks and stakeholders – patients, doctors, technology vendors, health systems, pharmacies, health plans, and policies into an integrated healthcare ecosystem facilitated by mobile communications. It can exchange critical health information through a single point of connectivity to deliver better health care to all the stakeholders irrespective of socio-economic status, geographies, and technicalities. A healthcare ecosystem will not only help the public healthcare organizations in India to build the necessary technology architecture and infrastructure to adapt the digital technology-driven healthcare business but also a standard practice to deliver quality health care to everyone whenever and wherever it is required 24 × 7.

CONCLUSION

An inclusive mHealth Ecosystem is not just about integration of technologies in a healthcare system, rather it is all about how to make the available health communication technologies more approachable to facilitate the integration of healthcare providers, patients, resources and processes to improve quality health care for all. It is a multidimensional concept which focuses on maximizing the capabilities and capacities of healthcare system to meet the clinical and operational needs of the deprived communities. The quality aspects of healthcare need to be addressed through interactive clinician involvement in the care giving process through an ICT enabled healthcare system. This will further leverage the healthcare organizations and institutions to increase their potential for delivering quality healthcare in more efficient ways. An mHealth Ecosystem in India can not only deliver an advanced, safe and patient friendly care environment to everyone but can also provide a more efficient output to the care givers through the synergies created by the modern communication technologies. The increased adoption of mobile communication technologies in Indian healthcare system will improve the quality and safety of healthcare and medication administration and will a play a proactive role in shifting towards an efficient, transparent, cost-effective patient care environment which is the vision of the new National Health Policy of Government of India implemented in 2017 (NHP, 2017).

Integration of the healthcare industry is required to change the current practices of healthcare in clinical setting. The emerging digital technologies have the potential to ensure better collaboration between various stakeholders in a healthcare system which can have a positive impact on the overall healthcare ecosystem. Advanced and proactive diagnosis, treatment and monitoring through robust and intelligent digital technology infrastructure can improve the efficiency of information and patient flow and can reduce waiting and treatment time thus delivering quality care in a timely manner which is the key requirement for any healthcare system in 21st century.

The increased use of digital technologies in Indian healthcare ecosystem will not only improve the patients' movement in a hospital system but can also accelerate and improve the treatment services and outcome. In coming days the hospitals and clinics will be more integrated and connected to the other aspects of a healthcare system. The advances in mobile communication technology will make the critical care services more patient-centric by automating and improving care delivery and diagnostic mechanisms which will further optimize the health care facilities for maximum comfort, care and efficiency.

ACKNOWLEDGMENT

The author(s) declared no potential conflicts of interest with respect to the research, authorship, and/or publication of this article. This research received no specific grant from any funding agency in the public, commercial, or not-for-profit sectors.

REFERENCES

Atun, R. A., & Mohan, A. (2005). *Uses and Benefits of SMS in Healthcare Delivery.* London: Imperial College.

Bhat, V. (2005). Institutional arrangements and efficiency of health care delivery systems. *The European Journal of Health Economics*, *6*(3), 215–222. doi:10.100710198-005-0294-1 PMID:15864675

Blaya, J. A., Fraser, H. S., & Holt, B. (2010). E-health technologies show promise in developing countries. *Health Affairs (Project Hope)*, *29*(2), 244–250. doi:10.1377/hlthaff.2009.0894 PMID:20348068

Carman, J. M., Shortell, S. M., Foster, R. W., Hughes, E. F. X., Boerstler, H., O'Brien, J. L., & O'Connor, E. J. (2010). Keys for successful implementation of total quality management in hospitals. *Health Care Management Review*, *35*(4), 283–293. doi:10.1097/HMR.0b013e3181f5fc4a PMID:20844354

Carroll, N., Kennedy, C., & Richardson, I. (2016). Challenges towards a connected community healthcare ecosystem for managing long-term conditions. *Gerontechnology (Valkenswaard)*, *14*(2), 64–77. doi:10.4017/gt.2016.14.2.003.00

Cooper, P. W. (PwC) & Global System Mobile Association (GSMA). (2012). Touching Lives through Mobile Health: Assessment of the Global Market Opportunity. Retrieved from https://www.pwc.in/assets/pdfs/publications-2012/touching-lives-through-mobile-health-february-2012.pdf

Copeland, B. (2018, October 22). What's ahead for the health care ecosystem? *The Wall Street Journal*. Retrieved from http://www.deloitte.wsj.com

Coyle, D., & Meier, P. (2009). *New Technologies in Emergencies and Conflicts: The Role of Information and Social Networks*. Washington, DC and London, UK: UN Foundation-Vodafone Foundation Partnership.

Curioso, W. H., & Michael, P. N. (2010). Enhancing 'M-health' with South-to-South Collaborations. *Health Affairs (Project Hope)*, *29*(2), 264–267. doi:10.1377/hlthaff.2009.1057 PMID:20348071

Duffy, J., & Holland, M. (2009). *The digital hospital of tomorrow: the time has come today.* A white paper by Health Industry Insights, an IDC company. Retrieved from http://www.healthindustry-insights.com

Gartner. (2012). *Forecast: Mobile Advertising, Worldwide, 2009-2016*. Retrieved from http://www.gartner.com/resId=2247015

Giles, R. (2012). *Envisioning the digital hospital: the future of healthcare*. Hewlett Packard Development Company. Retrieved from http://www.hp.com/go/healthcare

Global System Mobile Association. (2017). GSMA Connected Society & Connected Women Dalberg Global Development Advisors. Accelerating affordable smart-phone ownership in emerging markets. Retrieved from https://www.gsma.com/mobilefordevelopment/wp-content/uploads/2017/07/accelerating-affordable-smartphone-ownership-emerging-markets-2017.pdf

ICATT. (2010). *Computer-based Learning Program for Health Professionals in Developing Countries*. Basel: Novartis Foundation for Sustainable Development. Retrieved from novartisfoundation.org

Ivatury, G., Moore, J., & Bloch, A. (2009). A Doctor in your Pocket: Health Hotlines in Developing Countries. *Innovations: Technology, Governance, Globalization, 4*(1), 119–153. doi:10.1162/itgg.2009.4.1.119

Kaplan, W. A. (2006). Can the Ubiquitous Power of Mobile Phones be used to improve Health Outcomes in Developing Countries? *Globalization and Health, 2*(9), 21. PMID:16719925

Khokhar, A. (2009). Short text messages (SMS) as a reminder system for making working women from Delhi breast aware. *Asian Pacific Journal of Cancer Prevention, 10*, 319–322. PMID:19537904

Kobusingye, O. C. (2005). Emergency Medical Systems in Low and Middle Income Countries: Recommendations for Action. *Bulletin of the World Health Organization, 83*(8), 626–631. PMID:16184282

Krishna, S., Boren, S. A., & Balas, E. A. (2009). Healthcare Via Cell Phones: A Systemic Review. *Telemedicine Journal and e-Health, 15*(3), 231–240. doi:10.1089/tmj.2008.0099 PMID:19382860

Levin, Z. D., & Bertschi, I. (2018). Media health literacy, eHealth literacy, and the role of the social environment in context. *International Journal of Environmental Research and Public Health, 15*(8), 16–43. doi:10.3390/ijerph15081643 PMID:30081465

Lindquist, A. M., Johansson, P. E., Peterson, G. I., Saveman, B. I., & Nilsson, G. C. (2008). The Use of Personal Digital Assistant (PDA) among Personnel and Students in Healthcare: A Review. *Journal of Medical Internet Research, 10*(4), 31. doi:10.2196/jmir.1038 PMID:18957381

Marjanovic, S., Ghiga, L., & Knack, A. (2018). Understanding value in health data ecosystems: A review of current evidence and ways forward. *Rand Hand Quarterly, 7*(2), 3. PMID:29416943

Mechael, P. N., Batavia, H., Kaonga, N., Searle, S., Kwan, A., Fu, L., & Ossman, J. (2010). *Barriers and Gaps Affecting mHealth in Low and Middle Income Countries.* Policy White Paper. Columbia: Center for Global Health and Economic Development, Earth Institute, Columbia University.

Nahar, P., Kannuri, N. K., Mikkilineni, S., Murthy, G. V. S., & Phillimore, P. (2017). mHealth and the management of chronic conditions in rural areas: A note of caution from Southern India. *Anthropology & Medicine, 24*(1), 1–16. doi:10.1080/136484 70.2016.1263824 PMID:28292206

Nair, P., & Bhaskaran, H. (2015). The Emerging Interface of Healthcare System and Mobile Communication Technologies. *Health and Technology, 4*(4), 337–343. doi:10.100712553-014-0091-x

National Health Policy, Government of India. (2017). Retrieved from http://pib.nic.in/newsite/PrintRelease.aspx?relid=159376

Okpala, P. (2018). Balancing quality healthcare services and costs through collaborative leadership. *Journal of Healthcare Management, 63*(6), e148–e157. doi:10.1097/JHM-D-18-00020 PMID:30418376

Patnaik, S., Brunskill, E., & Thies, W. (2009). Evaluating the Accuracy of Data Collection on Mobile Phones: A Study of Forms, SMS, and Voice Calls. In *Proceedings of the International Conference on Information and Communication Technologies and Development* (pp. 74-84). Retrieved from http://hdl.handle.net/1721.1/60077

Patrick, K., Griswold, W. G., Raab, F., & Intille, S. S. (2008). Health and the Mobile Phone. *American Journal of Preventive Medicine, 35*(2), 177–181. doi:10.1016/j.amepre.2008.05.001 PMID:18550322

Phadke, A. (2016). Regulations of Doctors and private Hospitals in India. *Economic and Political Weekly, 51*(6), 46–55.

Planning Commission. (2012). Retrieved from www.planningcomssion.nic.in

Rajagopal, D. (2018, August 26). Not all is well with India's corporate hospital chains. *The Economic Times*. Retrieved from https://economictimes.indiatimes. com/industry/healthcare/biotech/healthcare/not-all-is-well-with-indias-corporate-hospital-chains/articleshow/65545784.cms

Ray, P. K. (2017). An integrated approach for healthcare systems management inIndia. In P. Mandal & J. Vang (Eds.), *Entrepreneurship in Technology for ASEAN*. Singapore: Springer; doi:10.1007/978-981-10-2281-4_6

Schulz, J., Decamp, M., & Berkowitz, S. A. (2018). Spending patterns among medicare ACOS that have reduced costs. *Journal of Healthcare Management, 63*(6), 374–381. doi:10.1097/JHM-D-17-00178 PMID:30418364

Shankar, P., Balasubramanian, D., Gurusimer, J., Verma, R., Kumar, D., Bahuguna, P., ... Kumar, R. (2017). Cost of delivering secondary-level health care services through public sector district hospitals in India. *The Indian Journal of Medical Research, 146*(3), 354–361. PMID:29355142

Shetty, B. (2018, May 10). Improving the healthcare ecosystem. *Business World*. Retrieved from http://www.businessworld.com

Singh, R. (2016). Integrated Healthcare in India – A Conceptual Framework. *Annals of Neurosciences, 23*(4), 197–198. doi:10.1159/000449479 PMID:27780986

Somvanshi, K. K. (2018, July 27). Five Paradoxes of Indian Healthcare. *The Economic Times*. Retrieved from https://economictimes.indiatimes.com/industry/healthcare/biotech/healthcare/five-paradoxes-of-indian-healthcare/articleshow/65159929.cms

Telecom Regulatory Authority of India. (2018). Report on Indian Telecom Services Performance Indicators, Quarterly Report - July-September. Retrieved from Retrieved from https://www.trai.gov.in/sites/default/files/PRNo114Eng28112018_0.pdf

The Bengal Chamber (BCC) & Price Water Cooper (PWC). (2018). *Reimaging the possible in the Indian healthcare ecosystem with emerging technologies*. Retrieved from https://www.pwc.in/assets/pdfs/publications/2018/reimagining-the-possible-in-the-indian-healthcare-ecosystem-with-emerging-technologies.pdf

Varshney, U. (2007). Pervasive Healthcare and Wireless Health Monitoring. *Mobile Networks and Applications, 12*(2-3), 113–127. doi:10.100711036-007-0017-1

Waldman, J. D., Kelly, F., Aurora, S., & Smith, H. (2004). The shocking cost of turnover in health care. *Health Care Management Review, 43*(3), 181. PMID:14992479

Zayyad, M. A., & Toycan, M. (2018). Factors affecting sustainable adoption of e-Health technology in developing countries: An exploratory survey of Nigerian hospitals from the perspective of healthcare professionals. *PeerJ, 6*, e4436. doi:10.7717/peerj.4436 PMID:29507830

ADDITIONAL READING

Androuchko, L., & Nakajima, I. (2004). Developing Countries and e-health services: Enterprise Networking and Computing in Healthcare Industry. HEALTHCOM. In *Proceedings of 6th International Workshop*, Geneva, June 28-29 (pp. 211-214). Retrieved from http://www.ieeexplore.ieee.org/xplore/login.jsp

David, K. A., Jennifer, M. K., & Phalen, J. M. (2006). What is e-health: Perspective on the evolution of e-health research. *Journal of Medical Internet Research, 8*(1), 30. Retrieved from http://www.jmir.org/2006/1/e4

Hubley, J. (1994). *Communicating health: An action guide to health education and health promotion*. London: Macmillan.

Kanungo, S. (2004). Research Directions for Studying ICT Interventions in Poor and Rural Areas in Developing Countries. In M. P. Gupta (Ed.), *Towards E-Government, Management and Challenge* (pp. 155–164). New Delhi: Tata McGraw Hill.

Mahapatra, A.K., & Mishra, S.K. (2007). Bringing the Knowledge and Skill Gap in Health Care: SGPGIMS, Lucknow, India Initiatives. *Journal of e-Health Technology and Application, 5*(2), 67-69.

Protti, D., & Catz, M. (2002). Electronic Health Record and Patient Safety: A Paradigm Shift for Healthcare Decision-Makers. *ElectronicHealthcare, 1*(3), 35.

Rao, R. V. (2012). Understanding Common and Specific Applications of E-Government: A Case from India. In Unnithan, C., & Fraunholz, B. (Eds.). *Towards E-Governance in the Cloud: Framework, Technologies and Best Practices. Proceedings of ICEG 2012*. Retrieved from http://www.iceg2012.com

World Health Organization. (1988). *Education for health: A manual on Health Education in primary health care*. Geneva, Switzerland.

KEY TERMS AND DEFINITIONS

Citizen Health Information System: A biometric based health information system which constantly updates health record of every citizen-family. The system incorporates registration of births and deaths, maternal and infant death reviews, nutrition surveillance among children and women.

Digital Health: The digitization of paper-based patient records/prescriptions to reduce the errors causes due to illegible handwriting and drug name confusion. It helps to detect anomalies and efforts in automating health alerts.

Digital Hospital: An ICT-based hospital that connects all of its digital medical equipment with a standardized program to increase the efficiency of the hospital operations, diagnosis, and treatment.

Health Governance: A synergy of building up healthcare capabilities, policies and business and care models to make ICT based healthcare services effective and quick.

Health Mobility: Mobility of mobile technologies used in healthcare business allowing the temporal synchronization of healthcare intervention delivery claiming people's attention.

Healthcare: The maintenance or improvement of health via the prevention, diagnosis, and treatment of disease, illness, injury, and other physical and mental impairments in human beings.

Healthcare Ecosystem: Basically known as an ecosystem of interconnected stakeholders in the healthcare system where each one takes initiatives to improve the quality of care while lowering the cost of the care.

Integrated Healthcare: It is an approach to deal with healthcare system networks and connections between different healthcare organizations with a focus to increase the continuum of healthcare delivery around patients and populations.

Mediphone: A tele-triage facility for immediate healthcare related acute minor ailment over phone. The service allows everyone to get medical advice by an expert team of doctors and qualified para-medical staffs.

mHealth: A general term for the use of mobile phones and other wireless technology in medical care to educate consumers about preventive healthcare services and for disease surveillance, treatment support, epidemic outbreak tracking and chronic disease management.

Mobile Technologies: Includes mobile phones, personal digital assistants, smartphones and handheld/ultra-portable computer devices having a range of functions and applications like photos and video (MMS), telephone and web access and various software application supports.

Mobile Technology for Community Health: The transformation of disease management by managing sample tracking, treatment registration and adherence, patient tracking, treatment reminders, alerts and reporting.

World Health Partners: A multi-level service delivery network which leverages the latest development in telemedicine and point-of-care diagnostic technology to improve access and quality of healthcare services.

Chapter 6

The Contribution of Technologies to Promote Healthy Aging and Prevent Frailty in Elderly People

Cristina Albuquerque
University of Coimbra, Portugal

ABSTRACT

In this chapter, the author discusses the contribution of technological achievements and ICT applications to prevent or reverse frailty in elderly people and to promote active and healthy aging. After a theoretical and political reflection about the issues associated to a new paradigm of aging in current societies, the author underlines the potentialities of technology as a complementary mechanism to achieve alternative and innovative responses as well as integrated and multidimensional policies and actions.

INTRODUCTION

The increase in life expectancy is unequivocally one of the most objective indicators of the social, scientific and technological development achieved in modern Western societies. The increment of medical knowledge coupled with an appreciable investment in the fields of technical support for diagnosis and social care-systems for elderly population have enabled, especially since the second half of the 20th century, not only to prolong life, but also to do so in conditions of greater dignity and quality. Nevertheless, despite these achievements, it is also undeniable that the expressiveness

DOI: 10.4018/978-1-5225-8470-4.ch006

of the current "double aging" phenomenon, currently with particular incidence in the Japanese and European contexts, also advocates a necessary multidimensional adaptation in living contexts and in current public policies. The main concerns are, in fact, related with how to protect and monitor dependent individuals, how to support family members and caregivers, and how to assure comprehensive ways to guarantee healthy and meaningful aging increasing social participation and preparing people across their lives to a better adaptation to retirement.

According to European data projections, by 2050, almost 140 million people will be older than 65 in Europe and will represent 16.7% of the World's total population (He, Goodkind, Kowal, 2016). In the same way the number of people aged 80 years old, and above, is projected to increase enormously in Europe, from 22 million in 2008 to 61 million in 2060 (European Economy 2, 2009), growing also, consequently, the risks of dependency or disability. The protection and care for elderly people are thus considered two of the most relevant social, political and health concerns in current societies. It is imperative to find processes to support their active, healthy and continued social and economic participation for as long as possible (Iyer & Eastman, 2006). For this purpose innovative, and integrated measures (social, economic, cultural and technological) are essential.

Indeed innumerable challenges, directly or indirectly associated with aging, are emerging in contemporary societies, particularly in terms of the labor market readjustment, the sustainability of health systems and social protection, the urban planning and the family organization. For example in what concerns the articulation between working time, leisure time and family time (especially when there are situations of elderly dependency to be considered). In the same way it is essential the adaptation of social institutions and their models of functioning, taking into account the changing profiles and expectations of the current and future elderly people and families. The concern with the situation of elderly dependency, for instance, has shown the growing need for long-term care provided by the family networks and community supports. To this extent dependency forces also the restructuring of the social, political and economic responses to the problem in order to assure quality of life and social inclusion for older people (Mollenkopf & Walker, 2007; Noll, 2007). Some of these challenges, and the answers that they necessarily imply, have even been addressed by various socio-political sectors as a difficult commitment to legitimize and manage in societies facing major issues of financial sustainability and global economic competitiveness.

So, new answers and innovative processes must be conceived. To that end, as it is argued along the chapter, support technology and ICT can play an important role if they are integrated in a multidimensional and complex action strategy towards aging. In fact, technological developments can give an important contribution, both to promote elderly's independent life and participation, and to assure gains in some aspects such as: reducing expenses of health and care systems; assuring lower levels of morbidity and fewer years of disability; providing individual solutions to frailty conditions or dependency problems; improving life standards; liberating families and care-givers; creating conditions to wider participation, high life standards and management of elderly people' home conditions (McLean, 2011; WHO, 2015).

As part of the 2020 Strategy, the current Digital Agenda for Europe is geared towards objectives more closely related to European competitiveness, economic efficiency and networking. In this context, the European Commission 2014-2020 has adopted the "Single Digital Market" as a priority line of action, aiming to contribute to improve the quality of life of European citizens, producing a differentiated impact according to their social characteristics, sphere of interests and economic activity. It is therefore proposed, for instance, to develop and update the digital competences of all European citizens to ensure that they can fully participate in the digital society and in the labor market; to strengthen the use of digital technologies in the field of health care by improving the reach and quality of services provided to citizens; to stimulate the dissemination of e-government solutions; to foster the creation and consumption of cultural content through the use of tools that not only increase the dissemination and distribution of such content, but also ensure adequate protection for its authors; to guarantee greater online security, in particular for the most vulnerable users, and to strengthen regional cohesion through the spread of internet access throughout Europe, covering rural and remote communities.

It is thus clear that in the European context and all over the world the investment in technological devices and ICT processes is a central pillar of political action allowing conceive greater economic efficiency and digital literacy, but also, new and adapted responses to the needs and expectations of specific populations.

Within this scope, to face the challenges of an aging society implies also to identify the opportunities that technological and socioeconomic innovation can produce in the quality of life of older and impaired people. In fact, the use of advanced technology and ICT devices can allow dependent, or frailty people, to stay at home even with medical problems under treatment. This self-sufficiency is today a widely underlined approach in social perspectives and political measures that has both cost reduction advantages and enhanced care quality and well-being (Stathopoulos, 2013). Additionally, the use of technologies can also contribute strongly to the so-called active aging by promoting larger connection opportunities and social and cultural possibilities of participation. Especially if, from a prospective outlook, we think about the characteristics of elderly people in the near future: more informed, more skilled, with higher expectations and more familiar with ICT. If we add to this scenario the mutations in the European' welfare model and the transfer of a set of care tasks, previously provided by public services, to citizens and families, it is possible to anticipate the potential of these new ways to intervene. Technologies can provide effectively, as several studies show (Swarte & Stephan, 2002; Sourbati, 2004; Leal & Bogi, 2014), new and relevant tools and processes able to enhance independency and to improve the quality of life, health and wellbeing of older people, contributing, like this, to the effectiveness of the so called "healthy aging" (WHO, 2015).

Considering this theoretical and political background the author underlines, in this chapter, the potentialities of technological achievements and ICT applications in promoting positive and healthy aging, and prevention, or minimization, of frailty in elderly people. In this context the advantages of ICT, allowing networking and the construction of innovative ways of integrated intervention on aging societies, are also reflected. This new perspective of intervention in the older ages is in fact coupled with a new research and political interest in innovative experiences that can guide an evidence-based definition of the main priorities for current public health and aging policies. The chapter is thus structured in three main parts: first, a theoretical reflection concerning the new scientific findings and political perspectives about the meanings and implications of active healthy aging and the prevention of frailty in elderly people; second, the contribution of technologies in promoting innovative and integrated measures in aging environments; third, the discussion of new research perspectives and challenges articulating technological advances and elderly people' needs and expectations in contemporary societies.

"HEALTHY AGING": A GUIDE TO AN INTEGRATED ACTION

The current 'Healthy Aging' political framework (WHO, 2015)[1] – that replaces the previous World Health Organization' conception of Active aging (2002) - underlines the process of developing and preserving, across live trajectories, the functional ability essential to enable wellbeing in older ages. Within this scope healthy aging pillars are linked with the creation of capability environments and opportunities to be and to conquest what people consider the most valuable life dimensions (Sen, 2009). In the same way they are associated with the construction, preservation or improvement of personal ability to: meet basic needs; learn, grow and make decisions; be mobile; build and maintain relationships; and contribute to society. The capabilities of the individual (that can be influenced by several factors such as age-related frailty, chronical diseases, etc.), the possibilities of the context (including the multidimensional impacts of poverty, the access to health or social care-systems, social policies, etc.) and the interaction between them are, thus, the interconnected bases of functional ability. In fact, it is currently consensual that the larger probability of illness resulting from the aging process is not only associated with the chronological age, but also environmentally conditioned.

The vulnerability of elderly people is largely associated with a complex myriad of factors such as: (1) the accumulation of metabolic waste and free radicals; (2) the exposure to accidents and "stressful" events; (3) the various diseases and disabilities, (4) the physical environment where the individual lives and lived before; (5) the social environment and involvement in cultural, religious and learning activities; (6) the healthy lifestyle regarding nutrition, physical exercise, sexual activity, sleep and leisure; (7) the cognitive, occupational and material resources; and (8) the attitude towards life (Fonseca, 2006).

Therefore, healthy aging is not necessarily associated with absence of diseases but mostly with the possibilities of controlling them adequately and promoting wellbeing across life. The main idea is thus to conceive aging as a process that begins at birth. Scientific data show, in fact, that good levels of physical and cognitive functionality are not deterministically linked with age. Considering this the WHO's Healthy Aging agenda (from 2015 to 2030) stresses the importance of crossed action of multiple sectors and considers elderly people diversity and the different cumulative impacts of advantage or disadvantage conditions across people's lives. In line with scientific evidences the Agenda also highlights the personal and environmental circumstances that influence differently life span: like sex, ethnicity, family, education, material conditions, among others (Blane, 2006; Marmot & Wilkinson, 2006; Michel, Dreux, & Vacheron, 2016; Øvrum, Gustavsen, & Rickertsen, 2014; Sowar, Tobiasz-Adamczyk, Topór-Mądry, Poscia, La Milia, 2016; Tobiasz-Adamczyk & Brzyski, 2005). Studies also show that standardized responses, disregarding the specificities of elderly people and territorial settings (urban, rural, depressed areas, etc.) have limited long-term effectiveness and can even promote increased health and social inequalities. For instance, at this level, technologies can assure more effective scalability procedures and models, as well as better adapted and personalized measures to specific target groups and environments (Boehler, Abadie, & Sabes-Figuera, 2014).

It is thus clear that healthy and active aging is currently a multidimensional social and political construct, engaging not only subjective and axiological perceptions about what quality of life means and which are the expectations and goals to achieve in an older phase of life, but also, the material and environmental conditions necessary to that end (Lee, Lan, & Yen, 2011). The political potentialities of this framework are however limited by the absence of a minimum consensual scientific agreement about the major dimensions (physical, mental and/or social) to take into account to understand more objectively the concept of healthy or "successful" (Rowe & Khan, 1997) aging and to design political orientations accordingly (Sowar *et al.*, 2016).

Research has revealed that healthy and active aging can be enhanced by developing structural intervention (friendly urban planning; smart healthcare and social-care facilities; open and diverse cultural initiatives; material inequalities reduction; lifelong learning and digital literacy, etc.) to build more positive living environments and enlarged capabilities across life span (Marmot & Bell, 2012; Braveman, Egerter, & Williams, 2011; Beard & Bloom, 2015). This implies however that different disciplines (medicine, architecture, urban planning, education, psychology, social work, etc.) learn to work synergistically and are willing to construct a shared knowledge and operational model. But this is indeed yet a big challenge to surpass.

The scientific discussion around healthy aging has been influenced until this moment by two different, and sometimes antagonistic, theoretical currents about aging: the bio-medical and the psychosocial perspectives. The first one values essentially the physical, mental and psychological functioning in older ages, according to comparable criteria, clinical indicators and etiology. The second one is more associated with life satisfaction, meaningful activities and relationships, and social engagement (volunteer work; associative participation; support to family; leisure and cultural activities; among others). So, in this psychosocial perspective, the models to appreciate objective and subjective indicators of "successful" aging are multidimensional and linked with capacities to be, to act and to have (Bryant, 2001; Kahana, Kahana, Kercher, 2003). In fact, a conception very connected with some recent sociological and economical reflections about human needs. These renewed and more complex discussions - like the one proposed by Manfred Max-Neef (1991), "the human scale development", and the capability approach developed by Amartya Sen and Martha Nussbaum (1993) – highlight the intimate connection between subjective and intersubjective perceptions of wellbeing and life value and the environmental possibilities to fulfil expectations and to develop adequate possibilities to be and to functioning.

Within this scope, one of the major challenges to face currently is to conceive policies and interventions that can link bio-medical criteria and psychosocial indicators, and even factors that surpass the strict boundaries of health although influencing it (lifestyle, social inclusion, religious norms, spirituality conceptions, family relationship and proximity networks, etc.), in order to design multidimensional, integrated, innovative and diverse responses (Beswick, Rees, Dieppe, Ayis, Gooberman-Hill, Horwood, et al., 2008; Illario, Vollenbroek-Hutten, Molloy, Menditto, Iaccarino, & Eklund, 2016).

Aging Well Across Life Span: The Prevention of Frailty in Elderly People

In fact, to understand the aging process, and the personal, familial and social impacts that it may involve, necessarily implies a complex analysis that concepts can hardly translate. For instance the notion of frailty (originally defined by Fried, Tangen, Walston, Newman, Hirsch, Gottdiener, *et al.*, 2001) acquired a growing interest in the last decades and became a central health (personal and public) issue associated with aging (Bergman, Ferrucci, Guralnik, Hogan, Hummel, Karunananthan, *et al.*, 2007).

Nevertheless it remains an unclear and non-consensual concept and an imprecise diagnostic criterion to guide epidemiological studies or even clinical practice (despite some operational and valuable efforts like the definition of the "phenotype of frailty" by Fried, and the "frailty index", developed by Rockwood and colleagues, 2005). Moreover, the various debates around frailty seem to be oriented by a double conception of normality versus pathophysiological characteristics, contributing to hide the vulnerability factors in between. The dimensions that should be included in the definition of frailty (a concept inherently multifactorial) are not yet in fact sufficiently precise and continue to promote a lot of controversial debates (Cesari, Gambassi, Kan, & Vellas, 2014). Even if almost everyone – policy makers, researchers, health professionals, caregivers - agree that frailty increase the risk of unfavorable or limited clinical recovery and produce several critical consequences on affected people, services, families and community. Additionally, the choice of the assessment methods and of the valued criteria to identify frailty (and in what domains) will have important and differentiated impacts on the personal and public financial spheres. For instance, the differentiated conception of functional loss as an outcome or as a part of frailty identification have relevant impacts in the ways to conceive, to prevent and to respond to it (Cesari et al., 2014).

It is thus essential to develop criteria to identify and screen frail individuals, especially the older ones, and to stratify risks. This can allow to prioritize actions and to promote integrated responses - medical, psychological and social -, as well as prevention and reversion programs (Beswick et al., 2008). In other words, it is important to make the term useful and more easily assessed to be considered in the design of preventive measures and to inform the development of strategies to reverse vulnerability and functional disability in elderly people. In fact, recent studies reveal that frailty can be reversed or delayed by early intervention or by promoting independence, active aging and participation strategies (Gill, Baker, Gottschalk, Peduzzi, Allore, & Byers, 2002). Although the imprecision of the construct, the current larger interest on it is effectively linked with its predictive validity and the

148

possibility, desired by individuals, families, labor market, politicians and clinicians, to avoid, or to retard the most possible, morbidity, hospitalization, severe injuries, dependency, long care periods, and death (Boyd, Xue, Simpson, Guralnik, & Fried, 2005).

For most authors frailty represent a condition of high vulnerability to adverse health conditions, multidimensional (cognitive, psychological or physical) decline, lower resistance to environmental and personal stressors, and functional deficits (Kaethler, Molnar, Mitchell, Soucie, & Manson-hing, 2003; Rockwood, Song, MacKnight, Bergman, Hogan, McDowell, & Mitnitski, 2005). More recently some scientific contributions stress the importance to consider a multidimensional conception of frailty, identifying the complex and differentiated connections between clinical-functional and socio-familial categories that can influence, in one way or another, health and wellbeing (Moraes, Lanna, Santos, Bicalho, Machado, Romero, 2012). To this purpose authors identify social conditions (e.g., socioeconomic status, social support, social engagement, and feeling of self-sufficiency), personal and familial circumstances (e.g., gender, race, education, employment situation, marital status or widowhood, familial support, care responsibilities, and access to health and social services), and clinical-functional factors namely associated with the phenotype of frailty. Moreover, the attitudes and behaviors of the people around elderly individuals can help to promote autonomy or to worsen dependence. In this perspective, being able to continue to live in their own home, for instance, is, for a large number of elderly people, an important factor of independency, emotional backup and wellbeing (Albuquerque, 2016; Albuquerque & Amaro da Luz, 2018).

In truth, public policies and health and social care systems should be diverse and oriented both to minimize and overcome adverse personal or social conditions across life, and to improve the functional ability of different profiles of elderly people (robust, dependent or frail). To this end, (new) technology devices and ICT processes can contribute to assure, as we argue in the next sector of this chapter, both the balance between independency, monitoring (of health conditions and mobility, e.g.) and support, and the design of innovative and more adapted measures and policies, multidimensional, coordinated and integrated, allowing to add "life to years, and years to life" (Jotheeswaran, Bryce, Prina, Acosta, Ferri, Guerra, et al., 2015).

This new paradigm of aging policies and intervention can imply however managing increasing expenses with services adaptation, new devices and pharmaceuticals. The current costs of the health care system will be almost impossible to uphold in the next decades, considering the ratio between elderly people and working population (one to one by 2050). So, the possibility to prevent or to screen frailty more efficiently would be, from a public health and social point of view, a way to reduce costs associated with institutionalization and hospitalization and, at the same time, to assure a better quality of life for elderly individuals and families.

Nevertheless, conceiving care under an integrated approach presupposes a major shift in health policies, in the traditional clinical models, in the processes of shared responsibilities between health and social professionals, in the care delivery supports, and in the conceptions of patient and of disease. The three pillars supporting this shift are: (i) the right to have clear information to make a decision; (ii) the right to have encouragement to make the right choice in a given situation; and (iii) the right to have the capacity to deliver the chosen option (EU, 2015). The increasing of the individual's responsibility in managing their own health condition and treatment is thus clear under this new paradigm and raises innumerous complex questions, for instance about the adequate information to do the right choices. The adaptation to patient needs and the necessary efficacy and efficiency of the responses, reducing health costs and increasing the quality of care, puts this way in the forefront of the reflection the need to increment the construction of new responses, engaging differently stakeholders, users and (new) technologies to enhance data sharing possibilities and to promote patient's empowerment and health literacy.

CONTRIBUTION OF TECHNOLOGIES TO ACTIVE AND HEALTHY AGING

The WHO's Global Strategy and Action Plan on Aging and Health (2016) sets clearly the commitment to achieve, from 2010 to 2030, healthier and longer lives for everyone as an investment in the future. Within this scope, some of the Strategy goals are to develop age-friendly environments, to align health systems to the needs of older populations, to develop sustainable and equitable systems for providing long-term care (home, communities, institutions), and to improve measurement, monitoring and research on Healthy Aging (WHO, 2016). To this purpose the Strategy prioritize not only the intervention in areas already supported by consolidated evidences, but also, other lacunar fields that need more robust data to inform renewed policies and health and social intervention.

In this perspective, for instance the conception of an integrated political framework and care-system for elderly people is recognized as a priority. Scientific evidences support in fact the idea, as we underlined in the previous section of this chapter, that the prevention of frailty and the promotion of healthy aging across life pathways suppose multidimensional and integrated responses. But to do so it is essential to transform the way to think about and to act on aging. The effective networking and coordination between key partners and services are, to that end, essential, as well as more coherent and equitable health and social policies. In other words, it is fundamental, in current aging societies, to develop a political and social framework that give effectively, beyond rhetoric, the possibility to live longer and successful lives, allowing elderly people to contribute actively to the construction of social environments and personal options.

The operability of this renewed paradigm, conceiving aging differently (more positive and prepared across life span) and diverse ways to intervene (more coordinated, less bureaucratic, less institutionalized, and more participated) raises however innumerous challenges to overcome. How to assure, in an effective and non-expensive way, the coordination and networking between currently disconnected partners? How to avoid enormous institutionalization costs and maintain, in a secure and screened way, the elderly people in their homes? How to increase, with controlled costs and good results, the quality of health services and, at the same time, elderly people' participation and social inclusion strategies?

Emerging technology has an enormous potential to answer adequately to these questions.

Acting Differently on Aging: Potentialities of Technologies to Prevent Problems and Innovate Answers

Many technological systems and devices allow currently the connection to family, neighbor networks, emergency services and daily supplies (e.g., food supply, laundry, shop), as well as the continuously monitoring of health indicators (e.g., tele-care devices, tele-therapy or tele-rehabilitation services). These devices allow not only to answer rapidly to an emergency situation but also to assure a higher quality of data gathered for medical support and diagnosis.

Tele-services are particularly relevant for frail and dependent elderly. The service of telehealth, for example, has the function of decentralizing care from hospital to home. Elderly people, or other patients, may be accompanied and consulted at home, for instance by videoconference, and have their vital signs (e.g., blood pressure, respiration, pulse, glucose, weight, ECG, among others) continuously monitored online. This is not only important to assure major health protection and quality of life for elderly people and families, but also to improve health services, both by providing rapid responses to patients' needs and expectations, and by liberating health services of enormous flux of patients requesting mere follow-up assessment.

The tele-alarm services (tele-assistance of first generation) are another possibility to support and monitoring dependent or frailty populations. By wearing a necklace, bracelet or some type of transmitter or micro sensor it is possible to trigger, if necessary, an alarm or an emergency call (e.g., HelpPhone). Like this, the user is permanently connected not only to an emergency service (24 hours functioning over 365 days), that can intervene and/or evaluate the situation immediately, but also, if chosen, to someone in the family or neighborhood (e.g., e-Neighbor service). These devices can inform about an abnormal pattern of behavior or urgent situation. Another type of monitoring alarms (tele-assistance of second generation) can be used to alert to intruders (in connection with police departments), environmental control systems (lighting and temperature), energy management services, time control for the use of medicaments, fire detection, leak detection of water or gas and control of doors, windows and curtains opening and closing. For instance, the I-Living is a device developed by the University of Illinois that allows through computer technology and wireless communication to provide a new form of independence to the elderly. It has the following features: Activity Reminder (e.g., notifies the user when is time to take medication), Vital Signal Measurement (measures vital signs and notifies the competent authorities if there is an anomaly), Personal Belonging Localization (finds objects that have been tagged), Personal Behavior profiling (detects signals of possible chronic diseases), Emergency Detection (in case of emergencies, e.g. the elderly immobilization for a long period of time, sends an electrocardiogram to the competent authorities).

Several investigations in the area of continuous monitoring of daily activities are still under way. The following may be mentioned: small electrodes to be placed in the textiles and which may help to monitor brain waves and sleep patterns; toilets that analyze urine and feces to early detection of diseases; mirrors that will allow to measure vital signs; toothbrushes that can analyze saliva; intelligent refrigerators that can evaluate stored foods and give information about their nutritional composition; contact lenses that help measure glucose and pressure levels in the eye; sensors that allow to identify in the car dangerous levels of pollution, among many others.

Also several robotic equipment's, with high levels of interactivity, have been developed as interfaces for elderly people' assistance and monitoring, either in functional forms of aid (e.g., health, rehabilitation), or psychological support (e.g., company). Some recent robotic experiences even allow, in a non-intrusive way, to develop many functions in the quest for user's social independence and well-being: observe and interact (if desirable) with the user; help in critical situations; perform various types of services (e.g., video conferences with clinicians, relatives and/ or friends); management of daily routines; management of money; recognition and prevention of threats or accidents; programs to stimulate reasoning and cognition; leisure activities (e.g., reading books); memory support (e.g., special dates and events; take medication; checking food; location of keys, eyeglasses, phone, remote control and other objects), and emergency calls (Albuquerque, 2016).

Prevention and Frailty Reversing Strategies Using Technological Applications

The elderly people independence is associated with the capacity to perform all, or the main activities essential to daily living despite age specific constraints. However, the individual conception of what "independent" life means differ a lot considering multiple interconnected factors, namely in relation with possibly existing health problems and other conceivably affected skills. Assuring a little more of mobility or access to automatic emergency calls is sometimes enough to increase the individual's feeling of autonomy, safety and self-confidence (Gaßner and Conrad, 2010, p.15). The technologies that provide some solutions to daily practices are, in this perspective (if all the ethical principles of privacy are assured), an important support to autonomy (Albuquerque, 2016). Considering this, technology advancements and devices can provide a relevant support in different life spheres (Gaßner and Conrad, 2010, p.17):

a) Social participation, networks and hobbies: elderly people frequently experience the loss of friends and phenomena of isolation and loneliness. The maintenance of communication, human closeness, social networks and active participation in society are major guarantees of good psychological health and general well-being. ICT technologies can help even elderly with mobility difficulties to maintain links with friends, family, associations, clubs, hobbies, and, like this, preserve, or even consolidate and recreate (new) forms of social and cultural engagement. The hobbies (games, arts, reading, walking, sport, collecting objects, etc.) are also important strategies for social interaction and self-development. At this level, ICT may create opportunities for elderly to maintain their traditional leisure activities, or even to find new ones, especially in cases of mobility restrictions and other hindrances. The possibilities at this level are enormous (e.g., virtual visits to museums, concerts, other countries, or create virtual communities) but they are not yet sufficiently explored;

b) Autonomy: Mobility and independence is intimately associated with autonomous life and sense of liberty. To move from one place to another, in home or outside, without insuperable physical burdens, or to be able to do some exercise is in fact an important factor of life quality. To provide assistive technologies able to neutralize mobility barriers and to potentiate the possibilities of elderly people are at this level essential. For instance, supports for driving a car, robots that can help the mobility at home, among other solutions that has been already tested and applied.

The so called "age-friendly homes" combine different digital solutions to assure independent and secure life adapted to older individuals' specific needs and health problems. The so called "domotics" consists in the automation of domestic dwellings assuring, by the use of multidisciplinary knowledge about quality of life, dimensions of comfort, communication and security in a sustainable manner. A noninvasive monitoring can be a great tool, because the mere opening of a refrigerator, a window or a door can be a problem for an elderly user. Currently there are many similar applications and projects, already implemented or in study. For instance, the automated beds are specific equipment's that allow the user to change them autonomously, as pleased, to read, to sleep, to get up and to watch TV; the cranes ceiling are adapted equipment's which allow locomotion (lift, throw or go to bathroom) with greater ease;

the automated cupboards and countertops allow height adjustments, thus enabling to reach them by any person in various situations; the internal lifts and elevators are essential to climbing stairs by people with reduced mobility; the automated toilet bowl is a device that eases the toilet use and cleaning, among many other examples.

The monitoring devices for personal objects are also a very important contribution of technologies to improve quality of life of dependent or frail elderly. In fact this advancement allows an even larger level of autonomy and the adequate answer to personalized needs. For instance, the footwear with GPS is particularly relevant for elderly people, especially if they suffer from Alzheimer's or other degenerative diseases with loss of memory. The GPS device is placed in the heel of an apparently normal shoe and if the user go beyond the geographic limit of his normal life context it triggers an alarm warning family, friends and professionals. Another example is the technological clothes. They were created by a group of scientists at the University of Ulster, in Northern Ireland, to help monitoring the elderly people physical conditions and needs (heart functioning; temperature or even check the timetable of public transports);

c) Learning and Education: being informed and assuring continuing apprenticeship is essential to prevent or reverse aging loss of competencies and even some degenerative diseases. Actual IC technologies, for instance internet, interactive television, mobile phones, handhelds, etc., provide new opportunities to be informed (e.g., e-newspaper), to continuing learning (e.g., e-learning courses), to stimulate the memory (e.g., interactive memory games) and to maintain/gain motivation and larger connections, even without leaving home or bed;

d) Social interaction devices: although video conferencing and internet does not replace personal visits it is a relevant option to assure elderly connection with friends and family members, especially if they inhabit faraway. If there are difficulties of typing an email or something similar, there are already applications that transcribe dictation text using voice recognition technology (e.g., Dragon Dictation). In what concerns the access to information, it is possible, through an electronic reader or even the personal computer, to access all kinds of information: newspapers, books and documents that can be stored to be read at any time. For leisure times there are several library services and programs of games that make players tunneling too, do exercise or dance by the use of motion sensors embedded in the body of the player. The use and exchange of digital pictures is also an innovative option for connecting.

The advantages of technology application to support autonomy and quality of life of elderly people are in fact unquestionable. In the same way technology can increase the possibilities of networking for professionals and services. However, to increase the possibilities of building integrated and multidimensional policies and intervention, directed to promote healthy and active aging and to prevent frailty, imply that professionals from different knowledge domains work together and share experiences and assessment results. Online platforms and IC technologies can facilitate enormously this process of shared learning and resource coordination in differentiated territorial scales.

Technological devices can also be very useful to map needs and to identify the existence, nature and distribution of explicit and potential concerns. In fact, computer tools can easily cross variables and mining data to reveal patterns and identify differential needs (in categorical and/or geographic terms). However, it is not enough to map the needs. It is essential to understand the expectations and the association between resources, contexts and people. What they objectively possess and what they need to possess, what they feel that they need to possess and what they don't identify as necessary, what they wish to possess and what and how they manifest it, the desire to benefit from a resource and the constraints (social, economic, cultural, axiological, religious, political or geographic) that determine the access to it and the use of it.

To promote innovative and coordinated intervention on aging is thus essential to identify or gain leverage resources (the use of social networks, even for political purposes, is a prime example) and to establish connections between the top and the bottom, the local and the national, the national and the international levels. That leads to what Adrian Worsfold (2011) calls a new buzzword, the "interoperability": the information is available across different groups and within different levels of access for their purposes. innovation in health care and social care systems for elderly people also imply to coordinate and to plan information and work processes with other professionals and services, neutralizing spatiotemporal barriers which may contribute to slowness and inefficiency of processes; to enhance intra and extra services participation dynamics, not just for users, but also for professional association; to improve the quality of information and research (including research-action and practice based learning), by promoting for instance the collaboration with universities and research centers (national and international), taking advantage of the knowledge produced by them and disseminating data and knowledge gathered and analyzed in the practice contexts; to potentiate the shared knowledge of international projects, practices and professionals, learning about new action models and assessing their applicability and dissemination possibilities; to ensure the information and knowledge sharing through quick access to government sites, legislation, databases, projects, organizations, mailing lists, social innovation methods and projects, research data and bibliographic references; to build networks via online discussion forums and communities of practice, and to potentiate participation dynamics in strategic health and social diagnosis, ensuring best practices and promoting sustainable changes, enduring and continuously assessed, as well as more innovative methodological processes of collection and data projection.

However, some problems and constraints must be reflected and overpassed in order to use, in the best way, the potentialities of technologies to promote healthy and active aging.

Issues and Problems

The articulation between technological development and the conception of an effective active aging and more innovative and efficient health care-systems is in fact a very important topic to explore in current societies. It can allow not only to respond and to prevent more adequately some of the new social and health risks, but also to fulfil elderly expectations (e.g., to rest in their own homes) without a major effort for families. The conciliation between work and family obligations could be, like this, facilitated. Additionally, after a considerable economic effort in the beginning, the introduction of technological devices in social and health care follow-up and alternative intervention would contribute, in a medium/ long term, to more efficient (economically and socially), accountable and effective responses. Nevertheless some critical questions must be reflected at this point.

The social isolation of some elderly people especially in urban areas is a very serious and increasing problem. The transformation of families' structure and the difficult conciliation between family and work obligations, added to the increased privatization, and sometimes inadequacy, of responses to elderly people' needs and expectations, sets the framework to a more profound and exigent construction of alternative and innovative responses.

The association of technological contributions to achieve differently the goals and processes of social care and health promotion, monitoring and support is at this level very pertinent, as it was possible to argue previously in this chapter. However, the introduction of technologies in the context of social care and health services may also, under certain circumstances, be a perverse obstacle to assure equal opportunities concerning citizens' access and fulfilment of rights. Considering this, the conception of public policies should imply a deeper reflection on the nature and meaning of inequalities in contemporary societies. In fact, digital inequality (Norris, 2001), may follow other income, health care, culture or education inequalities, which demands a social and "rhizomatic" global attention from politicians and professionals to the various dimensions of effective equality opportunities (Albuquerque, 2016).

Moreover, this reflection must not forget the importance of training and the effective access to technological tools and opportunities on nowadays information society, by each citizen. Technologies can, on one hand, increase the possibilities to address social exclusion, for instance by connecting citizens and creating platforms of information and participation, but, on the other, they can enlarge the possibilities of "digital divide" (Parrot & Madoc-Jones, 2008), "because the person does not have access to new technology or skills to use that technology" (Steyaert & Gould, 2009, p. 742). It is yet the case for many elderly people, especially if they live in rural or impoverished areas and regions.

Another critical point of analysis is related to safety and privacy. The guaranties of safety for elderly people are associated with their capacity to control the technological devices and to the evaluation of their reliability. For this, devices have to respect privacy and to be conceived as pertinent from the elderly people point of view, namely by understanding and addressing some of the fears of elderly people: burglary, falling, lacks of memory (e.g., lock the door, switch off the stove, taking medications), among others.

Finally, technology cannot be conceived as a panacea to solve all the problems of care systems, or the issues associated with adverse aging problems and inadequate lifestyles and conditions across life. Technology is only a tool or a possibility that must be conceived in an integrated and coordinated perspective with other political, economic, cultural and clinical measures. Thus, the main point is the reflection about how to define and operationalize multidimensional interventions that can promote real possibilities and opportunities to an active and healthy aging, not only in late years, but mainly, across all phases of life.

SOLUTIONS AND RECOMMENDATIONS

In what concerns the development and production of new devices and services allowing the growing of independent living, the participation, expectation and requirements of elderly people must be taken into consideration. For instance, the usability of devices by older people, many of them without technology knowledge and with particular restrictions on hearing, seeing and walk, are important aspects.

Additionally, old people are not a homogeneous group. Not only the experiential knowledge and expectations regarding technology are different, but also the personal characteristics and social, cultural and economic backgrounds (Miskelly, 2005; Sowar et al., 2016). Considering this, a technological standardized view is not sufficient, nor adequate. An adaptation to particular needs of elderly people is essential to allow the conception of really useful, effective and innovative answers and services.

As already mentioned, aging may condition many areas of personal and social life especially by producing specific constraints associated to the lack, or decrease, of mobility, vision and hearing, as well as a higher vulnerability for chronic diseases (such as diabetes, Parkinson's, dementia, cardiovascular problems), so there are major possibilities of co-morbidity and multi-morbidity situations (to suffer from multiple coexisting adverse medical conditions) (Gaßner & Conrad, 2010). These situations require the development of more adapted and sophisticated technology devices and systems, replying to more complex disease patterns and many different profiles of patients' needs and care expectations. In the same way the participation of individuals and families is essential to assure that the devices conceived to help dependent people are really adjusted to expressed or latent requirements, as well as to individual, familial, social and medical expectations and exigencies.

Like this, initiatives to provide public access to computers and internet, especially for those that don't have access to them at home, as well as skill training to use technologies properly, would be central goals for a renewed "public policy agenda on aging", working with current tools to promote renewed forms of support and social inclusion, in line with the WHO's Strategy (2016) and the European initiatives around Active and Health Aging (2015).

Additionally a more close proximity between academia and research centers, and social care and health care services is also a very important strategy to test new ideas and to produce new devices in larger quantities, reducing this way the costs associated. The use and availability of technological devices for all elderly people in need and willing to use them implies in fact the development of integrated policies and determination of clearer political and economic priorities. The costs of this type of technologies are still impossible to support for the majority of individuals, elderly people and families. So, new forms of articulation between policies of health, education and research, as well as innovative partnerships between services, centers of research and industry must be conceived.

The electronic devices promote, in a more explicit or implicit way, the osmosis of the private and the public spheres of life. So, the classical dilemma between the need of protection and security, and the preservation of liberty and privacy emerges. This dilemma, especially if we consider the characteristics of vulnerable populations (either by health conditions or by social and cultural factors), needs currently, considering the large and accelerated technological developments ongoing, a much more complex reflection and protection.

The ethical concerns about privacy, liberty of users, confidentiality and accountable use of information must effectively be reflected and translated into specific legislation of data protection. In the European Union a large step was assured in this domain with the publication of the Regulation (EU) 2016/679 of the European Parliament and of the Council of 27 April 2016 on the protection of natural persons with regard to the processing of personal data and on the free movement of such data, and repealing Directive 95/46/EC (General Data Protection Regulation).

The application of the Regulation (since May 2018) within all the European Union Area is, in fact, a major conquest assuring the protection of 'natural people' in the processing of personal data. Before, under the Directive 95/46/EC, the data protection norms in the European Union were fragmented, generating a sense of diffused risk and loss of confidence in the relationship between citizens and services in the European space and in the online activities. The larger warranties and homogeneity on data protection (setting out also 'the circumstances for specific processing situations' in each Member State) intends thus to facilitate the free flow of data, people and business in the European space and to protect, in a widespread and coherent way, the fundamental rights to privacy and liberty (at this level the right to erasure, or 'right to be forgotten' (article 17°), is particularly important and was reinforced). In the text of the Regulation is stated (point 4) that 'the processing of personal data should be designed to serve mankind. The right to the protection of personal data is not an absolute right; it must be considered in relation to its function in society and be balanced against other fundamental rights, in accordance with the principle of proportionality. This Regulation respects all fundamental rights and observes the freedoms and principles recognised in the Charter as enshrined in the Treaties, in particular the respect for private and family life, home and communications, the protection of personal data, freedom of thought, conscience and religion, freedom of expression and information, freedom to conduct a business, the right to an effective remedy and to a fair trial, and cultural, religious and linguistic diversity' (2016, p. 2).

Although all the regulation at this level the dangers associated to privacy violation in daily practices and concrete services, using sometimes arguments of attention and protection, as well as the possible inadequate use of medical and social information must be considered carefully. Effectively, there are a lot of examples of privacy violations and disrespect by the private space and choices of care in facilities and services for elderly people. The self-determination and participation of elderly people in the decisions about their life and about care procedures are essential to assure effective independence and respect for dignity. For the health and social professionals the choices of when and how to intervene, and what kind of data is relevant and who has access to, are issues particularly important.

A common concern that emerges when technology is associated with care is the possibility of losing the personal and "warm hands" support. Technology must be, in fact, conceived as a tool to potentiate responses complementary to personalized care. By liberating professionals and families from some care tasks, technological devices help to free human resources, currently with fewer time and availability to caring duties, to other priority personal supports. Additionally technologies can potentiate workforce and informal support improvement, both by promoting opportunities to learn with others, and by acquiring new training possibilities and renewed professional skills.

In this context, the networking process engaging different professionals, knowledge domains and services is essential to build new and more articulated measures and policies. This imply, however, to share languages, to overpass sterile and unreal frontiers between medical issues, social issues, and psychological issues, and to find a common understanding platform to reflect about and to act on aging problems in current societies, as well as to promote effectively healthy and active aging across life pathways. In the same way new partnerships between private and public stakeholders and services are fundamental to promote new responsibility models and shared projects in the field of aging nowadays traversed by new exigencies and new expectations of elderly people, families and professionals.

Technologies can facilitate this connection and the accomplishment of these goals by sharing diagnosis, assessment and experiences among distinct stakeholders. However, their efficacy is closely connected with the shift in the way to think and to act on aging currently: not only to maintain older individuals without diseases, but also, to promote their active participation in the construction of society. It is thus crucial the stimulus to path-breaking and cooperation in order to promote new forms of aging well and being healthier across life and in the last years of it.

FUTURE RESEARCH DIRECTIONS

Nowadays health and social care systems must transform themselves in order to cope with current demands tuned with new expectations in an aging and globalized society. In this context it is important to identify the renewed skills (including the digital ones), knowledge and principles of future health and social professionals. This will imply systemic adaptations on educational organizations, curricula and policies, but mainly a shift in health and care culture (EC, 2015).

The increment of research concerning criteria for frailty prevention or early intervention, and innovative resource-management to promote more efficient care systems, associating or not technologies, will help to minimize progressively the cost of later correction actions. Technology can help in this adaptation ensuring not only potentially better management processes, but also alternative responses to identified or latent needs of elderly people, families or professionals. Some research must however be done concerning the adaptability of some technological devices to medical and social conditions, as well as the impacts that they have potentially in personal relationships, social participation or isolation, family connection, emotional equilibrium, etc. In the same way, it is important to understand the consequences associated with the introduction of technologies on services and professionals, for instance, on the levels of motivation, processes of tasks management and levels of bureaucracy, networking processes, and accountability procedures, among others.

Likewise, research is needed to identify and assess best practices in the design and outcomes of innovative and integrated care systems. Larger evidence at this level can allow to understand and anticipate the needs of elderly people and to adapt professional action and services responses accordingly. Data would inform also political decision oriented to the integration of technological advances with social and health system, and the formal and the informal care processes, avoiding, or minimizing, balkanized, ineffective and large resources-consumption actions. Additionally, more scientific studies could identify and compare critical areas and needs, according to different territories, different population groups, different conceptions of health and disease (influenced for instance by religious convictions) and distinct subjective and objective expectations about a successful and active life. The conclusions would help to understand, for instance, different engagements of patients in clinical procedures and follow-up and different results of aging and treatment processes. Thus, this complex and interconnected research would be very pertinent to define more rational intervention plans, reducing over prescription, and engaging, with precise tasks and responsibilities, differentiated partners. And even, the understanding of how to promote health literacy, supporting and informing individuals' decisions. This is in fact a main field to investigate because the wellbeing literacy is a relevant trigger to an active and healthy aging prepared consciously since younger years.

CONCLUSION

Nowadays the promotion of active and healthy aging is not only a political orientation but a health and social requirement. The financial costs associated with long periods of hospitalization and the consequences of frailty and illness of older people stress the need to find innovative and more effective processes to respond to new needs, but also to prevent adverse effects of aging as early as possible. For this purpose, it is important to redefine the way of thinking and intervening on aging, considering it not only as the culmination of a process but above all as the product of a set of options and experiences along life-path.

The current political framework highlights the importance of keeping older people functional and contributing to the building of societies for as long as possible and in conditions of good health and well-being. This implies a transformation in the ways of understanding and intervening in the aging processes themselves, defining measures and policies that, in an articulated and integrated way, can intervene in different dimensions of quality of life.

Within this scope, learning to work together is fundamental, as well as defining new skills for current and future professionals and new disruptive responses framing technological discoveries as mechanisms of complementarity of changes that have to be necessarily holistic.

REFERENCES

Albuquerque, C. (2016). Social Care and Life Quality of Frail or Dependent Elderly: The Contribution of Technologies. *International Journal of Privacy and Health Information Management*, 4(1), 12–22. doi:10.4018/IJPHIM.2016010102

Albuquerque, C. P., & Amaro da Luz, M. H. (2018). The Potentialities of Local Innovation Ecosystems to Tackle Wicked Problems: The Case of Aging. *Technology Transfer and Entrepreneurship*, 5(2), 67–82. doi:10.2174/2213809906666181214 141821

Beard, J. R., & Bloom, D. E. (2015). Towards a comprehensive public health response to population ageing. *Lancet*, *14*. Retrieved from https://www.ncbi.nlm. nih.gov/pmc/articles/PMC4663973/ PMID:25468151

Bergman, H., Ferrucci, L., Guralnik, J., Hogan, D. B., Hummel, S., Karunananthan, S., & Wolfson, C. (2007). Frailty: An emerging research and clinical paradigm–issues and controversies. *The Journals of Gerontology. Series A, Biological Sciences and Medical Sciences*, 62(7), 731–737. doi:10.1093/gerona/62.7.731 PMID:17634320

Beswick, A. D., Rees, K., Dieppe, P., Ayis, S., Gooberman-Hill, R., Horwood, J., & Ebrahim, S. (2008). Complex interventions to improve physical function and maintain independent living in elderly people: A systematic review and meta-analysis. *Lancet*, *371*(9614), 725–735. doi:10.1016/S0140-6736(08)60342-6 PMID:18313501

Blane, D. (2006). The life course perspective, the social gradient, and health. In M. Marmot & R. Wilkinson (Eds.), *Social Determinants of Health* (pp. 54–77). Oxford: Oxford University Press.

Boehler, C., Abadie, F., & Sabes-Figuera, R. (2014). Monitoring and Assessment Framework for the European Innovation Partnership on Active and Healthy Ageing (MAFEIP). Second report on outcome indicators. *JRC Science and Policy Report*.

Boyd, C. M., Xue, Q. L., Simpson, C. F., Guralnik, J. M., & Fried, L. P. (2005). Frailty, hospitalization, and progression of disability in a cohort of disabled older women. *The American Journal of Medicine*, *118*(11), 1225–1231. doi:10.1016/j. amjmed.2005.01.062 PMID:16271906

Braveman, P., Egerter, S., & Williams, D. R. (2011). The social determinants of health: Coming of age. *Annual Review of Public Health*, *32*(1), 381–398. doi:10.1146/ annurev-publhealth-031210-101218 PMID:21091195

Bryant, L. L., Corbett, K. K., & Kutner, J. S. (2001). In their own words: A model of healthy aging. *Social Science & Medicine, 53*(7), 927–941. doi:10.1016/S0277-9536(00)00392-0 PMID:11522138

Cesari, M., Gambassi, G., van Kan, G. A., & Vellas, B. (2014). The frailty phenotype and the frailty index: Different instruments for different purposes. *Age and Ageing, 43*(1), 10–12. doi:10.1093/ageing/aft160 PMID:24132852

EC – European Commission (2015). *Innovation for Active & Healthy Ageing. European Summit on Innovation for Active and Healthy Ageing.* Brussels, 9-10 March 2015. Final Report.

EC – European Commission. (2016). *European Innovation Partnership on Active and Healthy Ageing.* Action Group A3, Renovated Action Plan 2016–2018. Retrieved from https://ec.europa.eu/eip/ageing/library/action-plan-2016-2018-a3_en

EC- European Commission, Information Society and Media. (2010). i2010: Information Society and the media working towards growth and jobs. Brussels.

European Economy 2. (2009). *2009 Ageing Report: Economic and budgetary projections for the EU-27 Member States (2008-2060).* Joint Report prepared by the European Commission (DG ECFIN) and the Economic Policy Committee (AWG). Luxembourg: European Commission - Directorate-General for Economic and Financial Affairs.

European Union. (2016). Regulation (EU) 2016/679 of the European Parliament and of the Council of 27 April 2016 on the protection of natural persons with regard to the processing of personal data and on the free movement of such data, and repealing Directive 95/46/EC (General Data Protection Regulation). *Official Journal of the European Union.*

Fonseca, A. (2006). *O envelhecimento. Uma abordagem psicológica.* Lisboa: Universidade Católica Editora.

Fried, L. P., Tangen, C. M., Walston, J., Newman, A. B., Hirsch, C., Gottdiener, J., ... McBurnie, M. A. (2001). Frailty in older adults: Evidence for a phenotype. *The Journals of Gerontology. Series A, Biological Sciences and Medical Sciences, 56*(3), M146–M156. doi:10.1093/gerona/56.3.M146 PMID:11253156

Gaßner, K., & Conrad, M. (2010). *ICT enabled independent living for elderly. A status-quo analysis on products and the research landscape in the field of Ambient Assisted Living (AAL) in EU-27.* Berlin: Institute for Innovation and Technology.

Gill, T. M., Baker, D. I., Gottschalk, M., Peduzzi, P. N., Allore, H., & Byers, A. (2002). A program to prevent functional decline in physically frail, elderly persons who live at home. *The New England Journal of Medicine, 347*(14), 1068–1074. doi:10.1056/NEJMoa020423 PMID:12362007

He, W., Goodkind, D., & Kowal, P. (2016). *An Aging World. International Population Reports*. Washington: U.S. Government Publishing Office.

Illario, M., Vollenbroek-Hutten, M. M. R., Molloy, W., Menditto, E., Iaccarino, G., & Eklund, P. (2016). Active and Healthy Ageing and Independent Living. *Journal of Aging Research, 2016*, 8062079. doi:10.1155/2016/8062079 PMID:27818798

Iyer, R., & Eastman, J. K. (2006). The Elderly and Their Attitudes toward the Internet: The Impact on Internet Use, Purchase and Comparison Shopping. *Journal of Marketing Theory and Practice, 14*(1), 57–67. doi:10.2753/MTP1069-6679140104

Jotheeswaran, A. T., Bryce, R., Prina, M., Acosta, D., Ferri, C. P., Guerra, M., & ... (2015). Frailty and the prediction of dependence and mortality in low- and middle-income countries: A 10/66 population-based cohort study. *BMC Medicine, 13*(138), 1–12. PMID:25563062

Kaethler, Y., Molnar, F., Mitchell, S., Soucie, P., & Manson-hing, M. (2003). Defining the concept of frailty: A survey of multi-disciplinary health professionals. *Geriatrics Today: Journal of the Canadian Geriatrics Society, 6*, 26–31.

Kahana, E., Kahana, B., & Kercher, K. (2003). Emerging lifestyles and proactive options for successful ageing. *Ageing International, 28*(2), 155–180. doi:10.100712126-003-1022-8

Leal, A.S.L., & Bogi, A. (2014). Network for the Market uptake of ICT for Ageing Well. In *Good Practices Handbook*. Project co-funded by the European Commission within the ICT Policy Support Programme.

Lee, P., Lan, W., & Yen, T. (2011). Aging successfully: A four-factor model. *Educational Gerontology, 37*(3), 210–227. doi:10.1080/03601277.2010.487759

Marmot, M., & Bell, R. (2012). Fair society, healthy lives. *Public Health, 126*(Suppl. 1), S4–S10. doi:10.1016/j.puhe.2012.05.014 PMID:22784581

Marmot, M., & Wilkinson, R. (2006). *Social Determinants of Health* (2nd ed.). Strasbourg: Oxford University Press.

Max-Neef, M. (1991). *Human Scale Development. Conception, application and further reflections*. New York: Apex Press.

McLean, A. (2011). Ethical frontiers of ICT and older users: Cultural, pragmatic and ethical issues. *Ethics and Information Technology, 13*(4), 313–326. doi:10.100710676-011-9276-4

Michel, J. P., Dreux, C., & Vacheron, A. (2016). Healthy ageing: Evidence that improvement is possible at every age. *European Geriatric Medicine, 7*(4), 298–305. doi:10.1016/j.eurger.2016.04.014

Miskelly, F. (2005). Electronic tracking of patients with dementia and wandering using mobile phone technology. *Age and Ageing, 34*(5), 497–499. doi:10.1093/ageing/afi145 PMID:16107453

Mollenkopf, H., & Walker, A. (2007). Quality of Life in old age. Synthesis and future perspective. In H. Mollenkopf & A. Walker (Eds.), *Quality of Life in Old Age* (pp. 235–248). Springer. doi:10.1007/978-1-4020-5682-6_14

Moraes, E. N., Lanna, F. M., Santos, R. R., Bicalho, M. A. C., Machado, C. J., & Romero, D. E. (2012). A new proposal for the clinical functional categorization of the elderly visual scale of frailty. *The Journal of Aging Research & Clinical Practice.* Retrieved from http://www.jarcp.com/1808-a-new-proposal-for-the-clinical-functional-categorization-of-the-elderly-visual-scale-of-frailty-vs-frailty.html

Noll, H. H. (2007). Monitoring the Quality of Life of the Elderly in European Societies. A social indicators' approach. In B. Marin & A. Zaidi (Eds.), *Mainstream Ageing: Indicators to monitor sustainable policies* (pp. 329–358). Aldershot: Ashgate.

Norris, P. (2001). *Digital divide: Civic engagement, information poverty and the internet worldwide*. Cambridge: Cambridge University Press. doi:10.1017/CBO9781139164887

Øvrum, A., Gustavsen, G. W., & Rickertsen, K. (2014). Age and socioeconomic inequalities in health: Examining the role of lifestyle choices. *Advances in Life Course Research, 19*, 1–13. doi:10.1016/j.alcr.2013.10.002 PMID:24796874

Parrott, L., & Madoc-Jones, L. (2008). Reclaiming information & communication technologies for empowering social work practice. *Journal of Social Work, 8*(2), 181–197. doi:10.1177/1468017307084739

Rockwood, K., Song, X., MacKnight, C., Bergman, H., Hogan, D. B., McDowell, I., & Mitnitski, A. (2005). A global clinical measure of fitness and frailty in elderly people. *Canadian Medical Association Journal*, *173*(5), 489–495. doi:10.1503/cmaj.050051 PMID:16129869

Rowe, J. W., & Kahn, R. L. (1997). Successful Aging. *The Gerontologist*, *37*(4), 433–440. doi:10.1093/geront/37.4.433 PMID:9279031

Sen, A. (1993). Capability and Well-being. In M. Nussbaum & A. Sen (Eds.), *The Quality of Life* (pp. 30–53). Oxford: Clarendon Press. doi:10.1093/0198287976.003.0003

Sen, A. (2009). *The Idea of Justice*. UK: Penguin Press.

Sourbati, M. (2004). *Internet use in sheltered housing. Older people's access to new media and online service delivery*. London: Goldsmiths College, University of London.

Sowar, A., Tobiasz-Adamczyk, B., Topór-Mądry, R., Poscia, A., & La Milia, D. I. (2016). Predictors of healthy ageing: public health policy targets. *BMC Health Services Research*, *16*(Suppl. 5), 289.

Stathopoulos, C. (2013). *DELIVERABLE D6.3 - Ethical and Social Best Practices on e-Accessibility. Value Aging*. TECNALIA. Retrieved from http://va.annabianco.it/wp-content/uploads/2014/09/07AGE03_D6.3_FINAL.pdf

Steyaert, J., & Gould, N. (2009). Social work and the changing face of the digital divide. *British Journal of Social Work*, *39*(4), 740–753. doi:10.1093/bjsw/bcp022

Swarte, V., & Stephan, C. (2002). *European Senior Watch Observatory and Inventory. A market study about the specific IST needs of older and disabled people to guide industry, RDT and policy. Case Studies*. Society and Technology Programme.

Tobiasz-Adamczyk, B., & Brzyski, P. (2005). Psychosocial work conditions as predictors of quality of life at the beginning of older age. *International Journal of Occupational Medicine and Environmental Health*, *18*(1), 43–52. PMID:16052890

WHO. (2015). *World Health Statistics 2015*. Global Health Observatory (GHO) data.

WHO. (2016). *Global strategy and action plan on ageing and health (2016-2020)*.

Worsfold, A. (2011). *Information for social care: A framework for improving quality in social care through better use of information and information technology*. Retrieved from http://www.differ.freeuk.com/learning/health/socialcareinfo.html

ADDITIONAL READING

Fairhall, N., Sherrington, C., Kurrle, S. E., Lord, S. R., Lockwood, K., Howard, K., ... Cameron, I. D. (2015). Economic evaluation of a multifactorial, interdisciplinary intervention versus usual care to reduce frailty in frail older people. *Journal of the American Medical Directors Association*, *16*(1), 41–48. doi:10.1016/j.jamda.2014.07.006 PMID:25239014

Gordon, A. L., Masud, T., & Gladman, J. R. F. (2014). Now that we have a definition for physical frailty, what shape should frailty medicine take? *Age and Ageing*, *32*(1), 8–9. doi:10.1093/ageing/aft161 PMID:24148267

Gregorevic, K. J., Hubbard, R. E., Lim, W. K., & Katz, B. (2016). The clinical frailty scale predicts functional decline and mortality when used by junior medical staff: A prospective cohort study. *BMC Geriatrics*, *16*(1), 117. doi:10.118612877-016-0292-4 PMID:27250650

Harrison, J. K., Clegg, A., Conroy, S. P., & Young, J. (2015). Managing frailty as a long-term condition. *Age and Ageing*, *44*(5), 732–735. doi:10.1093/ageing/afv085 PMID:26175349

Jegger, C.Futurage Group. (2013). Major drivers of health inequalities in later life and future research needs. *BMC Proceedings*, *7*(4), S5. doi:10.1186/1753-6561-7-S4-S5 PMID:24899923

Jopp, D. S., Wozniak, D., Damarin, A. K., De Feo, M., Jung, S., & Jeswani, S. (2015). How could lay perspectives on successful aging complement scientific theory? Findings from a U.S. and a German life-span sample. *The Gerontologist*, *55*(1), 91–106. doi:10.1093/geront/gnu059 PMID:24958719

Pak, R., & Mclaughlin, A. (2018). *Aging, Technology and Health. eBook*. Academic Press.

Rebola, C. B. (2015). *Designed Technologies for Healthy Aging*. In *Synthesis Lectures on Assistive, Rehabilitative, and Health-Preserving Technologies*. doi:10.2200/S00576ED1V01Y201404ARH006

KEY TERMS AND DEFINITIONS

Active Aging: The process and the outcome of a positive subjective wellbeing, good health (physical, cognitive, functional), social participation and security, enhancing the possibilities to act and to make choices as people age.

Digital Literacy: The capability to understand and to use technologies to communicate, to create, to interact and to evaluate information and actions.

Frailty: The state of increased and multidimensional vulnerability and the decline of the ability to cope with daily or acute stressors. It is normally associated with aging decline in functional domains of personal life.

Health Literacy: The capability to find, process and comprehend health information to make the appropriate decisions and to choose health services and resources accordingly.

Healthy Aging: The process, across life span, and the outcome of options and opportunities of good health (physical, mental, social) promotion in order to assure, in older years, an independent and high quality of life.

Innovation: The application of an original idea or invention that creates economic and/or social value.

Integrated Policies: Articulated policies concerning complex issues and interventions and that transcend the boundaries of established and dissociated policy fields. Various similar notions are also used: policy coherence, cross-cutting policy-making, concerted decision-making, policy consistency, and policy co-ordination.

Wellbeing: A sense, objective and subjective, of satisfactory conditions of existence: health, prosperity, security and protection, participation, emotions and links with others.

ENDNOTE

[1]   Present also in the European Health agenda, for instance in the Second Program of Community Action in the Field of Health 2008–2013: Together for Health.

Chapter 7
Managing End–of–Life Information in Palliative Care:
Between Discord and Conceptual Blends

Alexandre Cotovio Martins
Polytechnic Institute of Portalegre, Portugal

ABSTRACT

In this chapter, the author develop a sociological analysis of the role played by professional management of information about patients' end-of-life (EoL) processes in palliative care (PC). Thus the author will thus highlight the processes by which PC professionals manage private health information about patients in the frame of this type of care. Thus the author will show how managing information about prospective EoL trajectories by healthcare professionals is one of the major challenges in their daily work in PC wards. The author verifies that, in these contexts, patients and their families and members of the healthcare teams tend to have different experiential and personal careers in their relation with disease, the organization of care, and EoL trajectories, whose confrontation at the level of interaction produces complex effects in social processes that occur in daily activity contexts of PC.

INTRODUCTION

The sociological study of dying, death and bereavement is, as Exley (2004) states, a relatively recent field of study and can be dated back to the late 50's and early 60's of the XXth century. As Broom and Kirby (2012) argue, despite the fact that more recently we can verify the existence of a growth in sociological work on dying in palliative care units as a relational experience, little exploration exists about

DOI: 10.4018/978-1-5225-8470-4.ch007

the significance of contemporary family structures and relations in the process. These authors view the relative scarcity of sociological studies that include in their analysis the experience of dying - not only the experience of the dying person, but also of their close relatives -, as a significant gap in the sociological knowledge and understanding of the dying processes in palliative care. This is thus a field that, in the words of Broom and Kirby (2012), requires sociological investigation, in order to augment the standard focus on individual preferences in palliative care with sophisticated and nuanced understandings of the family contexts. Having precisely in mind the need to better understand the relationships between patients, their families and healthcare professionals in palliative care, in our research we addressed the specific social challenges to which health care professionals are confronted with in services of palliative care. We envisaged these challenges in its relation to the diversity of modes of experiencing end-of-life that patients and their families bring to the frame of healthcare. One of the main purposes of the research was, thus, to describe and analyse the ways by which healthcare professionals deal, in palliative care, with complexity in social situations, namely complexity caused by the confrontation, at the level of interaction, between different experiential and personal "careers" related to end-of-life care.

BACKGROUND: THE BODY AS A MATERIAL ANCHOR FOR COGNITIVE PROCESSES

In this Chapter, the author develops an exploratory analysis of the role played by distributed cognitive processes in palliative care, namely in the frame of specifically social problem-solving work developed by palliative care professionals. Palliative care is a specific form of healthcare, dedicated to promote comfort and quality of life for patients in advanced or terminal phase of chronic illness. In this type of care, the intervention of professionals needs to address frames of action which typically involve the private sphere of patients and their families. In these frames, one of the major elements which compose a significant part of the private sphere of patients is their body, namely the parts of it usually covered and protected from public scrutiny. Unveiling a part of what happens in this kind of frame is the purpose of this text.

In our analysis, we use the concept of *material anchor*, built by distributed cognition scientist Edwin Hutchins (2005), which allows to analyze and give centrality to the body of the patient as a particular material structure. Social actors in palliative care use this material anchors in the coordination of their actions, namely by coordinating internal (cognitive) structures with external (the body of the patient) structures. Material anchors play a relevant role in reasoning – or, in other words, in cognitive processes -, namely when social actors are in a situation which might not be easily apprehended through known cultural models, as it is frequently the case with patients and their families in end-of-life settings. In these cases, the blending of cognitive and material structures to stabilize reasoning emerges as a very relevant type of cognitive process. As Edwin Hutchins states,

The stability of (...) complex conceptual models is sometimes provided by their being embedded in conventional (culturally shared) well-learned and automatically applied internal mental structure. A conceptual model with these properties is a cultural model. (...). Other conceptual models achieve stability by virtue of being blended with an external physical medium. Problems that are too complex to hold in mind as a cultural model, and possibly some that are too complex to express at all in internal conceptual models, can be expressed and manipulated in material structure (Hutchins, 2005, pp. 1573-1574).

We are interested in envisaging the body of the patient as a material structure which is coordinated with cognitive processes in conceptual blending (Hutchins, 2005) for a set of intertwined reasons. In our previous research (Martins, 2015), we analyzed the specific social challenges with which health care professionals are confronted in palliative care. We verified that, in these contexts, patients and their families, and the members of the healthcare teams tend to have different experiential and personal careers (Glaser & Strauss, 2007, 2009) in their relation with disease, the organisation of care and end-of-life trajectories (Glaser & Strauss, 2007, 2009). The confrontation at the level of interaction produces complex effects in social processes that occur in the daily activity contexts (Martins, 2015). We observed also that professionals believe that this diversity, on the other hand, affects the comfort of people at the end of their lives, as it causes uncertainty around the definition and management of end-of-life and care trajectories (Martins, 2015). In this frame in particular we addressed the *hospital careers of illness* that characterise the end-of-life of many people during their aging process (Martins, 2015). These careers exert considerable importance in end-of-life processes, affecting the interaction around the terminal patient and the organisation of their terminal care (Glaser & Strauss, 2007). The hospital careers of illness include the different experiences that people undergo in their relationships with hospitals and healthcare professionals. For example, some patients repeatedly return to the same hospital. When this happens, the healthcare teams might react differently of the way they react when a "newcomer" arrives. The extent of the patient's familiarity with the hospital can also influence their reactions in the path towards death. One aspect of the effect of careers of this type in terminal situations is the conception of time, for example, in the acceptance or non-acceptance of death.

On the other hand, a central aspect of hospital careers of illness in palliative care is its close relation with the dying trajectories (Glaser & Strauss, 2007) of terminally ill patients. The concept of dying trajectory is quite relevant for our purpose, namely because it is referred to the close relation of observable physiological changes and social actor's perception and reasoning over them. As the seminal work on dying trajectories developed by Barney Glaser and Anselm Strauss puts it, dying trajectories have shape and duration, but these are not purely "objective" properties. According to the authors, "Neither duration or shape are purely objective physiological properties. They are both perceived properties; their dimensions depend on when the perceiver initially *defines* someone as dying and on his *expectations* of how that dying will proceed" (Glaser & Strauss, 2007, p.6). This relation between physiological transformations across a certain duration – that is, transformations in the patient's body and its observable signs – and cognitive elements of perception and expectation developed by different social actors can adequately be analysed as a process of conceptual blending (Hutchins, 2005; Thévenot, 1998), in which material and conceptual structures are tentatively coordinated.

The dying trajectories of patients (Glaser & Strauss, 2007; Martins, 2015) are also characterized by its close relation to critical moments in the frame of social interactions in palliative care (Martins, 2015). We define a *critical moment* as a situation where there is discord between the relevant actors in view of elements of uncertainty present in situations of palliative internment. The use of the term "critical" derives precisely from the nature of these situations, mobilising the critical competence and skills of social actors (Boltanski & Thévenot, 1999), aimed at reducing the uncertainty inscribed in these very situations and involving discord about dying trajectories (Martins, 2015; Glaser & Strauss, 2007).

The critical moments in which discord tends to emerge challenge to reason about distributed cognition in cases in which the stability of cognition is not guaranteed and the material anchoring of cognition becomes problematic. As a matter of fact, cognitive processes require a certain amount of stability in the representation of constraints, in order to operate. According to Hutchins, there are two main forms of achieving this kind of stability in conceptual models: "First, the conceptual models that anthropologists call cultural models achieve representational stability via a combination of intrapersonal and interpersonal processes. Second, the association of conceptual structure with material structure can stabilize conceptual representations" (Hutchins, 2005, p. 1574). As we will see the problem to which professionals in palliative care are confronted with (although obviously not lived by them in these terms) in situations of diversity about care and end-of-life trajectories is precisely the building of conceptual blends. These can articulate and stabilize the coordination of conceptual structures and material structures in a way that allows them to create common frames of understanding about specific situations, thus reducing uncertainty and social complexity in the management of end-of-life situations. In other words, since professionals cannot always achieve representational stability via a common model of understanding of end-of-life situations, they will often have to achieve it via the association of conceptual and material structure (the body of the patient in its end-of-life evolution).

With this analytical frame, it will be now developed a sociological analysis of the role played by professional management of information about patients' end-of-life processes in palliative care. This analysis will also highlight the processes by which palliative care professionals manage privacy and health information about patients in the frame of this type of care. The main objectives of the analysis are to show how managing information about prospective end-of-life trajectories by healthcare professionals is one of the major challenges in their daily work in palliative care wards and to describe and analyze how, in situations in which discord tends to emerge, the ability of palliative care teams to manage information about End-of-life trajectories becomes a crucial aspect of the quality of the care provided. The main findings of the project over which this chapter focuses upon may be of interest to help healthcare practitioners, as well as policy-makers in this area to rethink privacy and health information management issues in palliative care, connecting this approach to the overall frame of this book.

METHODOLOGY

Research Design

The research goal was to make a deep data-collection, in three phases: in the first one, through direct, non-systematic observation and exploratory interviews; in the second one, through ethnographic observation (twelve months), and in the third one, through in-depth interviews. Our population was constituted by professionals of medicine, nursing and social work in palliative care. We chose these professions because (i) professionals of each one of them work directly and in proximity (Martins, 2015) with dying patients and their families; and (ii) they were, at the time of data collecting, the most frequent professions in palliative care teams in Portugal. Thus, the sample is constituted by the professionals working in palliative care in the chosen hospitals at the time of the fieldwork process. Fieldwork was accomplished in two hospitals with socially contrastive publics, and according to two criteria: (p) the palliative care team of each one of them integrated the different professions to be observed; (q) they had socially contrastive publics.

The data contained in the field logs and interviews were, in the first stage, subject to an exploratory Categorical Content Analysis, based on the following positive discrimination criteria: i) the existence of relevant family relations (i.e. with observable influence in the contexts of action in palliative care wards) of patients under palliative hospital internment; ii) the existence of discord between relevant actors (patient, family, professionals) in view of elements of uncertainty present in situations of palliative internment. With this procedure, 59 households were identified as being involved in situations with the intended features. The interviews were made to the professionals who dealt with these households.

Data Collection

The analysis conducted herein was carried out on data collected under the project *Building paths towards death: an analysis of everyday work in palliative care*, reference PTDC/CS-SOC/119621/2010, financed by the Portuguese Foundation for Science and Technology (FCT). In particular the data obtained through twelve months of ethnographic observation carried out at two hospital internment units providing palliative care in Mainland Portugal and 37 in-depth interviews to professionals in palliative care – physicians, nurses and social workers (table 1). The ethnographic observation records were kept in "field logs", drawn up by two scholarship students contracted under the aforesaid project.

HOSPITAL CAREERS OF ILLNESS, DYING TRAJECTORIES, AND DISCORD IN PALLIATIVE CARE

Discord and Representations of End-of-Life

We observed that the emergence of discord is part of the dynamics of action present on a daily basis in various situations in the context of palliative care. This discord is not distributed by chance in the different observed situations, where some are more hazardous: a) the initial admission in palliative internment, b) the situations of discussion of the (im)possible hospital discharge of palliative patients and c) the situations of discussion of the end-of-life trajectory of the patients and related aspects. We also observed that divergence not only tends to arise in specific situations, but also takes on a variety of social configurations, as we have discussed elsewhere about discord in palliative care (Martins, 2015). Mostly, what is important to highlight here is the association of divergent cognitions to hospital careers of illness, in the

Table 1. Number and length of the interviews (in order of realization)

	Gender	Profession	Interview Length
Phase I (see below)	F	Nurse	2h11m00s
	F	Nurse	2h12m19s
	F	Physician	1h00m38s
	F	Physician	2h17m04s
	F	Nurse	1h11m38s
	F	Social Worker	1h33m00s
	F	Nurse	1h10m27s
	F	Social Worker	0h57m56s
Phase III	F	Nurse	1h58m50s
	F	Nurse	00h57m31s
	M	Nurse	00h41m09s
	F	Nurse	02h44m15s
	M	Nurse	00h59m26s
	F	Nurse	00h30m50s
	F	Physician	00h59m47s
	F	Social Worker	00h47m38s
	F	Nurse	00h42m11s
	F	Nurse	00h53m39s
	F	Nurse	00h39m45s
	F	Nurse	00h50m22s
	M	Social Worker	00h50m57s
	M	Nurse	00h34m01s
	F	Physician	02h02m01s
	F	Nurse	00h35m16s
	F	Nurse	00h22m54s
	F	Nurse	00h46m24s
	M	Nurse	00h35m13s
	F	Nurse	00h45m54s
	F	Nurse	00h44m35s
	F	Nurse	00h40m52s
	F	Nurse	00h31m35s
	F	Nurse	00h41m11s
	F	Nurse	00h45m16s
	F	Nurse	00h44m36s
	F	Nurse	01h12m17s
	F	Nurse	00h33m28s
	F	Nurse	00h50m14s

Source: (Author)

first place. The typical critical moments we identified here are clearly connected to regular points of these careers, observable in palliative care wards.

One of these typical situations goes on when the patients are admitted in the palliative care unit. The perception of professionals of palliative care about this is that many of the situations of discord and tension between them and the patients, or them and patient's families, or even between patients and their families are related to what they consider to be a *lack of information* over their condition. In their view, health care professionals in other hospital services (as for instance oncology wards) don't always say to the patients in what real physical condition they are and don't define in a clear way what is to be expected. They think this tends to create a lot of turbulence in the palliative care ward admission processes.

[The patients] were operated on, the doctor said that it was okay that he would live for the rest of his life and then he or she comes to the palliative care unit and then we have to work all this and that is where it becomes complicated, "- Look –we say -, your doctor, who operated you, told you that at that specific time, but unfortunately the disease has appeared again and has progressed and it's like this ..." "- Ah! But the doctor said he'd be fine for the rest of his life. Why is he here?", the family says. And that makes all things a lot more difficult, because the family and the patient are not prepared, and they often react very badly... both being sad or really don't wanting to believe what we're saying [Nurse, palliative care ward].

Sometimes families resist, despite the information we give them, sometimes they pretty much deny the situation. And sometimes they also think they do not need it, they do not need a certain intervention... Because they are not facing this need at the moment (...), but we have to deal with it in advance. And sometimes it is difficult to work with families at this level, even in palliative care. Because people always find that they can, somehow, deny things [Nurse, palliative care ward]. (Martins, 2018)

As we can conclude by reading these excerpts, the professionals tend to envisage these cases as situations in which interactional problems (as perceived by them) emerge from what they consider to be a - greater or lesser - deficit of information about end-of-life trajectories by patients and their families. As we shall see, one of the ways by which professionals try to solve these interactional problems is to inform patients and their families about what they consider to be their *real* condition, which is, their medically-defined end-of-life trajectory. Of course, thinking sociologically, we see that this process is one in which professionals try to define and stabilize end-of-life situations, namely by defining and stabilizing, at least in a way that avoids interactional troubles, the representations of patients and their families about the end-of-life process that they are living or to which they are closely related.

THE BUILDING OF FRAMINGS OF UNDERSTANDING: DEFINING AND STABILIZING REPRESENTATIONS

Information Management and Coordination of Actions

The relevance that palliative care professionals give to the building of stable representations of dying trajectories may be seized if we observe their staff reunions or if we ask them how they manage medical information about dying trajectories as a team. Both the reunions, changes of shift and the everyday activities of the team that require interaction with patients and their relatives are carefully monitored having the management of information about dying trajectories in mind. In other words, there is a strict coordination of actions among team members in order not to create any unexpected "incident" around perceptions and expectations on these trajectories. Besides, the management of medical information about the physical condition of the patients is considered a central aspect of work in palliative care by all the professionals we observed and interviewed. This means that, in order to define and stabilize the representations that patients and their families produce around dying trajectories, palliative care teams must firstly stabilize and coordinate accurately cognitive elements about each case between its members.

As a matter of fact, the management of this specific kind of information, as something that we could observe, is quite frequently an object of great attention in the reunions (generally weekly reunions) of the palliative care teams. Professionals try, in their meetings, to share their insights about "how much" the admitted patients and their families know about their "real" condition, what kind of expectations they are developing over the future trajectories and how they are reacting emotionally if they are aware of the nearness of dying. Of course, this means that, from the very first moment the patient is admitted, the team members try, through several delicate forms of interaction, to gather information around these points. We could also observe these close interactions between team members, patients and their families, which are widely meant to prepare decision-making processes in staff's reunions. Changes of shift constitute another kind of situation in which particular care is posed in this type of coordination: most professionals consider this a critical issue to be worked when shifts change, in order not to "break" the degree of coordination of the team over time.

Right from the start, it's very important for us to know what the patient knows, what the family knows, what the patient wants to know, what the family wants us to say and ... And this is not (hesitation)... Sometimes... We always make the admission but we don't always know immediately, it's not all unveiled in the admission and, therefore, we have to understand very well and to draw very well the profile of that family and that patient, you know? Before that we can, let's say, hum, act, say, and in a manner suited not to hurt the sensibility of anyone... and this makes all the difference. It's not easy to do! As we were seeing yesterday, sometimes the first approach is not easy, and yesterday we saw, when we were in our weekly reunion that the Doctor said "-That patient is in denial!" (Nurse)

Everyone has to know how to act for that family, everyone must have the same communication and strategies, everything ... because otherwise it's not worth it, if everyone does it their way it's not worth it. And the sharing of information is very important! Very important indeed! (Nurse)

If we don't pass on some kind of information [among us], then the language will be different, I will tell the patient one thing, the next one says another, the other comes, says another, and often the patient will explore this, asking you, then asking the other colleague to see if the answer is the same, hum, and if the information is the same, he knows, "Okay everything is the same, this team works all the same". (Nurse). (Martins, 2018)

Information and Cognitive Blending

The specific cognitive forms to which professionals call *information* about dying trajectories and which they try to manage for the already exposed purposes are conceptual blends which use is rooted in their daily activity (Hutchins, 2005; Thévenot, 1998). From this standpoint, dying trajectories can be analyzed as complex sets of conceptual blends that articulate medical concepts (right away concepts such as "signs" and "symptoms", but also complex definitions of organic disorders, etc.), scientific data collected through medical and technological mediations (such as CTs, X-Rays, blood samples, etc.), statistical data about survival rates, etc., and, in the most relevant cases, the *body* of the patient, as a material anchor in which specific medical concepts find root and cognitive support. The physiological evolution of the patient's body is the very basis for the definition of dying trajectories and reasoning about them by professionals (obviously, dying trajectories are not designated like this by health care professionals).

We already noticed that we could observe that there can exist quite a diversity in the definition of dying trajectories in palliative care wards, namely because actors bring to the core of these processes different personal and experiential careers (Glaser & Strauss, 2007; Martins, 2015) in their relation to end-of-life processes. Given the fact that dying trajectories are not exclusively "objective", the perceptions and expectations of social actors, with their specific and differentiated frames of reference developed over time, promote this diversity. But precisely, this is considered to be a problem by the health care professionals in the palliative care wards that we observed. Not the diversity in itself, but the uncertainty that they believe it can cause, because it is directly related with expectations which, in their view, can create situations of discord and consequent suffering to patients.

Yes, there are criteria, without a doubt. And even medical criteria, as a matter of fact, that indicates what to expect, isn't it? That indicates us. However, in terms of expectations [of those involved] it's different, you know? We have patients who are very ill and still have a very high expectation [about their future]. Very high. And we see that that person, hum, has a very marked asthenia, anorexia, easy fatigue and the person sees this but continues to think that she's still very well and that this is a fleeting condition (Nurse).

One typical situation occurs when a patient starts to do apneas, so to speak. Stop pacing, you know? So we see that he will not last long. This is an easy-to-see symptom, and the family members do see it, don't they? That he no longer breathes for a little bit, a few seconds and then that increases and goes on making longer and longer snouts until, until, until it stops. Maybe it will be the most visible and easiest symptom to see and which indicates that the situation is really nearing its end, you know?

In these cases, if the family is present, they sometimes call us: "- Oh, he stopped breathing", we try to explain that this is a natural process and a normal thing. "- You can stand close and you can hold his/her hand, but we will not intervene... We will not reanimate, we will not do anything, because there is no indication in this sense". We always have to talk to them and explain what's going on (Nurse). (Martins, 2018)

Believing that giving insights to the patients and their families about their "real" end-of-life trajectories is the right way to avoid both uncertainty and discord and some forms of suffering related to it, the observed professionals typically engage in a search for "informing" these actors about medically-designed trajectories. The process, on the other hand, involves sharing part of the conceptual blends that professionals use in their daily activity with patients and their families, be it in a lay translation made by professionals *ad hoc*. The process is not linear, nor always identical, not even immediate. On the contrary, it starts with the admission of the patient, and it is highly dependent on the tact (Breviglieri, 2008) of professionals to engage and try to alter, when they think it's necessary, the perception of those actors. Although the purpose is to share what is "really going on" with the body of the ill person and, expectedly, adjust and coordinate reasoning and expectations about end-of-life as much as possible. They think this can only be made with delicate, case-driven, smooth communication processes.

In the process, professionals bind general forms of medical representation of the ill body with local, particular references to that same body which may transmit, to the patients and their families, concise but effective anchors for them to understand medically-defined end-of-life trajectories. The body of the patient with its transformations becomes, thus, a fundamental support for cognition and a privileged *medium* used to build local forms of perception and communication in which professionals invest great part of their daily work, forms that are able to function as cognitive clues for the ill person and their families to interpret end-of-life processes as close as possible to medically-defined end-of-life trajectories.

Often before the apnea, the person starts with some rustling. Therefore, one of the symptoms [by which we perceive the person is entering in the terminal phase] is the person starting with rustling, also there is a certain tiredness, there is a difficulty to expel secretions, so this is one of the first signs, is the rustler. On the other hand, there is a great fatigue, sometimes it's a look into the void, the gaze, staring at the void, then, um, and the respiratory part, therefore, comes some dyspnea, some deep breathing with moments of apnea and therefore, these are usually the most important. The body cooling, it's also important. Umm. So these are, shall we say, the criteria, okay? More clinical ones, which are more visible and which are the most... It's the anuria too, when the person begins to collapse (Nurse).

It's one of those things that we have to be very careful about [talking to the family], it's precisely about the prognosis, it's precisely saying that, "- Look, there may be... it may be something that happens suddenly, because a blood vessel can blow", we have very complex situations here! "We can have something sudden, but it can be slow, progressive and calm. But we can always have oscillations" (Nurse).

We have patients who are doing well, perfectly well and who suddenly begin to get more tired one day, the next day they start to bed. It is important, and it depends on the patient that we have ahead, that we know how to talk and there are people who need to know what is going on and so we try to explain that this can happen to them, but it is normal and this situation: "- Look this can happen but is normal, don't be scared. For example, you can have blood in the stool, have constipation (...), but this may come from controlling the pain, morphine creates, for example, constipation but we are trying to correct this". Therefore, we must try to anticipate and inform the patient and the family of some situations that may happen. So this is a task that we have little by little to do throughout the day to prepare them...(Physician)

I think that no one is ever totally prepared for all kinds of things that happen here, but, um, and we slowly try to tell the evolution of things to the patient, how he is now, how he was tonight, how he was in the morning, if he is better, if he is worse; we also try gently to alert the the family: "- Look, this can get worse. We are not saying that it will get worse, but we have had others ... ", for example, giving an example of other cases, or of a particular pathology, saying it's normal, it's part of the pathology itself that something happens and we explain it to the family... For the family to be aware and not to be alarmed when they see a certain signal or a certain symptom that they were not used to until then, but, there it is, that's it, and we're trying to warn "- Don't be surprised if this or that happens" ... . Anyway, we're here to help and to explain, but let's say ... there, we give "warning shots", let's say it can happen, it may not happen, we'll go and talk to the family (Nurse). (Martins, 2018)

This kind of process is not, on the other hand, always one in which each professional approaches patients and their relatives and tries to "inform" them about their condition. As a matter of fact, there is a regular and more structured approach conducted by the team in order to discuss a set of themes which are considered to be relevant, naturally also with strong emphasis on the dying trajectories. We are talking about *family meetings*, reunions where the palliative care teams meet the patient's families, in order to discuss a number of selected themes.

Family meetings, or family conferences, are usually envisaged in the literature (*e.g.* in Lautrette, Ciroldi, Ksibi & Azoulay, 2006; Fineberg, 2005) of palliative care as intending to ensure the quality of care, working in proximity with the families, giving them support and even making them a *partner* in caring procedures. Of course, *informing* the families about their relative's medical condition and the related plan of care is a central aspect of these meetings, as we could observe in our ethnography of hospital wards. Within this information, the focus on dying trajectories and hospital careers of illness becomes a central aspect. Once again, this is a typical moment in which professionals try to "inform" patient's relatives about the characteristics of medically-designed dying trajectories, with its bodily signs, and of what families should *expect* – both in terms of the process and outcome of the trajectories, both in terms of the plan of care. Even though this plan is to be, at least tentatively, shared and negotiated with the family, the medical aspects associated to the dying trajectories largely structure the frame of negotiation and its limits - although that there are cases of discord and professionals don't always get the agreement of the families about their opinion.

In general, the family is looking for us. Trying to talk to us about it, to know where things are, whether it is soon or not, or what they can do or not, what they can talk to [the patient] or not, whether it is beneficial to bring food from home or not. (...) It has already happened, it has already happened in families that are in complete denial - and it is a bit extreme -, we are thinking that death is eminent and the family does not want to accept it and we think it can be very harmful for the patient himself to have his family there ... We seek comfort, rest and the family being around the patient saying, "- Get up!", "- Don't you spend so much time in bed!", "- Don't complain so much"... We've already had a case which was most unpleasant... in this case, we had to convene the so-called family conferences where, in a more direct way, we usually try to call the familiar to reality and to what is really happening and, normally, our doctor speaks very convincingly. It's also easier when you have a medicine diploma, which the family or the patient himself understands as relevant (Nurse).

We've had cases of users here who were not feeding for days and weeks and it was our option not to intubate, and the relatives were engaged in making a point about this and wanted and wanted and wanted and then, then... There we had to set up a family conference and try to explain our position, but they also mark theirs, right? We've had cases in which we have even had to intubate the patient voluntarily [by his request]. The annoying sometimes is when there is the case, for example, imagine that there are two sons, and there's one who thinks that the father should eat through ... And the one other says "-No"; sometimes it is very difficult to manage this.

SOLUTIONS AND RECOMMENDATIONS

Although the research here briefly and partially discussed cannot give yet any "solutions and recommendations", since it is in its beginning, its purposes are also practical. The study intends to contribute to the advancement of knowledge in the field of sociological studies over palliative care, namely in Portugal, by: 1) analyzing the role of discord and uncertainty in the frame of palliative care; 2) studying discord in its relations to the larger frame of careers of illness; 3) addressing the relations among these careers and End-of-life trajectories; 4) analyzing the ways by which palliative care professionals try to reduce discord and uncertainty in palliative care by composing a diversity of views and engagements around End-of-life.

It is considered that the main expectable achievements of the research are: (1) the advancement of knowledge in the area, substantiated by (a) an enlargement of the Portuguese Sociology of Health's field of study, which has produced, until this date, few studies about palliative care (let us note that palliative care is a recent field of work of in our country); (b) an improvement of our theoretical framework, previously established in our own sociological research, developed about palliative care, which will be upgraded by testing the concepts used in a field where we expect to see some of their limits and possibilities at work; (2) the production of socially useful information and knowledge (a) about some central conditions of professional action and judgement in palliative care, which may be useful for the reflection about practices of professionals in the field; (b) which may suit the needs of Non-Governmental Organizations and Public Agencies in this sector.

FUTURE RESEARCH DIRECTIONS

The results discussed here are only exploratory. The research on this issue needs to be deepened, namely giving more focus upon processes of cognitive blending, in order to try to build a more systematic analytical frame which can lead to (i) the establishment of a typology of the uses of the body as a material anchor by palliative care professionals in order to stabilize representations around end-of-life processes; (ii) the establishment of a more accurate typology of the modes of relation between medically-defined end-of-life trajectories and the palliative care patients' and their families' lay representations of end-of-life processes; (iii) draw a broader analysis of the palliative care internments' ecological aspects which are closely related with the cognitive processes that are taking place in end-of-life management by palliative care professionals.

CONCLUSION

In this brief chapter, it was given an account of the engagements in action of professionals of palliative care which involve a delicate management of information about the private, bodily sphere of the patients, The information is made in order to reduce uncertainty and appease disquietude and discord around situations of end-of-life care. There were highlighted situations in which discord tends to emerge and that challenge researchers to reason about distributed cognition in cases in which the stability of cognition is not guaranteed and the material anchoring of cognition becomes problematic. Health professionals in the observed palliative care wards try to face discord, and try to define and stabilize representations over the body of the patient, by blending conceptual and material structures. This blending may be suitable to reduce the diversity of perceptions of the actors at play, and thus, in their view, to avoid certain situations of discord about dying trajectories and correlated procedures of care. Having this in mind, it was also stressed the relevance that the building and the maintenance of the conceptual blends that result from these processes have in the organization of work in palliative care teams. Namely, in what concerns the management of the daily work of professionals in their relation with patients and their relatives, be it in the team's reunions, staff's shifts, individual contacts between staff and families and patients or family conferences.

The main purpose here was to describe how, when professionals deal with this specific kind of complexity, they try to blend conceptual and material structures which may be suitable to reduce the diversity of perceptions of actors at play and thus, in their view, to avoid certain situations of discord about the dying trajectories and correlated procedures of care. In other words, how they engage in sharing definitions of cognitive frames around the patients' body, which may stabilize, as much as possible, conceptual structures that are suited to reduce uncertainty in the development of care actions and thus promote patients' comfort in their end of life.

ACKNOWLEDGMENT

This research was funded by the Portuguese Science and Technology Foundation (FCT), in the frame of the projects PTDC/CS-SOC/119621/2010 and PTDC/SOC-SOC/30092/2017.

REFERENCES

Boltanski, L., & Thévenot, L. (2006). *On justification: Economies of worth*. Princeton, NJ: Princeton University Press. (Original work published 1991)

Breviglieri, M. (2008). L'individu, le proche et l'institution. Travail social et politique de l'autonomie. *The Information Society*, *145*, 92–101.

Broom, A., & Kirby, E. (2012). The end of life and the family: Hospice patient's views on dying as relational. *Sociology of Health & Illness*, *35*(4), 499–513. doi:10.1111/j.1467-9566.2012.01497.x PMID:22742736

Chandrasekharan, S., & Nersessian, N. (2011). Building cognition: the construction of external representations for discovery. *Proceedings of the Cognitive Science Society, 33*.

Exley, C. (2004). Review article: The sociology of dying, death and bereavement. *Sociology of Health & Illness*, *26*(1), 110–122. doi:10.1111/j.1467-9566.2004.00382.x PMID:15027994

Fineber, I. (2005). Preparing professionals for family conferences in palliative care: Evaluation results of na interdisciplinary approach. *Journal of Palliative Medicine*, *8*(4), 857–866. doi:10.1089/jpm.2005.8.857 PMID:16128661

Glaser, B., & Strauss, A. (2007). *Time for dying*. Aldine Transaction.

Glaser, B., & Strauss, A. (2009). *Awareness of dying*. Aldine Transaction.

Hutchins, E. (2005). Material anchors for conceptual blends. *Journal of Pragmatics*, *37*(10), 1555–1577. doi:10.1016/j.pragma.2004.06.008

Lautrette, A., Ciroldi, M., Ksibi, H., & Azoulay, E. (2006). End-of-life family conferences: Rooted in the evidence. *Critical Care Medicine*, *34*(Suppl), S364–S372. doi:10.1097/01.CCM.0000237049.44246.8C PMID:17057600

Martins, A. (2015). Building paths towards death: sociological portraits of discord in family relations of the elderly in palliative care. In J. M. Resende & A. C. Martins (Eds.), *The making of the common in social relations* (pp. 6–21). Newcastle Upon Tyne, UK: Cambridge Scholars Publishing.

Martins, A. (2018). Viver e morrer no hospital: retratos sociológicos do desacordo nas relações familiares dos idosos em cuidados paliativos. In J. Resende & C. Delaunay (Orgs.), Democracia, promessas, utopias e (des)ilusões: Dilemas e disputas nas arenas públicas (pp. 123-139). Carviçais: Lema de Origem.

Thévenot, L. (1986). Les investissements de formes. In L. Thévenot (Ed.), *Conventions économiques* (pp. 21–71). Paris: Presses Universitaires de France.

Thévenot, L. (1990). L'action qui convient. In P. Pharo & L. Quéré (Eds.), *Les formes de l'action. Sémantique et Sociologie* (pp. 39–69). Paris: EHESS.

Thévenot, L. (1997). Un gouvernement par les normes. Pratiques et politiques des formats d'information. In B. Conein & L. Thévenot (Eds), Cognition et information en société (pp. 205-241). Paris: Éditions de l'EHESS (Raisons pratiques 8).

Thévenot, L. (1998). Pragmatiques de la connaissance. In A. Borzeix, A. Bouvier, & P. Pharo (Eds.), *Sociologie et connaissance. Nouvelles approches cognitives* (pp. 101–139). Paris: Éditions du CNRS.

Thévenot, L. (2001). Pragmatic regimes governing the engagement with the world. In T. Schatzki, K. Knorr-Cetina, & E. von Savigny (Eds.), *The practice turn in contemporary theory* (pp. 56–73). Brighton, UK: Psychology Press.

Thévenot, L. (2006). *L'action au pluriel. Sociologie des régimes d'engagement*. Paris: Éditions La Découverte.

Thévenot, L. (2009). Governing Life by Standards: A View from Engagements. *Social Studies of Science*, *39*(5), 793–813. doi:10.1177/0306312709338767

ADDITIONAL READING

McNamara, B. (2004). Good enough death: Autonomy and choice in Australian palliative care. *Social Science & Medicine, 58*(5), 929–938. doi:10.1016/j. socscimed.2003.10.042 PMID:14732606

Milberg, A., Torres, S., & Ågård, P. (2016). Health Care Professionals' Understandings of Cross-Cultural Interaction in End-of-Life Care: A Focus Group Study. *PLoS One, 11*(11), e0165452. doi:10.1371/journal.pone.0165452 PMID:27880814

Ochs, E., & Kremer-Sadlik, T. (Eds.). (2013). *Fast-Forward Family: Home, Work, and Relationships in Middle-Class America.* Berkeley, Los Angeles, London: University of California Press.

Okely, J. (1994). Thinking through fieldwork. In A. Bryman & R. G. Burgess (Eds.), *Analyzing Qualitative Data* (pp. 18–34). New York: Routledge. doi:10.4324/9780203413081_chapter_1

Pino, M., Parry, R., Land, V., Faull, C., Feathers, L., & Seymour, J. (2016). Engaging Terminally Ill Patients in End of Life Talk: How Experienced Palliative Medicine Doctors Navigate the Dilemma of Promoting Discussions about Dying. *PLoS One, 11*(5), e0156174. doi:10.1371/journal.pone.0156174 PMID:27243630

Silverman, D. (1993). *Interpreting Qualitative Data - Methods for Analysing Talk, Text and Interaction.* London: Sage Publications.

Stokoe, E. (2011). Simulated Interaction and Communication Skills Training: The' Conversation-Analytic Role-Play Method. In C. Antaki (Ed.), *Applied Conversation Analysis: Intervention and Change in Institutional Talk* (pp. 119–139). New York: Palgrave Macmillan. doi:10.1057/9780230316874_7

Walczak, A., Butow, P. N., Tattersall, M. H. N., Davidson, P. M., Young, J., Epstein, R. M., ... Clayton, J. M. (2017). Encouraging early discussion of life expectancy and end-of-life care: A randomised controlled trial of a nurse-led communication support program for patients and caregivers. *International Journal of Nursing Studies, 67,* 31–40. doi:10.1016/j.ijnurstu.2016.10.008 PMID:27912108

WHO. (2011). *Palliative care for older people: better practices.* Copenhagen: WHO.

Zimmerman, C. (2012). Acceptance of dying: A discourse analysis of palliative care literature. *Social Science & Medicine, 75*(1), 217–224. doi:10.1016/j. socscimed.2012.02.047 PMID:22513246

KEY TERMS AND DEFINITIONS

Career: Personal and experiential trajectories of relation with healthcare services and professionals, illness and disease, death and other situations and conditions, developed over time by individuals.

Cognitive Blending in Palliative Care: Process of binding general forms of medical representation of the ill body with local, particular references to that same body.

Conceptual Blend: A cognitive strategy which encompasses combining mental processes with material objects that can support cognition in complex, unstable situations.

Critical Moments: Situations where discord between relevant actors arises in view of elements of uncertainty present in different palliative care occurrences.

Dying Trajectories: The objective transformations of the sick body over time and the subjective views that different (namely patients and their families, but also health professionals) social actors build upon them, in end-of-life situations.

Hospital Careers of Illness: The objective trajectories of patients and their families over time in hospital facilities (for instance, the transition between wards or services), which are related to the subjective experience of these trajectories, also developed over time.

Medically Defined Dying (or End-of-Life) Trajectories: The objective transformations of the sick body over time as grasped through medical teams, when mobilizing medical knowledge.

Palliative Care: Healthcare provided to chronic, seriously ill and terminal patients, usually intending to promote comfort and quality of life in a context in which curing the patient isn't possible.

Chapter 8
The Hidden Face of Medical Intervention

Samuel Beaudoin
Université Laval, Canada

ABSTRACT

In health promotion discourses, access to medical care is presented as a universal remedy. As a result, ethical considerations are often limited to the issue of equitable access. Yet focusing on access to healthcare hides the issue of access to data needed for scientific development. Putting into place a system for saving lives involves population health monitoring and is founded on scientific rationality. This chapter refocuses political attention from medical intervention to what makes it possible. In doing so, the underlying ethical issue shifts from a concern with universal access to healthcare—considered a right from an equity standpoint—to a discussion of the options and consequences of a type of government based on science. The author puts forward the idea that it is not because it is technically and scientifically possible to do something that it should be done. To illustrate this argument, the chapter discusses the example of The Lancet's project on stillbirths (2011-2030) taken up by the WHO.

INTRODUCTION

This chapter is part of a broader debate on the relations between science, ethics and politics. It takes up both Nikolas Rose's (2007) suggestion to take the social critique of medicalization a step further, and Jonathan Glover's (2017) ethical challenge to go beyond the categorical imperative to save lives. Our aim is to inspire a discussion of the certainties currently surrounding equitable access to healthcare and to reveal what is hidden behind medical intervention so as to open a space for reflection.

DOI: 10.4018/978-1-5225-8470-4.ch008

This chapter is based on the results of research and analyses (Beaudoin, 2018). Its objectives are related to three analytical shifts concerning how politics, ethics and science are intermingled and used by experts and researchers. The first shift aims to refocus political attention from medical intervention to what makes it possible. The second is a shift in ethical focus from the issue of equitable access to a discussion of the options and consequences of a type of *government based on science¹*. The third shift is an invitation to reexamine the processes of knowledge production, moving from unlimited data production to an ethic of research restraint.

This chapter therefore seeks to reveal what is hidden behind medical interventions. There are two main arguments. First, that access to medical care hides access to data needed for scientific development. Second, that equitable access to medical services hides the standardization of the conception of human life. Finally, following the discussion on solutions and recommendations, a third argument concerns the future of research and suggests that the unlimited production of data on the human body and life hides the failure of progress, which is the very justification for universal coverage. Before examining these proposals, the context will be presented in which some of the main underlying ideas were developed.

BACKGROUND

In 1942, William Henry Beveridge published *Social Insurance and Allied Services* in which he developed the idea of universal state-covered social protection for the whole population and for all social risks. Better known as the Beveridge Plan, it proposed a guarantee not only to life, but to a healthy life, associated with the right to health. This model was implemented in England after the Labour Party was elected in 1945, and was thereafter exported throughout the world (Foucault, 2001a). The Beveridge Plan directly influenced the organization of health services in many countries. However, the creation of the World Health Organization (signed in 1946 and taking effect in 1948) under the United Nations charter (ratified in 1945) took the project of universal social protection to a worldwide scale, stating that "The health of all peoples is fundamental to the attainment of peace and security" (WHO, 1948, p. 1) and "The enjoyment of the highest attainable standard of health is one of the fundamental rights of every human being without distinction of race, religion, political belief, economic or social condition" (WHO, 1948, p. 1). The goal of the WHO is "the attainment by all peoples of the highest possible level of health" (WHO, 1948, p. 2). To achieve this, the WHO considers as a matter of principle that "Unequal development in different countries in the promotion of health and control of disease […] is a common danger" (WHO, 1948, p. 1) and that "The health of all peoples [...] is dependent upon the fullest co-operation of individuals and States" (WHO, 1948, p. 1). Henceforth, no political party could disregard health issues and expenses, since the WHO Constitution states that "Governments have a responsibility for the health of their peoples which can be fulfilled only by the provision of adequate health and social measures" (WHO, 1948, p. 1). On this basis, since the end of the Second World War, there has been a shared vision of what population health and individual well-being should be (Rose, 2006).

To truly grasp the breadth and depth of this new collective project, the WHO's principle-based definition of health is worth examining: "Health is a state of complete physical, mental and social well-being and not merely the absence of disease or infirmity" (WHO, 1948, p. 1). The underlying assumption is that this state is good and desirable for all individuals and for all peoples. The essential condition for the "fullest attainment of health" is "the extension to all peoples of the benefits of medical, psychological and related knowledge" (WHO, 1948, p. 1), to which the WHO adds the primary importance of an "informed opinion and active co-operation on the part of the public" (WHO, 1948, p. 1). In other words, and not without irony, the key to happiness would lie with the medical and psychological sciences, designated henceforth as saviors of bodies and souls. This program is promoted by experts and achieved through the active participation of people in their own *government*. In this chapter, both the nature of this idealistic conception of health and the scientific expansionism which it entails will be highlighted, and the ways in which this shared vision is approached as an imperative to be achieved, not an issue to be debated, will be questioned.

This chapter suggests that the propositions that constitute this shared vision—for example, universal social protection, the right to health, improved health, complete well-being, equality between individuals and between groups of people, scientific knowledge, informed public opinion, active public participation—are precisely at the core of what it means to be governed today. These propositions are in fact mechanisms by which individuals and populations can be known, administered and managed. This is not just a matter of ideas or ideals. It is a way of thinking about the world and those who inhabit it that generates ways of acting. Both ideas and the actions they generate are deeply ingrained in scientific reasoning. Hence, statistical analyses and taxonomical classifications are scientific practices which have a direct impact on people (Hacking, 2003, p. 210 ; Hacking, 2007, p. 286). This way of counting, classifying and ordering belongs to the *form of scientific rationality* within which a whole range of projects operate. Because of their scientific overtone, these projects are generally presented as progress or development, especially when compared to other worldviews. One such global project which aims is to reorganize reproduction practices is used here as an illustration.

190

This example is drawn from *The Lancet*'s project on stillbirths (2011-2030). In keeping with its Constitution, the WHO claims its legitimacy from progress in the medical sciences. *The Lancet*, is a British journal, reputed for its influence in the field of biomedical research and practices. Its influence can be seen in the fact that the WHO's *Every Newborn Action Plan* (ENAP) (with UNICEF) came out of *The Lancet*'s series *Every Newborn* (2014), itself the continuation of earlier series entitled *Neonatal Survival* (2005) and *Stillbirths* (2011). These were followed by the series *Ending preventable stillbirths* (2016), which came out after the action plan. To understand how the political and the scientific discourses and practices are intermingled, the propositions contained in the project on stillbirths will be analyzed, including the underlying vision, the aims, and the action plan developed for its implementation[2].

"What world do we want for every mother and every newborn baby?" is the question asked by *The Lancet* in a short editorial for the 2014 series *Every newborn* (Samarasekera and Horton, 2014, p. 108). Their answer is as follows: "We want one [a world] in which they [every mother and every newborn baby] are given the best chance to not only survive but also thrive" (Samarasekera and Horton, 2014, p. 108). And they add: "The requirements for such a world are laid out in this Series and accompanying action plan" (Samarasekera and Horton, 2014, p. 108). As it turns out, the related action plan is also the WHO's action plan for 2014. It has two goals: 1) ending preventable newborn deaths, and 2) ending preventable stillbirths (OMS, 2014, p. 7). These goals are part of the "unfinished agenda" of the Millennium Development Goals for women's and children's health. They are also part of a post-2015 vision for global health. The WHO defines this vision as "A world in which there are no preventable deaths of newborns or stillbirths, where every pregnancy is wanted, every birth celebrated, and women, babies and children survive, thrive and reach their full potential" (OMS, 2014, p. 7). These goals are part of *The Global Strategy for Women's, Children's and Adolescents' Health (2016-2030)* of the United Nations Secretary-General (UN 2015) and part of the mission of the United Nations Population Fund (UNFPA): "Delivering a world where every pregnancy is wanted, every childbirth is safe and every young person's potential is fulfilled" (UNFPA, 2017). Here is a moral position which gives legitimacy to political goals which *The Lancet* announces will be achieved by 2030, and the WHO, by 2035 (with intermediary targets set for 2020, 2025 and 2030). The idea is summarized under the banner: "a world converging within a generation" (Jamison et al., 2013, p. 194 ; Mason et al., 2014, p. 465 ; OMS, 2014, p. 7).

In 2011, in an effort to make their vision a reality, the *promoters* of *The Lancet* (with the support of all the authors associated with the series on stillbirths) sent out a call to action (Lawn et al., 2011, p. 7). To support their mission, they sought to mobilize the global public health community, individual countries, local communities and families. They recommended a series of ten actions to prevent stillbirths in an effort to remove obstacles to their science-based vision (Bhutta et al., 2011, p. 1527). Meanwhile, the WHO pursued its action plan which "calls upon all stakeholders to take specific actions to improve access to, and quality of, healthcare for women and newborns within the continuum of care" (WHO, 2014, Key messages). It is the notion of "continuum of care" which should retain our attention here, as it supposes the capacity to ensure equitable access to healthcare and medical treatment for every woman and newborn, with the explicit goal of protecting, or even saving them. The promoters posit that the healthcare process, called the continuum of care, opens the way for the control of reproduction from the beginning (prenatal care) to the end (postnatal care) (Horton and Samarasekera, 2016, p. 515). What is at the origin a scientific endeavor based on medical interventions (with the legitimacy provided by scientific rationality), becomes a political project when expanding its field of application to virtually all women and all newborns around the globe. This shift from science to politics is well illustrated by the hidden face of medical intervention, and more broadly, by its aspiration to save and improve human lives.

ISSUES AND PROPOSALS

Access to Healthcare Hides Access to Data for Scientific Development

In the public health literature, ethical considerations are often limited to the issue of equitable access to healthcare. The point being made here is that focusing on access to care masks the issue of access to data needed for scientific development. This is the case, for instance, with population monitoring, which is a set of interventions that seem to offer obvious benefits in addressing what is defined as a problem, particularly a public health problem. Monitoring relies on examination procedures and these procedures feed into databases. Such procedures result in the identification of various groups identified according to their potential risk, in this case, the risk of having problems during pregnancy. Once these groups are identified and monitored, they can be managed. Management then entails another series of procedures to reach targeted objectives. These *monitoring mechanisms* have an unpredicted effect in so far as they contribute to normalizing people. As such, they correspond to what Ian Hacking (2007) identifies as an engine of organization and control, which are the result of engines of discovery (counting, quantifying, creating norms and the associated *quantifying mechanisms* and *prevention mechanisms*). This engine of organization is a direct component of scientific knowledge (Hacking, 2007, pp. 306, 310–311). Knowledge can be called scientific to the extent that standards (for example around stillbirths and perinatal bereavement) are based on results that have been produced with the intention of aiming for truth. In other words, *intervention mechanisms* simultaneously make it possible to collect data in a scientific way and to manage certain types of people. The politics is located in the will to manage people, to shape them in a way that their action can be influenced and guided. This is how people can be governed. In other words, putting a system in place that saves human lives, in every country around the globe, is predicated on the form of scientific rationality (in that it calls for counting, quantifying, and normalizing so as to identify groups at risk), and directly influencing people's conduct so as to guide them towards political goals (a healthy and prosperous population).

This shift in attention from medical interventions to that which makes them possible, highlights the scientific rationality that produces "truth" about the world and those inhabiting it. This attention to scientific rationality, in turn, is useful in better understanding the complexity of what is hidden behind the *benevolence* generally associated with access to healthcare. Surprisingly, perhaps, the aim of the project is not just about saving women and newborns and preventing stillbirths, but "saving and counting" (Lawn et al., 2011, p. 5). Medical intervention and health prevention require this quantifying of the events of human life, beginning, in this case, with the numbers of stillbirths. The promoters of *The Lancet* are aware of this, and in their priority research themes they include data for action and follow-up (i.e. monitoring): "Count stillbirths, including through household surveys, sentinel surveillance systems, and strengthening of routine vital registration" (Lawn et al., 2011, p. 6). Moving from research to public policy, WHO's Action Plan strategy number 5 aims to "Count every newborn through measurement, programme-tracking and accountability" (OMS, 2014, p. 20). In addition to counting the living and the dead, health promoters also seek "Improved data [...] to enable tracking of the content and quality of antenatal and intrapartum care" (Samarasekera et al., 2016, p. 4). Indeed strategic objective number 2 is to "Improve the quality of maternal and newborn care" (OMS, 2014, p. 20). Thus, taking action to save women and newborns is a dual process involving both prevention and measurement.

The benevolence of saving lives therefore has two sides: a humanist side and a neoliberal one. On the one hand, is the conviction that man's vocation is to fight the natural order by protecting the weak and caring for the sick; and on the other is the evidence that medical morality is a benevolent morality, in the technical sense of calculating risks and benefits (Fagot-Largeault, 2010, pp. 3-4). This two-sided benevolence requires monitoring mechanisms, both as a system that saves lives and as an underlying system for ongoing measurement. It is through these connections that the reasons behind examination procedures are revealed.

Examination procedures are mechanisms for monitoring population health that aim to create knowledge —according to Michel Foucault's (1975) analyses—that is, to make visible and build a certain type of scientific object (Foucault, 1975, pp. 219-224). The stated goal of examination procedures—that is protecting the health of women and children—has a somewhat hidden motive: to build data collections. According to Foucault's analyses, it is examination procedures that have allowed for the epistemological unlocking of medicine (Foucault, 1975, pp. 217-219). Hacking (1990) specifies that "pathology became the study of unhealthy organs rather than sick people [thus the study of the object of science, not of political subjects]. One could investigate them in part by the chemistry of the secretions of living beings – urine, for example" (Hacking, 1990, p. 164). Data collection therefore involves measuring organisms: the body, its organs and its substances, such as urine, blood and mucus membranes. But data collections are not limited to case examinations, nor to data on individual organs. Data collections aim to get at the population level (the species, the population and its processes of fertility, birth, illness and death). They provide the material for research and statistics, demographic and epidemiological analyses. But, as has been shown, here is the space for an invisible shift; one from examination procedures and monitoring mechanisms intended to produce knowledge, document individual cases and build population databases, to mechanisms of power; that is, the use of knowledge to act on choices and claims. In this case, some of the effects of power are to normalize people and regulate the population (Foucault, 1975, pp. 217-227 ; Foucault, 1976, pp. 177-198). This is how the use of scientific rationality can lead, for instance, to a woman who not only accepts but requests medical interventions (blood tests, urine tests, ultrasounds, etc.) throughout her pregnancy. She wishes to be monitored and seeks medical interventions during childbirth because she believes that this is the only way to give birth to a healthy baby.

This analytical shift provides some perspective on the promotional argument of access to medical care. The promoters of *The Lancet* consider access to medical care as the ideal solution: "Most stillbirths are preventable with health system improvements: Stillbirths are preventable through high quality antenatal and intrapartum care within the continuum of care for women and children" (Samarasekera et al., 2016, p. 2 –Headline messages). However, this type of universal access is not a result of science; it calls for public policies as tools to plan and manage. WHO's Action Plan strategy number 3 aims to "Reach every woman and newborn to reduce inequities.

Having access to high-quality healthcare without suffering financial hardship is a human right" (OMS, 2014, p. 20). Thus, public policy is the vehicle that is used to influence behavior. Yet influencing behavior is not a scientific project, it is a political project which calls for deliberation. The right to health and equitable access to high-quality care say nothing about that. In fact, they imply obligations, or rather appropriate behaviors, which are rarely made explicit. The implicit pact of the right to health is as follows: provide your urine, your blood, your tissue samples, let us see though your body and soul, let us record and organize your life events (for example your reproductive life: conception, pregnancy, childbirth, death) and in return your health will be guaranteed. Reproductive health (for example, a desired pregnancy), obstetrical health (such as a safe birth) and population health (for example, reduced rates of mortality and stillbirths). This right to health, which appears "natural," is not. Yet neither is it a coercive mechanism, for nobody is forced to receive medical care. Instead it is an incentive by which one is encouraged to give. The rationale behind this incentive is to improve oneself, in both the humanist and the neoliberal senses. In the humanist perspective to improve oneself is to be a better person, a better mother, one who cares for her child to be. In the neoliberal perspective to improve oneself is to make sure that what has been received is increased, that a healthy child will contribute to the figure of a good mother. In other words, to improve oneself is to be counted so that we count for others. This is what the promoters of *The Lancet* call "a right to be counted, survive, and thrive wherever they are born" (Mason et al., 2014, p. 455). As the final sentence of *The Will to Knowledge* reminds us, the irony of this device is that it makes us believe that our freedom depends on it (Foucault, 1976, p. 211).

Clearly, the hidden face of access to care is access to data. A health system that aims to ensure access to medical care is also a health system that needs to ensure access to data. In this sense, the benevolence that claims to give every woman and newborn access to medical services has to create conditions for the examination process, since it is through examination that data can be collected. Every woman and newborn becomes an object for knowledge and simultaneously an object of power (Foucault, 1975, p. 224). Moreover, although access to medical care is part of the healthcare continuum, what is really at stake is ongoing access to data. This is what makes ongoing monitoring possible, without any objection from those directly concerned, because they see it as a way to improve their health capital. So, access to care is a strategic incentive to gain access to data. And access to data in a system based on scientific evidence has to be funded, since such procedures have a cost. Funding, however, is not an ethical issue, but a highly political one, because medical research entails access to technology.

It is important to understand that management procedures—that is, population health monitoring mechanisms—are adapted to fit examination procedures which increasingly involve technology, as do their recording devices (notes, audio recordings and spreadsheets). In the process of putting a system in place to save every woman and newborn not only are all cases to be counted, but they are recorded in a comparative system which implies means to compare.

Here it becomes clearer that the hidden side of access to medical care is much more than access to data per se. It is the integration of individual data into cumulative systems and calculations (Foucault, 1975, p. 223). It is by creating a comparative system that it becomes possible to measure global phenomena, to describe groups, to characterize collective realities, to estimate the gap between individuals, and to see how they are distributed in the "population" (Foucault, 1975, p. 223). And these population-level regulations are centered on the body-as-species, on the body as it is affected by the requirements of living beings and as a support for biological processes (Foucault, 1976, p. 183). Management procedures for administering high-risk groups are developed in the fourfold context of access to data, of data integration into cumulative systems, of building a comparative system and of population regulation, all of which suppose financial means and political will.

Scientific research is dependent on political and financial contexts and, in turn, uses procedures that define the type of persons targeted by interventions. Within a strictly economic logic (maximizing gain and reducing losses), the result of the pregnancy must be positive. In this logic, women's behavior has to be closely monitored so it can be modified for a wanted child to be conceived, for it to grow normally, and for it to be alive at birth. It is only in this way that a healthy child will be raised and will thrive.

Equitable Access Hides the Standardization of Conceptions of Human Life

An argument has been made that refocusing political attention away from medical intervention to what makes it possible reveals the inadequacy of centering ethical considerations solely on universal access to healthcare, as a right within an equity perspective. To do justice to the complexity of the issue, ethical questions cannot be confined to whether equal access has been achieved, since the issue of access to medical care, and the hidden issue of access to data, both merit inquiry. The ethical issue therefore must be shifted away from equitable access to a discussion of available options, their cost, and the consequences for a government based on science.

This second shift is important because the scientific and political project of *The Lancet* regarding global prevention of stillbirths, among other examples (suicide for instance), may be less a program to be carried out than a project to be questioned. The questioning could for instance bear on the kind of people produced by such policies and the type of government it promotes. Seeking to eradicate stillbirths, as if it were a scientific imperative, is in fact a project that implies a certain way of governing people. Regardless of how it is presented, there is plainly a political dimension.

A while ago now, in his 1986 book entitled *Risk Society*, Ulrich Beck (2003) summarized the impact of medicine acting in the name of health. When speaking for itself, biomedicine says it is in the service of health. But in fact, it has created entirely new situations and has changed the relationship of man with himself, with illness, with suffering and death, it has changed the world (Beck, 2003, pp. 435-436). The promoters of *The Lancet* embrace the usual definition of medicine as serving health, but they also embrace the project of changing the world: "*The Lancet* [...] retains at its core the belief that medicine must serve society, that knowledge must transform society, that the best science must lead to better lives" (The Lancet, 2016).

When the project of *The Lancet* is considered from the perspective of consequences, it is easier to understand its promoters' insistence that preventable stillbirths must be ended. A child who is stillborn has not survived and therefore cannot thrive. This presents a problem for a worldview in which lives must be saved and each person must accomplish his or her full potential. In this sense, a stillborn child and stillbirth are the antithesis of human reproduction and childbirth. It may seem natural to defend such an ideal against whatever threatens it, but it is actually a very specific philosophy of action, as summarized by Anne Fagot-Largeault (2010):

Medicine is inherently philosophical, as I have stated elsewhere. The philosophy inherent in the medical act can be summarized in three simple proposals: 1/ there is evil in the world; 2/ there is a remedy for it; 3/ we must use the remedy; even if the efforts to address the problem are in the end negligible, they must be pursued, "for honor's sake." The first assertion contains a host of metaphysical implications, the second implies an epistemology and methodology of sciences and techniques, and the third involves morality. (Fagot-Largeault, 2010, p. 2, our translation)

In the case at hand, this philosophy inherent in the medical act implies that stillbirth is an evil in the world, which is preventable[3] and must be solved. Given these philosophical claims, medicine must have scientific and technical means of prevention and intervention to solve preventable stillbirth, both being justified by a morality of benevolence. In an effort to normalize this ideal, the promoters of *The Lancet* and the WHO propose incentives, and point out what should be done and what should not.

As Jonathan Glover (2017) has argued, the death of fetuses and newborns is bad mainly because of how it affects those around. Both direct and indirect reasons are used to explain why stillbirth is considered unacceptable. Among the direct reasons are arguments about the sanctity of life, that birth is a blessing and death at the beginning of life is more unacceptable than at any other age. But these arguments do not hold for all circumstances. If stillbirths are considered a problem, and a public health problem at that, ideally a pregnancy should be wanted and the child to be born must be normal and healthy. The project of *The Lancet* of preventing stillbirths, taken up by the WHO, includes the promotion of contraception and the possibility of abortion. Therefore, the death of fetuses and newborns is bad less in and of itself than because of its impacts (for example on parents or on society). It would appear that life or death can be given according to circumstances. Among the effects that justify stillbirths as bad are the loss of a number of human lives for society, the loss of resources for the State, the psychosocial burden and the direct and indirect economic costs. This is how health promoters come to view grief—a psychosocial burden believed to accompany stillbirth—as something to be prevented and to be acted upon. *The Lancet*'s series *Every Newborn* (2014) is very enlightening: "The cost of inaction devastates families and societies, causing a substantial drain on human capital, through death, disability, poor growth, and lost potential for development and economic productivity" (Mason et al., 2014, p. 456). So not taking action, not preventing stillbirths, is seen to have a devastating effect on families and societies, conveyed in language that is *a priori* economic (depleted resources, human capital, development, economic productivity) with both qualitative (death, disability, human development, lost potential) and quantitative connotations (mortality, morbidity, poor growth). This is a contemporary version of what Catherine Rollet refers to as less suffering for families and more resources for the State (Rollet, 1998, p. 121). She explains that this political calculation is the corollary of mortality measurements: "Once mortality was measured with numbers, whether absolute or proportional, one could reason about human lives in economic terms. The notion arises from the number of lives that can be saved" (Rollet, 1998, p. 121, our translation). This helps to explain why the promoters of *The Lancet* want to put an end to stillbirths and the related perinatal bereavement.

This raises many questions which are far removed from scientific queries. Is saving lives, helping grieving parents and fulfilling the potential of each person intended to avoid a quantitative depletion of resources and an alteration of the quality of the products of conception? Is ending preventable stillbirths mostly about resource planning, waste management, preventing loss (stillbirth as a pure loss)? Is it about minimizing the effects of a system for regulating and channeling reproductive life (the direct and indirect costs of stillbirths)? Is benevolence but a thin varnish covering economic and political calculations?

While it may seem counterintuitive, there are many secondary benefits to stillbirths. This recalls the ironic formula found in a short text by Karl Marx [circa 1861-1863] (1970) on the secondary benefits of crime. The project on stillbirths developed by *The Lancet* and its continuation by the WHO (2014, with UNICEF), the UN Secretary General (2015) and UNFPA (2017) contribute to scientific research, university courses, academic publications, expertise, national and international public policies, employment for doctors, nurses, midwives, statisticians, archivists and more. These activities help to develop new health infrastructure, awareness campaigns, television series, on-line stories and best-sellers; they mobilize community organizations, citizen activism, solidarity marches, and more. These secondary benefits require funding for research, prevention and medical interventions, which involves participation by many partners as well as a public and private insurance system. Many bridges are built between government by science and finance, employment training, infrastructure, business, law and more, each of which is in a position to export and implement the project of preventing and ending stillbirths around the world. This is how stillbirths are useful to society. The reality of this paradox is that these actions in no way put an end to the fragility of life, that stillbirths cannot be ended today or in the future, and that this project has an unlimited duration, not only because life cannot be totally controlled, but because so many secondary beneficiaries thrive on it.

In the project initiated by *The Lancet*, those whose behavior must be modified, those whose antithetical behaviors and conceptions must be discredited to justify the implementation of "modern" practices, see themselves associated with "fatalism" or "beliefs" (Lawn et al., 2011, p. 2 ; Samarasekera et al., 2016, p. 6). The promoters assert that "fatalism impedes progress in stillbirth prevention" (Samarasekera et al., 2016, p. 5). In fact it impedes the normalization of the category "preventable stillbirth" and is in direct opposition to the wish "to eliminate all preventable stillbirths and close equity gaps" (Lawn et al., 2011, p. 7). It is also in conflict with the *ideal* taken up and promoted by the WHO. This explains why one of the priority research themes of *The Lancet*'s global research program on stillbirths and its implementation in low and medium income countries is to "Assess effective and sustainable mobilization of communities at scale for behavior change and care seeking" (Lawn et al., 2011, p. 6). This aligns with strategic objective number 4 of the WHO's Action Plan that states the need to "Harness the power of parents, families and communities" (OMS, 2014, p. 20). In well-meaning language, the aim is to export and put in place a doctrine. To try to structure how people think and act by producing the conditions for prevention and medical intervention.

This is how equitable access to medical care for preventing stillbirths or equal access to health services for bereaved parents hides a much deeper project; that of standardizing conceptions of human life. Stillbirth has to be created as something, as an object, so it can be eliminated, solved, ended, and so that a world can be made in which all women, around the world, can have access to prenatal care, a safe birth and a healthy baby. As Hannah Arendt (1972) said, every time you hear people talking about the grand goals of politics, such as building a new society where justice will reign, or waging a war to end all wars, or spreading democracy around the world, a specific way of thinking is at play (Arendt, 1972, p. 106). Arendt (1972) calls this an old attempt to avoid the disappointments and fragility of human action by doing something that has a beginning and an end, whose laws of motion can be determined and whose innermost content can be revealed (Arendt, 1972, pp. 106-107, our translation). Hacking (1990) talks about the "taming of chance". This sort of project suggests that it is possible to master all forms of life and thus to elude their fragility.

Once fully implemented, *The Lancet*'s supranational governmental project will determine the space of possible human experience. It will shrink it to the point that only what can be controlled remains. For an unlimited period of time, throughout the world, and in the most private areas of people's lives, it will impose a standard conception of human life. But one can ask, are uncertainties not part of life itself, of suffering and death? Is a life without risk and suffering not a diminished life? Are stillborn babies (like those who commit suicide) really pure losses for humanity and for those who experience or are connected to them? Or are they in fact losses for the State and experts?

SOLUTIONS AND RECOMMENDATIONS

Access to medical care is presented in health promotion discourses as the solution to all problems. The promoters of *The Lancet* consider that the ten interventions recommended for reducing stillbirths[4] are based on "sufficient evidence to recommend for implementation in health systems" (Lawn et al., 2011, p. 4). Yet this is not as clear as it might seem. In fact, the authors of the article that lies behind this assertion have a more nuanced view. There is a considerable distance between the affirmative stance of the promoters who consider that there is enough evidence to implement the interventions, and the many precautions presented by the authors (Bhutta et al., 2011, pp. 1533-1534). The latter highlight a lack of information, the need to do more targeted research to fill gaps, the urgency of developing data collection instruments, and the limitations of the studies being conducted, which make it difficult to formulate a definite opinion on the true effectiveness of the proposed interventions. The leap from a lack of information to "sufficient evidence" is an impressive one. Population health monitoring mechanisms may be first and foremost means for addressing and redressing a lack of information: "A major recommendation of this report, and of preceding reviews, is for stillbirth measurements to be included in all existing surveillance sites with pregnancy detection and outcome tracking" (Bhutta et al., 2011, pp. 1533-1534). The issue is critical because that report was the source identifying the conditions for the scientific legitimacy of medical and preventive interventions.

One example of medical interventions aimed at preventing stillbirths is the normalization of professional assistance during childbirth and of caesarean sections, particularly in countries where it is not already the case, and where the rates of stillbirths are highest: "These are the areas of the world [South Asia and sub-Saharan Africa] where, if the median proportion of births attended by a skilled delivery assistant were 100% rather than 50%, or if the median caesarean section rate was 20% instead of 3%, most of these tragedies would not have happened" (Mullan and Horton, 2011, p. 1291). The normalization of skilled delivery assistance (most often in a hospital setting) and the normalization of caesareans are not just solutions; they are new problems. Ironically, the fight to end stillbirths leads to new problems to be managed. As Hans Blumenberg put it "the progress of knowledge doesn't unburden the future from problems but rather increases them as the legacy of the present and its supposed 'successes' for the future" (Blumenberg, 2010, p. 151).

Furthermore, when a pregnancy ends in stillbirth, other problems arise. Autopsy provides a good example here. One of the advocated interventions in *The Lancet* program is access to autopsy, considered helpful in the grieving process because "Every parent whose baby has died wants to know why it happened" (Lawn et al., 2011, p. 6). In other words, "failure to offer autopsy denies parents a chance to understand the cause of their baby's death" (Flenady et al., 2016, p. 693). To be clear, autopsies are examination procedures that seek to establish cause of death and, as such, trigger population health monitoring mechanisms. This access to data becomes a means for establishing statistics (for example, rates of stillbirth by cause of death), forming high-risk groups (such as poor women with gestational hypertension), and assessing population-level progress (for example, in reducing rates of stillbirth) for statistical and demographic regulation or as an indicator of the quality of healthcare. But for parents an autopsy will, at most, identify a cause of death and tell them how their baby died. However, consenting to an autopsy in no way guarantees that they will find out "how did my baby die?" because "the proportion of unexplained stillbirths is high" (Flenady et al., 2016, p. 691). How high? In 2016 *The Lancet* answered: "The categories other unspecified (up to 46%) and unexplained (up to 76%) showed the widest variation and highest proportions" (Flenady et al., 2016, p. 693). How then can the promoters of *The Lancet* claim to end preventable stillbirths, particularly in high-income countries when up to three quarters of them are unexplained? Preventing what cannot be determined seems a very strange project indeed. What is more, the proportion of unexplained stillbirths appears to be increasing (up to 60% in 2007 according to Smith and Fretts (2007, p. 1716) and 76% in 2016, see above), not decreasing[5]. The idea that access to an autopsy can help in bereavement when a high proportion of parents will not get answers to their questions, either before or after the autopsy, is baffling.

These are but a few examples (for others, see Beaudoin, 2018) which demonstrate that the medical interventions that are recommended as solutions are often based on sparse and unreliable data, the result of non-existent data collection systems, different equivalence conventions and ambiguous definitions. The point here is not to resolve these difficulties, but to understand how women and newborns are nonetheless governed by the underlying form of scientific rationality. Our analysis (Beaudoin, 2018) has identified the discursive strategies and argumentative techniques used by the promoters of *The Lancet* (for example Lawn et al., 2011, and Samarasekera et al., 2016) who skirt these issues, exaggerate or downplay the numbers and, in doing so, encourage a shift from description (there are 2.6 million stillbirths per year around the world) to prescription (we must end preventable stillbirths around the world by 2030), a target by no means obvious.

The main questions then are: should scientific rationality be subject to certain limits? Should certain fields of life be protected from its grasp? With such questions, public interest and politics are reconnected in examining the place of science and what can and must lie outside its control.

FUTURE RESEARCH DIRECTIONS

Having shown how access to healthcare and the perspective of equitable access implies a range of structuring consequences, and having raised the ethical issue of the limits of science and scientific rationality (its extension into all spheres of human life and private life as well as its extension around the globe), the production of knowledge can be examined from a different angle. Rather than the unlimited production of data on human bodies and lives, an ethic of restraint is suggested.

First, one can ask whether it is true progress to accumulate unlimited quantities of data and evidence, to continually develop new policies for managing an increasing number of problems, to put in place an unending number of technical interventions that take us all in the same direction (however accessible and equitable). The argument made here is that it is not. As Michel Serres (1991) says: however wise an idea may be, it becomes horrible if it is the only one. It would be dangerous if the hard sciences were to convince us that they are the only way to think. Or the only way to live (Serres, 1991, p. 188, our translation). Blumenberg's (2010) position is convincing that "the notion that science must constantly grow, not only in the yield of its results but also in the effort of its actors, would, from the perspective of its early programmatic thinkers, not be progress but failure" (Blumenberg, 2010, p. 151). Could the unlimited production of health data and universal access to medical care, such as with *The Lancet*'s project on stillbirths, hide such a failure, the failure of progress?

Would it not be more sensible to restrain ourselves from forging ahead, to take the time to understand, to deliberate and to arrive at a shared opinion concerning what we want? It is not because we have the scientific and technical means to do something that it must be done. On the contrary, there is time to think about what we are doing and to exercise restraint. The first step, for both researchers and politicians—their public responsibility so to speak—may be less to produce evidence or to encourage specific behaviors than to show restraint concerning what we need to know and why we are doing research. To paraphrase Serres (1991), science will become wise when it holds back from doing all it is capable of (Serres, 1991, p. 188).

The use of scientific data raises the issue of criticism in research, since researchers are expected to operate within limits imposed by scientific imperatives. Hence, the usual approach to critiquing policy, for example, addresses only the question of who produces what and who is targeted. Such critique can improve a policy, stimulate reflection on categories, and possibly review equivalences. This type of critique through producing new data does not, however, examine the operations that lie behind these questions and how they are formatted.

In this chapter, the scientific and political rationality of *The Lancet*'s project on stillbirth have been investigated. Rather than produce new data on childbirth, the analysis has instead focused on the articulation of arguments and the rhetoric of advocates. Three research programs could be developed as follow-up and are given below as examples.

The first is an extension of the research and analyses already underway (Beaudoin, 2018). It would involve studying the project of *The Lancet* on stillbirths until 2030, both nationally and internationally. Internationally, *The Lancet* and WHO publications (and those of other UN agencies) could be followed to document the dynamic that has been identified, specifically the "intended biopolitics" (targets set for reducing rates of stillbirth for 2020, 2025, 2030) and the "subversive biopolitics" (the lifespan and the spread of the category stillbirth and the indicator of stillbirth)[6]. At the national level, the mechanism could be studied at different steps, from scientific research to global policies and then to national policies. The connections between studies and the project on stillbirths published in *The Lancet* (since 2011), the global policies of the WHO (since 2014) and the UN (since 2015) and the implementation, or not, of the recommendations could be analyzed, for example in the Quebec government's upcoming perinatal policy, scheduled to come out after 2018.

The second research program would be to broaden the range of examples. This would expand the reflection beyond the notion of preventable stillbirth to encompass avoidable mortality in a wider variety of cases. There are many potential examples, one particularly interesting case being suicide as a preventable premature death. Not only are both stillbirth and suicides considered preventable, but their effects on their close kin, however different, are understood to involve a shock that makes grieving imperative, more than for other types of deaths.

A third research program is related to the connections between a government based on science and the crucial issue of funding. This would involve another analytical shift so as to confront the problem of how science produces government. Clearly, the promoters of *The Lancet* want to create the space for action, present and future. However, they are dependent on funding mechanisms. Systematic analyses could therefore be conducted on the connection between funding mechanisms and medical intervention, health prevention, and quantification of life events. One possibility would be to explore the potential links between research and medical publications, global health policies, increased demand for evidence, the *Bill & Melinda Gates Foundation*, digitization (and electrification) around the world, and the production of wealth. This would help to reveal the implications of the type of scientific project at work, and to which Michel Foucault was referring when he said "we need to produce truth in order to produce wealth" (Foucault, 1997, p. 22, our translation).

CONCLUSION

This chapter has examined the hidden face of medical intervention. The journey has taken readers on "the road less travelled" to look from afar at three sides of the same mountain, to speak like Martin Heidegger (1958, pp. 5-6). First is the idea that access to medical care cannot be considered in itself but must be linked to better access to data needed for scientific development (and for results-based funding). Second is the idea that equitable access to medical care simultaneously results in standardized ways of thinking about human life and normalized ways of addressing its fragility, for all people around the world. Third is the idea that an unlimited production of health data may be less a sign of progress than an expression of failure, since the multiplication of information to be managed, of problems to be prevented and resolved, of interventions to provide, lead to infinite management and standardization. The central issue is to identify the limits one would wish for scientific rationality and the strength of its grasp on human life. Some brief concluding remarks will help to identify some options that arise out of these proposals for a shared vision that has developed since the end of World War II.

First, social protection would involve limiting the space given to science, to remove certain areas of life from its control, to deny the medical and psychological sciences any special role (granted by the WHO in 1946) in defining what human life is, or should be, or in defining evil, disease, health or well-being.

Second, social protection would ensure restraint in taking action when science and technology spontaneously try to expand; it will refrain from exporting premade models and solutions throughout the world; and it would circumscribe and limit medical interventions to a narrower sphere.

Third, revisiting social protection would guarantee a space for public discussion and debate, a space for public mediation on issues of life and death, a political sphere where building shared norms would not rely solely on the medical sciences or a definitive medical morality, but would be the result of an ethical consensus (Foucault, 2001b, p. 1199).

Finally, the arguments made here, of course, are against neither science nor medicine, but against their intrusion into all spheres of human life (even the most private) and their unchallenged expansion across the globe. This is what was questioned with *The Lancet*'s project on stillbirths, and its promotion by the WHO.

May these proposals be the subject of lively debate.

ACKNOWLEDGMENT

The author wish to thank Marie-Andrée Couillard for her attentive reading and judicious comments, as well as Mary Richardson for her translation from French to English. The author also wish to thank the editor, Cristina Albuquerque, and the anonymous reviewers for their constructive criticism and helpful suggestions.

REFERENCES

Arendt, H. (1972). *La crise de la culture. Huit exercices de pensée politique.* Paris, France: Gallimard.

Beaudoin, S. (2018). *Être gouverné. Entre science et politique* (Unpublished doctoral dissertation). Université Laval, Québec, Canada.

Beck, U. (2003). *La société du risque. Sur la voie d'une autre modernité.* Paris, France: Flammarion.

Bhutta, Z. A., Yakoob, M. Y., Lawn, J. E., Rizvi, A., Friberg, I. K., Weissman, E., ... Goldenberg, R. L. (2011). Stillbirths: What difference can we make and at what cost? *Lancet, 377*(9776), 1523–1538. doi:10.1016/S0140-6736(10)62269-6 PMID:21496906

Blumenberg, H. (2010). Care Crosses the River. Stanford, CA: Stanford University Press.

Fagot-Largeault, A. (2010). *Médecine et philosophie.* Paris, France: Presses Universitaires de France. doi:10.3917/puf.fagot.2010.01

Flenady, V., Wojcieszek, A. M., Middleton, P., Ellwood, D., Erwich, J. J., Coory, M., ... Goldenberg, R. L. (2016). Stillbirths: Recall to action in high-income countries. *Lancet, 387*(10019), 681–702. doi:10.1016/S0140-6736(15)01020-X PMID:26794070

Foucault, M. (1975). *Surveiller et punir. Naissance de la prison.* Paris, France: Gallimard.

Foucault, M. (1976). *La volonté de savoir. Histoire de la sexualité 1.* Paris, France: Gallimard.

Foucault, M. (1997). Il faut défendre la société. Cours au Collège de France (1975-1976). Paris: Gallimard.

Foucault, M. (2001a). Crise de la médecine ou crise de l'antimédecine. In M. Foucault (Ed.), *Dits et écrits II. 1976-1988* (pp. 40–58). Paris, France: Gallimard.

Foucault, M. (2001b). Un système fini face à une demande infinie. In M. Foucault (Ed.), *Dits et écrits II. 1976-1988* (pp. 1186–1202). Paris, France: Gallimard.

Glover, J. (2017). Questions de vie ou de mort. Genève: Labor et Fides.

Hacking, I. (1982). Biopower and the avalanche of printed numbers. *Humanity & Society*, 5(3-4), 279–295.

Hacking, I. (1990). *The Taming of Chance*. Cambridge, UK: Cambridge University Press. doi:10.1017/CBO9780511819766

Hacking, I. (2003). "Vrai", les valeurs et les sciences. In J.-P. Changeux (Ed.), *La vérité dans les sciences* (pp. 201–214). Paris, France: Odile Jacob.

Hacking, I. (2007). Kinds of People: Moving Targets. *Proceedings of the British Academy*, 151, 285–318.

Heidegger, M. (1958). Essais et conférences. Paris, France: Gallimard.

Jamison, D. T., Summers, L. H., Alleyne, G., Arrow, K. J., Berkley, S., Binagwaho, A., ... Yamey, G. (2013). Global health 2035: A world converging within a generation. *Lancet*, 382(9908), 1898–1955. doi:10.1016/S0140-6736(13)62105-4 PMID:24309475

Lawn, J. (2011). *Stillbirths – An Executive Summary for The Lancet's Series*. Retrieved from https://www.thelancet.com/series/stillbirth

Marx, K. (1970). Bénéfices secondaires du crime (Translated from the German, circa 1861-1863). In D. Szabo (Ed.), *Déviance et criminalité* (pp. 83–85). Paris, France: Armand Colin.

Mason, E., McDougall, L., Lawn, J. E., Gupta, A., Claeson, M., Pillay, Y., ... Chopra, M. (2014). From evidence to action to deliver a healthy start for the next generation. *Lancet*, 384(9941), 455–467. doi:10.1016/S0140-6736(14)60750-9 PMID:24853599

Mullan, Z., & Horton, R. (2011). Bringing stillbirths out of the shadows. *Lancet*, 377(9774), 1291–1292. doi:10.1016/S0140-6736(11)60098-6 PMID:21496920

Rollet, C. (1998). Lorsque la mort devint mortalité. In C. Le Grand-Sébille, M. F. Morel, & F. Zonabend (Eds.), *Le fœtus, le nourrisson et la mort* (pp. 105–126). Paris, France: L'Harmattan.

Rose, N. (2006). *The Politics of Life Itself: Biomedicine, Power, and Subjectivity in the Twenty-First Century*. Princeton, NJ: Princeton University Press.

Rose, N. (2007). Beyond medicalization. *Lancet*, 369(9562), 700–702. doi:10.1016/ S0140-6736(07)60319-5 PMID:17321317

Samarasekera, U. (2016). *Ending preventable stillbirths – An Executive Summary for The Lancet's Series*. Retrieved from https://www.thelancet.com/series/ending-preventable-stillbirths

Samarasekera, U., & Horton, R. (2014). The world we want for every newborn child. *Lancet, 384*(9938), 107–109. doi:10.1016/S0140-6736(14)60837-0 PMID:24853598

Senellart, M. (2004). Situation des cours. In M. Foucault (Ed.), Sécurité, territoire, population. Cours au Collège de France (1977-1978) (pp. 379-411). Paris: Gallimard.

Serres, M. (1991). *Le Tiers-Instruit*. Paris, France: Gallimard.

Smith, G. C. S., & Fretts, R. C. (2007). Stillbirth. *Lancet, 370*(9600), 1715–1725. doi:10.1016/S0140-6736(07)61723-1 PMID:18022035

The Lancet. (2016). *The best science for better lives*. Retrieved from https://www. thelancet.com/about-us

United Nations Population Fund. (2017). *Delivering a world where every pregnancy is wanted, every childbirth is safe and every young person's potential is fulfilled*. Retrieved from https://www.unfpa.org/about-us

United Nations Secretary-General. (2015). *The Global Strategy for Women's, Children's and Adolescents' Health (2016-2030)*. New York: United Nations.

World Health Organization. (1948). *Constitution of the World Health Organization*. Geneva: World Health Organization.

World Health Organization. (2014). Every newborn. An Action Plan To End Preventable Deaths. Geneva: World Health Organization; United Nations International Children's Fund; Committing to Child Survival.

ADDITIONAL READING

Desrosières, A. (2014). *Prouver et gouverner. Une analyse politique des statistiques publiques*. Paris, France: La Découverte.

Feher, M. (2007). S'apprécier, ou les aspirations du capital humain. *Raisons politiques*, 28, 11-31. (Translation: Feher, M. (2009). Self-Appreciation; or, The Aspirations of Human Capital. *Public Culture, 21*(1), 21–41. doi:10.1215/08992363-2008-019

Memmi, D. (2011). *La seconde vie des bébés morts*. Paris, France: Éditions de l'École des Hautes Études en Sciences Sociales. doi:10.4000/books.editionsehess.1794

Ong, A., & Collier, S. J. (Eds.). (2008). *Global Assemblages: Technology, Politics, and Ethics as Anthropological Problems*. Malden, MA: Wiley-Blackwell.

Rottenburg, R., & Merry, S. E. (2015). A world of indicators: the making of governmental knowledge through quantification. In R. Rottenburg, S. E. Merry, S. J. Park, & J. Mugler (Eds.), *The World of Indicators. The Making of Governmental Knowledge through Quantification* (pp. 1–33). Cambridge: Cambridge University Press. doi:10.1017/CBO9781316091265.001

Skorucak, T. (2015). *Le courage des gouvernés: une éthique de la vérité et de la désobéissance – à partir de Michel Foucault et Hannah Arendt* (Unpublished doctoral dissertation). Université Paris-Est, France.

Sokhi-Bulley, B. (2011). Governing (Through) Rights: Statistics as Technologies of Governmentality. *Social & Legal Studies*, 20(2), 139–155. doi:10.1177/0964663910391520

St-Amant, S. (2015). Naît-on encore? Réflexions sur la production médicale de l'accouchement. *Recherches familiales*, 12(1), 9-25.

Wahlberg, A., & Rose, N. (2015). The governmentalization of living: Calculating global health. *Economy and Society*, 44(1), 60–90. doi:10.1080/03085147.2014.983830

Woods, R. (2009). *Death before Birth. Fetal Health & Mortality in Historical Perspective*. Oxford: Oxford University Press. doi:10.1093/acprof:oso/9780199542758.001.0001

KEY TERMS AND DEFINITIONS

Benevolence: A way of thinking and acting that involves not only caring for, protecting, and fighting to save and improve lives through access to medical care, but also counting life events, population monitoring, and risk-benefit calculations using data needed for scientific development.

Form of Scientific Rationality: Forms of reasoning and operations that underpin scientific practice, and which come to be viewed as natural and self-evident. For example, the forms of reasoning in statistical analyses ad taxonomical classification as well as defining, counting, agreeing on equivalences, and creating standards for measuring.

Government: A way to manage people, to shape them so that their thoughts and actions, present, and future can be influenced and guided, including the conduct of oneself.

Government Based on Science: A type of government in which power is exerted through science.

Intervention Mechanisms: Target mechanisms that identify what must be aimed for and what must be avoided through techniques that direct people's choices towards standards based on scientific evidence.

Monitoring Mechanisms: Mechanisms that enable researchers to access data, which in turn triggers examination and management procedures, as well as techniques for encouraging and discouraging certain types of conduct.

Prevention Mechanisms: Mechanisms intended to have an upstream effect on what must be stopped or adjusted by creating standards.

Promoters: Experts who use discursive strategies and argumentative techniques in order to trigger mechanisms for government based on science, thus perpetuating the form of rationality.

Quantifying Mechanisms: Mechanisms aimed to establish what exists in the form of numbers; to count, calculate and measure by constituting people (or things) as research objects and based on equivalence conventions.

ENDNOTES

[1]   Terms in italics are defined at the end of the chapter.

[2]   Based on second hand data, from two main sources: first, the three *The Lancet*'s series on the project of stillbirth (*Stillbirths* (2011), *Every Newborn* (2014), *Ending preventable stillbirths* (2016)); second, WHO documentations, mainly the WHO Constitution (1948) and the WHO Every newborn Action Plan (2014). The material was treated following content analysis in order to make replicable and valid inferences by interpreting and coding the data. See Beaudoin (2018: 55-68) for further details on the research and analysis methodology on which this chapter is based.

[3]   At least partially, after the 28th week of gestation.

[4]   The ten recommendations for ending stillbirths are: "1.Periconceptional folic acid fortification; 2.Prevention of malaria with insecticide-treated bednets or intermittent preventive treatment with antimalarials; 3.Syphilis detection and treatment; 4.Detection and management of hypertensive disease of pregnancy; 5.Detection and management of diabetes of pregnancy; 6.Detection and management of fetal growth restriction (including caesarean section or induction, if needed); 7.Identification and induction of mothers with 41 weeks of gestation or more; 8.Skilled care at birth and immediate care for neonates; 9.Basic emergency obstetric care; 10.Comprehensive emergency obstetric care" (Bhutta *et al.* 2011: 1527, panel 2).

5   Blumenberg, taking the long view, sees nothing surprising in this: "At the time of Descartes and long thereafter there were – for clear reason, certainly – no 'unexplained' cases, no diagnoses refuted by autopsy. In the meantime, the share of such cases grows constantly – certainly also by refining the means to verify the total stock of the attacking 'properties of disease' " (Blumenberg [1987] 2010: 151).

6   This takes up Hacking's distinction: "The intended, overt biopolitics never worked – *and that is the rule*. But the subversive biopolitics set the stage of categorization in which we still live" (Hacking 1982: 289). Foucault also said that all governmentality is necessarily strategic and programmatic. It never works. But we can only say it never works by comparing to the programme (Foucault 1979, in Senellart 2004: 405).

Chapter 9
Healing Cultural Personae With the Media Dream:
Using Jungian Compensation to Foster ICT Coherence

Stephen Brock Schafer
Pacific Rim Enterprises, USA

ABSTRACT

Issues of cultural morality and health in a mediated reality of simulated illusion may be addressed with Jungian principles. The psychological dynamics of interactive images projected as media images correspond with psychological dream images as defined by Carl G. Jung. Therefore, images in the media mirror patterns of energy and information in what Jung called the collective unconscious. Dream dynamics may be used to address global political hacking, cyber warfare, and neuromarketing with ICTs.

INTRODUCTION

As we experience a paradigm shift into a media age, Information and Communication Technologies (ICTs) are altering the psychological parameters of human reality. Ongoing exposures relative to global political hacking, cyber warfare, neuromarketing, and consequences of mediated lies have made it abundantly clear that issues of cultural morality and health in a mediated reality of simulated illusion must be vigorously addressed and researched for years to come. The psychological dynamics of interactive images projected as media images correspond with the psychological

DOI: 10.4018/978-1-5225-8470-4.ch009

and structural dynamics of dream images as defined by Carl G. Jung. If this is true, images in the media—media dreams or Archetypal Representations (AR)—mirror patterns of energy and information in what Jung called the collective unconscious.

Jung called dream images archetypal representations (AR) because they are relatively conscious projections of unconscious quantum/archetypal energy patterns that he called "archetypes". Long before scientists began the study of quantum electrodynamics (QED), Jung discovered that these archetypes of the unconscious as well as their projections into "conscious" dimensions as AR have dramatic structure. Current cognitive research verifies that—indeed—the cognitive unconscious has the framework of metaphorical drama and that these story patterns may be correlated with energy patterns in the nervous system. (Lakoff, George, 2008, p. 23) Jung pioneered research on the healing dynamics of dreams. In doing so, he discovered the "moral" dynamics of illusion. This is highly significant relative to human navigation of the mediated age of illusion with which humanity is presently faced. Such verification suggests that Jungian genius may be effectively applied to the illusions of the Media-sphere which have suddenly manifested as cyber-warfare and political hacking. Unfortunately, Jung's genius has not been appreciated. Instead, if media morality is considered at all, Sigmund Freud's faulty model has been exalted. (Curtis, Adam, 2009)

Yes. Quantum, neurobiological, and media dimensions can be correlated. Therefore, human cognitive structure is susceptible to healing with the use of media biofeedback. Fundamental to Jungian healing with dream analysis is the principle that dreams "have a purpose," and that the dream purpose is the discovery of meaning—with the help of biofeedback provided by a psychiatrist—through "compensation" or harmonization of conscious and unconscious psyche. Jungian compensation is a process (the Amplification Method) that defines an essentially coherent psychic state. Recent research on coherence confirms that coherent states "heal" and such harmonious states can be evoked with specific feedback technologies. Abundant research confirms that *coherent* psychological states increase emotional and perceptual stability as well as alignment among the physical, cognitive, and emotional systems. (McCraty & Childre, 2010) Our hypothesis is that the images projected by information and communication technologies (ICTs)—the media dreams of a population—are subject to psychological analysis and compensation in-order to disclose and address unconscious sources of psychological stress in contextual collectives. In other words, computational biofeedback that creates coherent states of being becomes the measurable quintessence not only of *healthcare management but of generating and maintaining a global culture of conscience.* (Schafer, Stephen Brock, 2018; Schafer, Stephen Ed. 2017; Schafer, Stephen, 2012)

Research and discussion about the psychological influence of the media are both longstanding and off-target. It is only recently that research has focused on the QED neurobiological nature of this influence, and—even now—Jung's research on dream analysis has never been applied to the discussion. Carl Jung discovered that providing compensational feedback to help patients understand the symbolic meaning in their dream images can lead to insight as to the causes of subconscious problems. According to Jung, dream images are "archetypal projections" of subconscious "functional" (thinking, feeling, sensing, intuiting) energy and information patterns. Because such projections display dramatic patterns that are essentially recursive, unconscious meaning can be accessed because it is mirrored in the projected symbolic images. Archetypal projections are much like pixel projections in which meaning resides both in the images projected and in the computer programs that pattern the pixels. Thousands of Jung's clinical observations demonstrated that gradual insight as to the symbolic meaning in a series of dream images has the capacity to "compensate" for cognitive dissonance; i.e. the compensational process leads to alteration in cognitive energy patterns. These altered patterns are defined by their harmonious frequency. This is possible due to the dramatic-semantic structure of energy patterns in both conscious and unconscious cognitive dimensions. This compensational, "amplification method" depends upon a psychiatrist's empathetic feedback which consists of metaphorical amplification relative to symbolic meaning embedded in dream images. Therefore, the amplification method constitutes a biofeedback language that can be simulated with ICTs.

A new era for research on quantum cognitive processes supports Jungian empirical observations relative to the nature of *Archetypes of the Unconscious*. Essentially, unconscious archetypes are quantum energy patterns that seem directly correlated with ICTs. Like archetypes, ICTs are energy configurations that are projected as recursive dreamlike images which share the fundamental patterns of narrative and metaphor. Dr. George Lakoff has already addressed the subject of creating a computational model of narrative (Lakoff & Narayanan, 2010), and the recent discovery of quantum vibrations in neural "microtubules" (Hameroff & Penrose, 2014) tends to validate the measurability of connections among quantum, neural, and functional scales. Related ongoing research can be listed *ad infinitum* under the headings of virtual realities, neural networks, computational anthropology, cloud computing, data mining, and machine intelligence. The MIT Technology Review recently reported that researchers strive to create the "source code" for studying culture as a formal computational concept. (Aiello, Schfanella, & State, 2014). Advances in brain-scanning technologies makes study of neural processes possible (Trafton, Anne, 2014), and rapidly evolving methodologies such as *Particle based simulations (physX flex)* (2014) and "superconducting spintronics" pave the way for next-generation computing. (Kirk, Tom, 2014).

Arguably, to this point, Stephen Kosslyn's *Image and Brain* (1994) has been the primary source for information about how the brain processes imagery. But recently, Anne Trafton (2014) has pointed out that a new brain-scanning technique called magnetoencephalography (MEG) allows scientists to see when and where the brain processes visual information. MIT researchers combined fMRI and MEG data to reveal which parts of the brain are active shortly after an image is seen. Every time the eyes are opened, visual information flows into the brain, which interprets what is being seen. Now, for the first time, MIT neuroscientists have noninvasively mapped this flow of information in the human brain with unique accuracy, using MEG. This technique, which combines two existing technologies, allows researchers to identify with precision both the location and timing of human brain activity. Using this new approach, the MIT researchers scanned individuals' brains as they looked at different images and were able to pinpoint, to the millisecond, when the brain recognizes and categorizes an object, and where these processes occur.

"This method gives you a visualization of 'when' and 'where' at the same time. It's a window into processes happening at the millisecond and millimeter scale," says Aude Oliva, a principal research scientist in MIT's Computer Science and Artificial Intelligence Laboratory (CSAIL). Oliva is the senior author of a paper describing the findings in the Jan. 26 issue of *Nature Neuroscience*. Lead author of the paper is CSAIL postdoc Radoslaw Cichy. Dimitrios Pantazis, a research scientist at MIT's McGovern Institute for Brain Research, is also an author of the paper

Such technological advances have spawned an array of research in AI, simulation, and robotics that, from the historical perspective, are absolutely surreal. A constant stream of research papers is being reported relative to such subjects as, *The curious evolution of artificial life*, (2014); *On the origin of robot species: robots building robots by "natural selection"* (Saffell, Nick, 2015); and *A robot just passed the self-awareness test* (Geere, Duncan, 2015). Virtual reality applications extend in every direction ranging from military training to video game play: *Creating massive virtual worlds for [military] training.* (2015); *Playing games might help AI advance* (Knight, Will, 2015); and *Immersive media: to the holodeck and beyond* (Boyd, Frank, 2015).

However, such spectacular research on AI and Robotics is significantly flawed. First, it is based almost entirely on mental processes without inclusion of the importance of the human heart. Second, the purposes of these corporate dreams seem dedicated universally to profit via marketing and overwhelmingly to military uses. (Galeon, Dom, 2016; Creating massive virtual worlds for training, 2015; Dionisio, John David N., Burns, William G. III, and Gilbert, Richard, 2013; Freedberg, Sydney J. JR., 2015; Dooley, Roger, 2015a and 2015b; Zaltman, Gerald & Zaltman, Lindsay, 2008)

Largely due to decades of research by the Institute of Heartmath and its global network of colleagues, this trajectory of research is changing. Heartmath researches the effects of coherence in a holistic QED environment. Currently, research extends from the influences of coherence on the multi-functional human organism (McCraty, Rollin & Childre, Doc, 2010), on groups (Morris, Steven M., 2010), and on the planetary geosphere (McCraty, Rollin, Atkinson, Mike, Stolc, Victor, Alabdulgader, Abdulla A., Vainoras, Alfonsas, Ragulskis, Minvydas, 2017). Most relevant to the current argument advocating coherence as a cognitive principle for designing quality E-ICTs, is the longstanding research on the phenomenon that has become known as the Maharishi Effect.

The Maharishi Effect establishes the principle that individual consciousness affects collective consciousness. Nearly 50 scientific research studies conducted over the past 25 years verify the unique effect and wide-ranging benefits to the nation produced by the Maharishi Effect. These studies have used the most rigorous research methods and evaluation procedures available in the social sciences, including time series analysis, which controls for weekly and seasonal cycles or trends in social data. (Refer to: Scientific Research on Maharishi's Transcendental Meditation Programme—Collected Papers 98, 166, 317-320, 331, and 402.) Research shows that the influence of coherence created by the Maharishi Effect can be measured on both national and international levels. Increased coherence within the nation expresses itself in improved national harmony and well-being. In addition, this internal coherence and harmony generates an influence that extends beyond the nation's borders, expressing itself in improved international relations and reduced international conflicts. (Orme-Johnson, D. W., ND).

Though simulation models are rapidly evolving, they are still inferior to "real" human interaction. Historical attempts to model psychological processes with computers have been catastrophic (Curtis, Adam, 2002). However, due to spectacular advances in ICT sophistication, speed, and memory capabilities, advanced artificial intelligence models that provide compensational feedback may actually provide more effective information and communication than highly intuitive-empathetic psychiatrists. At least, such AI could make psychiatric therapy more widely available and less expensive. Most important, this paper argues that such advanced models can be designed to be non-manipulative in-order to preserve human autonomy. Such autonomy can be preserved due to the underlying motives and cognitive dynamics of Jungian healing therapy and the insights of Dr. George Lakoff.

If the characteristics demonstrated with compensation, coherence, and such phenomena as "Flow" and Maslow's "peak experience" are similar (McCraty & Childre, 2010; Jung 1933, p. 21 & p. 26; Kendra, Cherry, 2015a; Cherry, 2015b), it may be stipulated that Jungian compensation is essentially the same thing as coherence. The characteristics of coherence include self-realization, meaningful insight, functional harmonization, strong concentration and focused attention, feelings of serenity and loss of self-consciousness, timelessness, being focused on the present, feelings of personal power over situation and outcome, increase in personal awareness and understanding, generation of positive emotions that are intrinsically rewarding, and feelings of at-one-ness (atonement) with the world.

Extensive research by the Institute of Heartmath has proven that coherence has a cognitive signature that can be measured, projected as sine waves, and used as feedback to increase harmonization of bioenergetic systems. In other words, the Heartmath process compensates for cognitive dissonance and is measurable with technologies like EmSense.

The longstanding observation that "harmony heals" is no longer a platitude. It is a cognitive axiom that has been tested and proven. Biofeedback procedures employed by Jung and the Institute of Heartmath lead to increased cognitive coherence and neurobiological harmonization which has a multi-functional healing affect. In terms of reliable quality e-healthcare, it is critically important to understand that both processes are non-manipulative—driven by a subject/patient's contextual, largely unconscious predispositions rather than more limited externally imposed controls; i.e. in both systems, insight/coherence is achieved according to the unique (contextual) psyche (both conscious and unconscious input) of the subject rather than any externally imposed expectations.

BACKGROUND

Scientific expectations are often colored by personal and collective prejudices, and such impositions in the ICT design process would reduce the quality of e-care and destroy both its reliability and credibility. A glaring example of the difficulties involved with such external imposition has been explored in the BBC documentary, *The Century of Self* (Curtis, Adam, 2002), which reported on the mid-twentieth century effort of researchers to computerize healthcare. Due to the scientific materialism of the era and the difficulty of programming the unconscious, theoreticians and designers of healthcare computer programs totally ignored the existence of the "unconscious" as a factor in mental dissonance, neurosis, and psychosis. Eventually, efforts to diagnose psychological-emotional illness relied almost entirely on personal report questionnaires. A basic premise of Behaviorism was that the unconscious did not exist, and such prejudice in psychological research has had longstanding negative effects.

We now understand that the Behaviorist premise is blatantly false, and Behaviorism has fallen into disrepute. From the current perspective based on sophisticated neural imaging and the use of artificial intelligence algorithms, Behaviorism lacks both credibility and reliability. By definition, this discipline has no interest in any discovery of meaning for the purpose of healing the cognitive unconscious.

However, the attitudes behind this simplistic Behaviorist view of human cognition have become strongly framed in the collective unconscious and have persisted into the present day. One need only mention the fact of the existence of unconscious reality to provoke outrage from many. Beyond psychology, many researchers and the mass of humanity have incorporated the simplistic scientific-materialistic view into their cognitive reality—in-spite of vast evidence to the contrary.

Gradually, the prescient genius of Carl Jung (not to be confused with Freudian theory) is becoming highly practical—especially with regard to the function and potentials for ICTs. Jung uses the term "context" to describe a principle for personalizing the healing process and compensating for generalized disharmony and prejudice. That disharmony and seeming chaos exists in dimensions of the cognitive unconscious is not surprising. However, the research of Byron Reeves and Clifford Nass (1996) informs us in *The Media Equation* that humans in all demographics perceive media content as "real"; i.e. having psychological/social behavioral parameters. The many conclusions documented by Reeves and Nass about the fact that media technologies and ICTs have socially recognizable personality have proven invaluable in Microsoft 's efforts to create more user-friendly hardware and software. However, viewed from the Jungian perspective—media as archetypal representation—how humans perceive the media dream becomes highly significant. From Jung's perspective the media is, indeed, real. The media dream constitutes experience as real as the waking dream, and humans navigate these dreams according to discovery of meaning imbedded in "living" symbols. Most important, Jung demonstrates how the chaos of the unconscious can be harmonized with the process of Compensation.

Given proven psychological advertising practices such as defining target group personality with focus groups, changes in corporate perspectives regarding the "reality" of media, the rapid development of social media with its sophisticated algorithms, and longstanding refinement of Myers-Briggs concepts of personality profiling that are based on Jungian principles, applying Jung's principles to the analysis of media dreams should be relatively easy. Specific to ICTs, the research of Reeves and Nass strongly recommends that, "Media should be able to adapt to the personality of the user." (1996, p. 106)

Case records of Jungian theory and practice are voluminous and cover a period between 1916 and 1945. The book, *Dreams*, translated by R.F.C. Hull, (1974) provides both a clinical record and history of Jung's publications. In addition to records of Jungian therapy, extensive research has demonstrated that coherence/harmony has numerous "healing" consequences that are essentially contextual and couched in meaningful insight. A very few of these research studies are cited in the following list:

- **Stress reduction** (McCraty & Childre, 2010; Barrios-Choplin, McCraty, & Cryer,1997; McCraty, R. and D. Tomasino 2006; Childre, D. and D. Rozman 2005; Luskin, Reitz, Newell, Quinn, & Haskell, 2002))
- **Improvement of major depression and post traumatic syndrome** (Zucker, T.L., et al. 2009; Ginsberg, J.P., Berry, M.E., Powell, D.A. 2010; Karavides, MK, Leehrer PM, Vaschillo V, et al)
- **Neurocardiology** (Armour, J.A., and Ardell, J.L., 2003; Armour, J.A., 1994; Frysinger, R.C. and Harper, R.M., 1990)
- **Improvement of compassion, empathy, training and retention problems in children** (Knox, Lentini, & Alton, 2012)
- **Decision making of entrepreneurs, and enhanced learning** (Gillin, Lapiri, McCraty, Bradly, Atkinson, Simpson, & Scicluna, ND; Bradley, Raymond Trevor, 2006)
- **Psychological effects of compassion vs. anger** (Rein, Atkinson, & McCraty, 1995).
- **Athsma** (Lehrer P, Vaschillo E, Lu SE, et al. Heart rate variability biofeedback: effects of age on heart rate variability, baroreflex gain, and athsma. *Chest. 2006; 129(2): 278-284.*
- **Diabetes** (Lindmark S, Wiklund U, Bjerle P, Eriksson JW. Does the autonomic nervous system play a role in the development of insulin resistance? A study on heartrate variability in first degree relatives of Type 2 diabetes patients and control subjects. *Diabet Med.* 2003;20(5):399-405.
- **Improvement of personal, social, and global health** (McCraty & Childre, 2010; McCraty, R., 2002a; McCraty, R., 2002b)

If—as demonstrated above—coherence and compensation are the same things, ICTs programmed with Jungian principles of contextual compensation (the Amplification Method) in conjunction with mediated biofeedback methods, can contribute to the achievement of coherent personal and collective states

Most interesting of Jung's prescient contributions to cognitive health is the realization that fractal dream dynamics of the microcosm seem to be based on universal frequency patterns of the macrocosm as represented by QED field theory. In opther words, modern QED echoes the alchemical axiom that, "As it is below, so it is above". This idea has both abundant mythic precedent and widespread modern scientific acceptance. Most specifically, Jung says that, "Disruption in the spiritual life of an age shows the same pattern as radical change in an individual." (Jung, p. 202) Also, "A people presents only a somewhat more complex picture of psychic life than the individual." (Jung, p. 210) That is to say, what are currently understood as bio-electrical patterns are shared by individuals and groups in a QED unified field of energy-and-information. Based on symbolic content, mediated images are essentially bio-electrical patterns that—like dreams—provide potentials for meaningful insight. This suggests that, in-order to achieve curative insight, the key to navigation of the *unconscious psyche* resides in the correspondences (based on algorithmic recursions of isometric form) that may be mediated between digital software and the archetypal representations that the software projects. Jung also observed that because the psychic process has a quantitative aspect, the conservation of energy in the physical world is analogous to "compensation" by the psyche. Accordingly, "No psychic value can disappear without being replaced by another of equivalent intensity." (Jung, p. 209) Another way to say this is that dissonant psychic values can be replaced by coherent psychic values.

More recently, cognitive research has verified many of Jung's most important principles and empirical observations—in particular, the realization that the cognitive unconscious is energy that has dramatic structure and personality. (Jacoby, Yolande, 1973, pp. 82-83; Lakoff, George, 2008; Reeves & Nass, 1996) More implicitly, like dream images, archetypal representations appear to provide the entire substance of human reality and meaning in the form of memories, fantasies, sensory perceptions, and all the experiences of "real life." (Lakoff, 2008, pp. 14-15) Explaining the cognitive dynamic, Lakoff says, "Conscious thought is *reflective*, like looking at yourself in a mirror." (p. 9) Researching cognitive patterns of the unconscious, Lakoff has demonstrated that the bio-energetic cognitive unconscious has dramatic structure. Both Jung and Lakoff use the terms narrative-metaphorical to discuss cognitive patterns. However, the term drama is a more useful descriptor, and—in this paper—drama is used interchangeably with the term narrative-metaphorical to discuss the cognitive neurobiological architecture that consists of "functions" or psychic domains (thinking, feeling, sensing, and intuiting).

Lakoff is explicit as to the neuro-biological process by which metaphor frames human values. (Lakoff, 2008, p. 95) From the standpoint of ICTs, this is important because metaphor and coherence constitute the programmable dynamics of the amplification process leading to the achievement of measurable coherent states. Lakoff defines the two fundamental family metaphors that determine conservative values (The Strict Father Metaphor) and progressive values (The Nurturant Parent Metaphor). Such narratives and metaphors with which we identify at subconscious levels determine human value systems, the human worldview, human choices, and human actions. Lakoff observes that without reference to cognitive narratives, humans cannot know others. Without these unconscious narrative-metaphorical reference points, people cannot even know themselves. (Lakoff, 2008, pp. 33-34) Essentially, humans—both personal and collective—refer their identity and their very existence to subliminal dreamlike cognitive dramas. It may follow that the discovery and projection (conscious realization) of coherent subliminal meaning can change human reality on a scale appropriate to the challenges created by the realization that reality is a mediated illusion. Lakoff's goal is, "To make the cognitive unconscious as conscious as possible, to make *reflexive* decisions *reflective*." (2008, p 34) This would make a good premise for creating and maintaining reliable privacy and health information management.

These ideas raise questions as to the existence of structural parallels between psyche as understood by Carl Jung and the emergent media sphere or what some call the *Metaverse*. The media sphere has been defined as a collective ecology of the world's media including newspapers, journals, television, radio, books, novels, advertising, press releases, publicity and the blogosphere; imagery plays a part in all mediation whether it is broadcast, published, or auto-induced in the mind's eye. If structural parallels exist, it may be possible to analyze the images of the media-sphere according to Jungian methods for accessing subliminal meaning in-order to diagnose and heal "contextual" collectives. (Schafer & Yu, 2011; Schafer, 2011; Schafer, 2012)

The word Metaverse is a portmanteau of the prefix "meta" (meaning "beyond") and the suffix "verse" (shorthand for "universe"). Thus it literally means a universe beyond the physical world. More specifically this "universe beyond" refers to a computer-generated world, distinguishing it from metaphysical or spiritual conceptions of domains beyond the physical realm. In addition, the Metaverse refers to a fully immersive three-dimensional digital environment in contrast to the more inclusive concept of cyberspace that reflects the totality of shared online space across all dimensions of representation. (Dionisio, John David N.; Burns, William G. III; and Gilbert, Richard, 2013).

FOSTERING PSYCHOLOGICAL COHERENCE WITH ICTs

Jung based his method of dream analysis on his observation that dreams have dramatic structure and—like drama—"dreams speak in images" (Jung 1933, p 26) that have purpose and meaning. (Jacoby, pp. 58-59) The AI tools for accessing meaning such as Google Scholar, Microsoft Academic Search, PubMed and JSTOR are advancing apace; but, historically, these programs have been limited by objective search methodologies such as keywords and other information that is clearly categorized like the publication date. These AI tools do not address subjective meaning.

Meanwhile, advances in image quality and recognition are experiencing a quantum leap that—if Jungian principles are taken into account—addresses a more subjective meaning. Though images don't need to be realistic to be meaningful (Reeves & Nass, 1996, p. 85), enhanced realism obviously contributes to the sense of "perceived reality." Among many examples, Facebook is developing technology—a blend of artificial intelligence and machine-learning—that will be able to help blind people "see" images by enabling computers to distinguish what is in a picture. (Lee, Dave, 2015) Also, exploiting the graphics-rendering software that powers sports video games, researchers at MIT and the Qatar Computing Research Institute (QCRI) have developed a system that automatically converts 2-D video images of soccer games into 3-D. (Hardesty, Larry, 2015) Creation of sophisticated graphic imagery is, perhaps, the most relevant trend toward understanding the mediated dream as reality. The digital conversion of 2-D to 3-D serves as a significator verifying the prognosis that, in accordance with numerous advances in imaging technology, the "Metaverse" has already become an alternative human reality:

Reality is a dream, so understanding the unique dimensions of the Jungian dream becomes very practical. As to the meaning of dreams, *The Allen Institute for Artificial Intelligence* is working toward the goal of teaching computers to find meaning in the thousands of research papers published each year. The Institute has developed a new tool called *Semantic Scholar* that can search through millions of computer science papers. "The tool, launched [recently], features ways of refining searches based on information extracted from the text of papers." The objective is to create AI that can automatically highlight important new trends or discoveries and draw conclusions from them. (Knight, Will, 2015). In Jungian terms, meaning is intrinsically contextual, so—in-order to discover meaning—the *text* in academic papers should be understood as having contextuality as well as having semantic/dramatic structure. George Lakoff has further defined contextual representations in terms of the key family metaphors mentioned above. Understanding the family metaphors that have their source in neurolinguistic patterns could increase the reliability and quality of e-healthcare.

Perhaps it is unnecessary to remind the reader that metaphor has mathematical pattern and proportion and that this proportionality is the basis for Fourier Transforms, sophisticated AI algorithms, and contextual meaning. Notwithstanding the long and varied analysis of Aristotle's writing, his definition of analogy—one type of metaphor—may be reduced to the following idea. Aristotle demonstrated the mathematical pattern of analogy; i.e. the semantic form of analogy is expressed, "A is to B as C is to D" (life is to old age as day is to evening). The mathematical formula for analogy is $A/B = C/D$. Therefore, as old age (B) is to life (A), so is evening (D) to day (C). (Garrett, Jan, 2007) Using this formulation, the nature of old age as the "unknown" may be contemplated in terms of metaphorical resonance. Both formulations are about fractional proportion, and it is accurate to say that metaphorical proportionality is infinite in its potential to express fractal reality, but at the same time it is computational.

By the term "fractal", contextuality can be assumed. Jung observed, "That numbers have an archetypal foundation is not, by the way, a conjecture of mine but of certain mathematicians." (Jacoby, p.115f citing *Synchronicity*, par. 870) As all mathematicians know, Pythagoras discussed the personality of numbers. (Hall, Manly P. 2003, pp. 206-221) Also, throughout his book, *The Philosophical Scientists* (1985), David Foster refers to physicists such as Sir Arthur Eddington, Sir James Jeans, Bertrand Russell, and A. N. Whitehead who reached a consensus that, "The stuff of the world is mind stuff—an idea centered around symbolic data as a general interpretation of what [is meant] by mathematics". (p. 27) Perhaps these many observations could benefit designers of ICTs within the modern context of mediated dreams.

The entire mathematical edifice is based on proportional correspondences by which meaning is discovered in terms of "unknowns". What sometimes seems forgotten by even the most brilliant researchers is that "correspondence"—a fundamental research dynamic—is another type of metaphor upon which maps of all types (roadmaps, genetic maps, star maps) are based. Metaphors are contextual fractions which—according to their resonance—harbor infinite possibilities for discovery of multi-dimensional meaning.

Psychology has always been an important element in advertising; but, increasingly a new breed of neuro-marketer is emphasizing cognitive research with observations such as, *The Secret Behind Retail Customer Experience Success is Brain Science.* (Yohn, Denise Lee, 2015) and *The TMI Effect for Pictures Can Reduce Your Sales.* (Dooley, Roger, 2015a) As indicated in the recently published book, *Metaphoria*, which discusses the function of "deep metaphors" in marketing to unconscious cognitive dimensions of target groups, neuro-marketers are increasingly aware of the importance of thought-pattern recognition which corresponds to image-pattern recognition. The authors' conclusions emerge from their own research, but—as in much current research—fundamental Jungian principle pervades the discussion:

The psychologist Carl G. Jung argued that archetypes are patterns, symbols, and images that represent basic qualities of mind inherent in and shared by every person, regardless of culture. Hence archetypes are universal and operate in what Jung called our "collective unconscious." (Zaltman, Gerald & Zaltman, Lindsay, 2008)

As it turns out, deep metaphors are essentially Jungian archetypes, but the discussion relative to marketing—though it addresses morality—does not do justice to the fundamental Jungian dynamic of contextuality nor the Jungian objective of healing that is correlated with the discovery of meaning.

While neuro-marketers explore the deep psychology of sales, the military explores simulations and augmented realities with military morality: *Marines explore augmented reality* (Freedberg, Sydney J. Jr., 2015); *Creating massive virtual worlds for training* (2015); and *US Army: computer simulations improve lethality* (Kowal, Erik, 2015). According to Jung, such simulations are contextual images, and according to Reeves and Nass, they are perceived as real. Immediately, the hotly contested question of whether media can make viewers more violent is resolved. The answer is, certainly! Mediated experience is perceived as real, and real experience alters the shape of archetypal patterns.

Given the rapid pace of advancement in AI and machine intelligence, neuro-marketing, and virtual worlds for military training, this paper argues that the possibility of fostering coherent psychological states with ICTs should provide a foundational mandate upon which all serious research on information and communication technologies should be based.

IF A CULTURE HAS DREAMS

If a culture has dreams, perhaps its media dreams could communicate messages to contextual populations to warn them of existing or impending psychosis. If heeded, media dreams might provide meaningful insight that provokes the collective psyche into coherent psychological states and contributes to changing the collective psyche from *reflexive* to *reflective*. But that's nonsense! Or is it? Is the American Dream nonsense? Are the values upon which the dream is based nonsensical? Are hopes and goals meaningless? What happens when a culture's dreams become debased? History tells us. The society degenerates and dies. We all have a vague notion of what caused the decline and fall of Rome or of Babylon. We know something about the values—the dream—upon which Rome was founded, but most of what we know is only the outer expression of its inner psychological disharmony—its tyrants, its aggressive militarism, or its murderous entertainments in the coliseum. And how do we know about this debouche of Rome's psyche? We know about Rome because we have access to some of its media dreams—parchment and print, histories and drama. In their day, Roman citizens observed the decline, wrote and spoke about it to their contemporaries. Symptoms of the decline in the Roman dream could be observed in its media. Its media served as a bridge to span the gap between dimensions of Rome's psyche. Its media disclosed Rome's psychological corruption and foretold its inexorable decline. The citizenry did not respond. The great empire and the great dream faltered and died.

History repeats itself, and some say that the same meaningful message is being mediated to the American empire, but today's media-sphere is considerably different. The modern technological media is even more dreamlike than parchment and its paraphernalia is far more pervasive. Perhaps the modern *media dreams* seen darkly in TV drama, film, social media, I-phones, and the nightly news also reflect symbolic metaphorical significance relative to the psychological stresses that could lead to collapse of global systems. If a culture were a patient on Carl Jung's couch, Dr. Jung might use his amplification method of dream analysis to guide his contextual patient into a more coherent psychological state.

Understood as Archetypal Representations that, according to Carl G. Jung, are projections into conscious psychic dimensions from quantum-level unconscious dimensions, the Media-sphere provides a wealth of data for understanding cultural motives and the psychological dynamics at work during the Paradigm Shift in worldviews. In Jungian principle, dreams are archetypal representations that can be analyzed with the language of symbolism in-order to access contextual meaning that exists in unconscious cognitive dimensions. Such cognitive insight as to meaning can results in the creation of a coherent functional state-of-being that can be viewed as a wave pattern on a monitor. Providing media biofeedback relative to changing degrees of coherent states has proven to have demonstrable healing power. (McCraty, Rollin & Childre, Doc, 2010; Jacoby, Yolande, 1973; Jung, Carl G., 1933) Inducing coherent functional states with global media biofeedback has the power to heal personal and collective Psyche by fostering insight as to the meaning of its symbolic images. (Schafer, Stephen Brock, 2018, p. 373)

Media dreams also have a prophetic function much like the function of the science-fiction genre. As sci-fi award winner, A. A. Attanasio, has said, "Science fiction becomes science fact." (Schafer, Stephen Brock, 2018, p. 10) Those old enough to have eyes that see, can confirm the fact, and sci-fi ranging from *1984* and *Brave New World* to *"I Robot"* illustrate the truth of Attanasio's proclamation.

According to Carl G. Jung, dreams are projections from quantum unconscious dimensions into conscious dimensions where the language of symbolic images can be interpreted. In the language of dream analysis, Jung would have described the science-fiction film genre as a prospective (future oriented) dreamscape of Archetypal Representations that has a wealth of psychological data for-the purpose of understanding cultural motives, incoherent repressed cultural psychology, and the psychological dynamics at work during the Paradigm Shift of reality worldviews. In Jungian principle, dreams can be analyzed with the language of symbolism in-order to access and heal incoherent individual and collective psychic states. Insight as to the meaning of symbols in images is curative. If the pixel patterns of science fiction be understood and analyzed as the media-dreams of collective personae, they could provide in-depth meaningful insights that throw light on the cultural life-paths being explored during the paradigm shift. (Schafer, Stephen Brock, 2018, p. 435)

The significance of this hypothesis may be immediately construed from the nightly news where Fox news creates a reality of its own and MSNBC strives to synchronize the illusions with fact. It is in this unprecedented context that the destructive potential of mediated lies, cyber-warfare, and mediated delusion become very clear. Projections in the news inform us about the critical survival issues that humanity is struggling with. If we have eyes to see, survival issues may be addressed effectively. For example:

Leaders of a culture serve as Archetypal Representations (AR) that reflects character strengths and fatal flaws in the Collective Persona of the culture. Analysis of leaders as AR goes well beyond statistical polling models. Applying the cognitive principles of contextual Drama and Identification provides keys to psychological insight into cultural values, motives, and pathologies generated from the collective cultural unconscious. Beyond marketing and polling, these dramatic dynamics provide keys to healing of the collective unconscious. But instead, strategists in the giant industries of neuro-marketing and video games, are applying these cognitive dynamics for the limited manipulative purposes leading to profit and blasphemy. Due to the psychological power of the media, if these trends continue, the Democratic free society and human dignity itself will come to an end. Rhetorical applications to marketing manipulation and political propaganda have the potential to influence society in matters no less important than presidential elections. (Schafer, Stephen Brock, 2018, p. 473)

How does this relate to ICTs for healthcare and Social Services? First, it suggests that the unconscious electro-magnetic human psyche of the planet has enormous influence on planetary evolution; and, second, that it can be diagnosed and treated with compensational procedures. So, the digital software of ICTs should be programmed according to Jungian principles of compensation and coherence in-order to provide meaningful insight to users, ameliorate chaotic disharmony, and foster coherence in the media dream. ICTs are, perhaps, the most authentic of media dream—the keys to the Kingdom.

The Paradigm Shift is a fundamental change from a materialistic to a metaphysical worldview that has its expression in the technological Media-sphere or Media-dream. (Schafer, Stephen Brock, 2016 b & c) The Metaphysical concept called The Dweller on the Threshold is a tool for "fine-tuning" a Culture of Conscience. It is well known that the quantum reality is nothing like the perceived human reality; therefore, the psychological factors in a quantum reality are counter-intuitive to human inhabitants of their perceptual reality. Nevertheless, the cognitive unconscious can be accessed, analyzed, and harmonized using media-dreams according to Jungian dynamics of dream analysis. Mediated images serve as archetypal representation that reflect unconscious cognitive content, so media content can be analyzed in-order to access unconscious collective psychosis and to foster healing with mediated biofeedback. Analysis of current media dreams in the U.S. political domain divulges the symbolic Dweller on the Threshold. (Schafer, Stephen Brock, 2018, p. 501)

The metaphysical concept of the *Dweller* may be understood as an initiatory threshold—a bridge that must be crossed by the human family in order to achieve enlightenment. Metaphorically, media dreams are like a bridge--a way across, a connective passage, a span. Our use of bridges is essentially unconscious. We don't usually think about it. So it is with all languages—media that bridge the gap between conscious and unconscious meaning. Within the nervous system—which is, itself, a bridge—synapses bridge neural networks in-order to structure the human worldview. Since this worldview is being altered by quantum leaps, it is critical that we understand and make use of the bridging dynamic in-order to correlate the flow of cognitive traffic and to harmonize it.

Just as the loss or injury of a synapse can cause physical or emotional disability, ignoring bridges can be catastrophic and have multidimensional impact. After the collapse of the bridge in Kare, Minnesota, USA, information about bridge collapse was omnipresent in the American media sphere. The subject of collapsing bridges was popular in venues ranging from the nightly news to the history channel. Bridges were discussed, analyzed, and featured on talk radio, nightly comedy shows, and the Internet. These media dreams advised us that in many cases of sudden and unexpected failure, there existed a relatively small flaw or crack at some structural point within the bridge. That flaw contributed to increased pressure and stress on other points. In other instances of collapse, erosion or "scour" around bridge foundations was the nemesis. But always, the collapse came as a result of excessive displaced *stress* on the integrated structural components of the bridge. Inspections can be missed, small cracks can be overlooked, and even more obvious problems like scouring can be neglected because they exist unobserved beneath the surface of the water. Inevitably over time, even minor flaws unbalance the complex distribution of stress factors in the architecture of a bridge and lead to structural collapse.

Inexorably, the collapsed bridge story and metaphor becomes a symbol for meaningful insight—the collapse of a nation's infrastructure. If we think of collapsed bridges in terms of Jungian symbolism, they become dream motifs in the contextual "American" media dream. So, as an aspect of the media dream, the collapsed bridge (an archetypal representation) becomes a metaphor—a dream symbol—that evokes meaning in other psychologically contextual dimensions. Small structural cracks that create stress become meaningful as psychological stress points. Underwater scour becomes meaningful as repressed emotion; and, in each case, the pressure that creates stressful incoherence in the unified bridge structure translates to the metaphorically related context of pressures that create incoherence in the unified field of the national psyche.

Expanding the bridge metaphor to the arena of biology which includes bridging mechanisms such as synapses, permeable membranes, and chemical processes, these bio-bridges mediate the energies and life-forces of the physical body—individual, collective, and planetary.[1] In the individual person, wrinkles in the forehead, telltale discoloration or swelling under the eyes, lesions on the skin, and bloating of the body may signify that excessive stress is being placed on kidneys, heart, or the endocrine system. Such symptoms portend the failure of the whole physical system. A society may have similar symptoms: high rates of heart disease, diabetes, aids, cancer, and obesity may indicate that the collective persona is sick and that there is a serious threat of total collapse. In the case of the global organism, deforestation, air pollution, the catastrophic loss of biodiversity, and melting of the polar icecaps signify stresses existing at deeper systemic levels which—like scour—go unrecognized and unattended.

The bridge metaphor may be expanded to psychologically functional (emotional-psychological) realms. The principle purpose of Jungian dreams is that they bridge the gap between *Functions* of conscious and unconsciousness (mental, emotional, sensory, & intuitive) and provide the potential for compensation in-order to restore coherent states. In other words, dreams bridge or mediate information among psychic states of being—personal and collective unconscious states via dreams to personal and collective conscious states. Correctly interpreted, dreams tell the story of internal stresses that threaten the harmony and balance of the coherent psyche. Like the symbolism of dreams, the outer signs and symbols such as cracks in bridge girders, bags under the eyes, obsessive-compulsive disorder, neurotic behaviors, gradual inflation of currency, or recurrent economic "recessions" are all symbols that mediate a story in the language of symptomatic stress that can be understood as symbols of infrastructural weakness. With the help of a psychiatrist—or perhaps ICTs—a patient can decode the dream messages in-order to heal or re-integrate the outer expression of the persona.

The media sphere constantly warns us that we are presently experiencing the collapse of our global financial system. Metaphorically, this corresponds directly to a collapse of "values." Therefore, the media dreams based on this motif can be understood as a warning about the dangers of incoherence relative to our global value systems. If these dreams result in meaningful insight, they will compensate for the consequences attributed to incoherent values that foster fear, greed, aggression, destruction, sub-optimization, economic rapacity, and the devaluation of life. Instead, media dreams could foster meaningful insight and a transition to more coherent value systems characterized by harmony, mutual respect, honesty, and the value of life. A plethora of film-media dreams already do this, and they do it without sanitizing real problems. Just a few current examples of this positive approach are, *The Green Zone, The Insider, Sully, Total Recall, the Terminator series, I Am Legend, Thirteen Days, Remember the Titans, Elysium, The Day After Tomorrow, Kingdom of Heaven, the Bourne series, The Legend of Bagger Vance, Gandhi, Avatar*, and many more. Such media dreams have proffered contextual insights about our collective values for some time. Even such seemingly negative film dreams such as *A Nightmare on Elm Street, Angel Heart, No Country for Old Men, and DaVinci's Demons* have insightful value.

At local, national, and international levels, economic chaos and stress are media markers that emphasize priorities. Metaphorically, this means that the stress and chaos of human values are priorities, yet the priorities are not yet couched in terms of psychological awareness. If the psychological basis for the media were better understood and reported, it might result in cultural *reflection* rather than *reflexive* fear. In dreams, the outer symbolic forms always reveal symptoms of interior stresses that need correction. So, Jung's understanding of dream dynamics is much more sophisticated than simplistic "feel good" approaches. The compensational objective of Jungian dream analysis is to neutralize even the most objectionable patterns such as torture and malice, famine and genocide and to harmonize them with coherent alternatives that are contextual.

As it contemplates an "information society for all," Europe's *Information Society* reminds Europeans that, "While Information & Communication Technologies can reinforce social inclusion, offering new opportunities for many people currently excluded from today's society, we must make them accessible to everyone if we are to avoid creating a new divide between the "digital haves" and "have-nots." (Europe's Information Society, 2011) This is a commendable notion, but the scope of the perceived issue is far too narrow. The true scope of any issue related to modern information technology is universal and encompasses the psychological impacts of the global media on both "digital haves" and "have nots", and this entails its electromagnetic impacts on the unified field of energy and information.

Perhaps a culture's interactive imaging media—including ICTs, the Internet, film, and video games—can serve the function of the Jungian psychiatrist who assists a *patient* to access unconscious meaning, to reframe the cognitive unconscious of contextual collectives, and to foster coherent psychological states. Advances in sophisticated algorithms support this possibility. The following are just a few examples:

- A robot just passed the self-awareness test (Geere, Duncan, 2015)
- A better way to design brain inspired chips (Simonite, Tom, 2015)

- Why neural networks look to thrash human Go players for the first time (Anonymous, 2014)
- AI revolution—road to superintelligence (Urban, Tim, 2015)
- Virtual reality startups look back to the future (Parkin, Tim, 2014).

Like the dreams of an individual, contextual media dreams provide a potential for meaningful insight. Within the unified dream field, the various media sources (website "likes", blogs, television, social networks, film, video games, etc.) and their audiences (defined as target groups) provide context. Not only can ICTs reinforce social inclusion, if they are *reflective* they can foster deep meaningful insights within contextual user groups. Within each group resides the potential for meaningful insight that leads to harmony, coherence, and psychological healing. Increasingly, as ICTs incorporate design and methodology that fosters collective coherence, our global value structures will become more harmonious and sustainable.

PSYCHIC CONTEXT

Coherence and compensation depend on context. Jung defines the term "contextual" in terms of a patient's personality profile as in Myers-Briggs profiles.[2] Jungian context goes beyond the orthodox use of the term and incorporates the entire multi-functional psychic content of an individual or a target group. Dream symbolism serves as the "lighted stage" of *Global Workspace Theory* (Baars, 1997) and serves to delimit and ground parameters of psychological need for meaning. "Compensation" corresponds to "coherence," and may be achieved by degree. In-order to reiterate and expand concepts, Jungian dream analysis assumes that dreams have a contextual purpose that can be discovered during sessions in which the psychiatrist provides contextual feedback to patients who have various degrees of mental disorder. The generic "purpose" of the dream medium is to establish harmony between conscious and unconscious psychic states of the contextual patient, and the Jungian *Amplification Method* is the process whereby a patient achieves insight as to the cause of psychic disharmony. A representative example of this process is provided by Khodarahimi, Siamak (2009). Empirical research verifies that achieving meaningful insight can be curative. However, the idea that meaningful insight can lead to relatively coherent outcomes should not be limited to the treatment of mental disorder. The compensational dynamics of meaningful insight apply equally to creativity, learning, education, and transcendent states such as self-realization in Abraham Maslow"s *Peak Experience* (Kendra, Cherry, 2015a) and the *Flow experience* (Kendra, Cherry, 2015b). It would seem that we have sufficient grounds and good reason for hypothesizing the existence of correspondence between the dynamics of Jungian dreams and the dynamics of media dreams.

- Individual cognitive dynamics = collective cognitive dynamics
- Dream images are projections from unconscious psyche (energy & information) & ICT images are projections from unconscious software (energy & information)
- Narrative-metaphorical structure is a common denominator in:
  - Dreams emerging from the personal and collective unconscious psyche
  - Neurobiological patterns
  - Frames of the cognitive unconscious
- Structure of Jungian dreams = structure of media dreams
- Jungian compensation = coherence
- Individual psychic context = target group context
- Individual dreams have a purpose = media dreams have a purpose
- Meaningful collective purpose = meaningful psychic harmonization and coherence

Indeed, Information and communication technologies are central to modern life, and—like all breakthrough media—ICTs are changing not only the cultural conversation and the human worldview, but—perhaps—the Earth's electromagnetic field. *The Global Coherence Monitoring System* (IHM, 2009) initiated by the Institute of Heartmath has been established to explore fluctuations in the magnetic fields generated by the earth and ionosphere in-order to discover whether the earth's field is influenced by or reflected in human heart-rhythm patterns or brain activity and whether this field can indicate earthquakes, volcanic eruptions and other planetary events. (Institute of Heartmath, 2007) It may be stipulated that media—by stimulating thought, emotion, and other functions—causes electromagnetic changes in individual electromagnetic fields. It may also be stipulated that ICTs are a fundamental aspect of the global technological media; however, that ICTs influence an electromagnetic-psychological field in which psychological pathologies of cultural personae can be diagnosed and ameliorated requires some discussion. The book, *Exploring the Collective Unconscious in a Digital Age* (Schafer, Stephen, ed., 2017), deals with issues relevant to these questions.

Also relevant to these questions is the book, *Amusing Ourselves to Death.* (1985) Neil Postman, contrasts the effects of print and television media—the ICTs of their day—on the cultural conversation, and concludes that the new technology of television is seriously inferior for many important cultural purposes—especially serious purposes like education and government. Though his book was published in 1985, just before the Internet and a plethora of digital applications became commonplace, now is a good time to revisit his conclusions in-order to consider the direction that ICT research should take.

Postman ridicules the idea that—as a medium—television can be used to support a literate tradition aimed at discovery of meaning or to do anything but entertain. He argued that to view television as a medium relevant to the consideration of serious matters is a serious error. Postman's basic assumption is that each medium has its own epistemology—its contextual personality—defined by its structure and the messages it mediates. This idea is essentially Jungian and suggests the relationship that exists between contextual media and the archetypal representations they promote. He asserts that data or information alone is not the solution to cultural problems and that collateral learning is the way that enduring attitudes are formed. (p. 144) He argues that there is little public understanding of what information is and how it provides meaning and gives direction to a culture. (p. 160) Postman limits his argument to discussion of differences in the structure of the print medium and television thus implying issues of cognitive framing. However, in 1985, research on the cognitive unconscious was nascent and—notwithstanding Gestalt and the work of Jung—research on the cognitive impact of images had not been generally upgraded to the current need. "Mind's eye" images and internal representations were explored more fully in Stephen M. Kosslyn's *Image and Brain*. (1994) In 1992, Postman wrote, *Technopoly: the Surrender of Culture to Technology*, where he defines "Technopoly" as a society which believes that technical calculation is in all respects superior to human judgment. (Postman, 1992. p.51) He observed that, "Information has become a form of garbage, not only incapable of answering the most fundamental human questions but barely useful in providing coherent direction to the solution of even mundane problems." (p. 69) Postman is right, and his allusion to the importance of psychological coherence in mediation establishes his prescience. However, the technology Postman refers to is the mind-based sophistry mentioned above. If the influence of heart-coherence is introduced into the technological format, technological potentials for meaningful discovery expand exponentially.

As fundamental television epistemology, the profound impact of images on the personal and collective unconscious and issues of electromagnetic impact and influence on the cognitive unconscious were unheard of in 1992. Even with the advent of PCs, the Internet, and the vast array of imaging media applications available today, research on the impacts of imagery as cognitive reality lag far behind the need to know. Though advertising methods have always manipulated the unconscious, advertisers didn't really understand the cognitive complexity of what they were doing. They were limited to the principle of unconscious associations without understanding the neurological processes. The PBS documentary, *The persuaders* (Goodman, Barak, Dretzen, Rachel, Rushkoff, Douglas, Soenens, Murial, and Fanning, David, 2004), explores advertising that ranges from discovery of the "buy code" residing in the cognitive unconscious through high concept adds, and political advertising. Given this comprehensive exploration of the history, motives, successes, failures, and trends in advertising, it becomes clear that industry understanding of cognitive processes has been rudimentary. Today's neuromarketing exemplars know a little more than their forerunners. Based on some knowledge of psychology, one of these, Susan Weinschenk says:

We are multichannel [multi-functional] in many ways, right? We can listen and see at the same time. However, if you overload that too much, then we're not going to be paying attention. So, if you're showing me something on the slide and there's movement and there's animation going on while you're saying something, it's unlikely that I'm really listening to you anymore. (Dooley, Roger, 2015)

As mentioned above, though it was published in 1996, early in the cognitive revolution, the revelations of another book, *The Media Equation* by Reeves and Nass, are consistent with the most recent research on the cognitive unconscious. Their hypothesis was that—at unconscious levels—people perceive media as real and treat it in socially meaningful ways. Indeed, research discloses that people of all demographics treat media as if it is real; i.e. as if it has personality (p. 6-7). Reeves and Nass conducted thirty-five experiments, and all of them verified the media equation. Some of their findings are that, "Perceived reality does not depend on verisimilitude." (p. 85) Even line drawings are rich in personality. As long as the drawings have eyes and mouths or appear to be alive, they will evoke psychologically rich responses from viewers. (p. 85) All such "social" interfaces have a personality and evoke social responses. Also, these responses apply to "anything that presents words to a user, including LCD panels, toaster ovens, televisions, word processors and workstations." (p. 97) "Personality can be perceived in the most minimal of places—a simple English sentence." (p. 85)

At unconscious levels, ICTs are perceived as having social personalities, and this is directly relevant to multi-functional understanding of personality and the cognitive unconscious expressed by Jung and Lakoff. Increasingly, a prime virtue of ICT epistemology is that—like dreams—they are geared to problem solving whether the target group consists of consumers, students, or patients. This orientation could be extended to psychological problem-solving with relative ease. As we have seen, users perceive media in terms of personality. ICTs should be designed to take advantage of this fact in-order to satisfy the unconscious expectations of its target groups. One possibility is that the personality of ICTs should be consistent with culturally defined personalities of problem-solvers such as consultants, priests, or teachers but not limited to their contextual ideologies. In other words, ICT personalities should have coherent character. In-order to foster a coherent media experience,

ICT software should project—insofar as possible—the persona of a contextual problem-solver with a very broad and progressive mind—one that has discovered coherent meaning. Moreover, George Lakoff's argument is that people influenced predominantly by the Nurturant Parent Metaphor tend to have a progressive social orientation characterized by empathy, mutual respect, and balance which is consistent with American democratic values. It goes without saying that civilization benefits by progressive social skills—not by anti-social skills that often (but not always) characterize a Strict Father orientation. Lakoff says:

We have reached a point where our democracy is in mortal danger—as is the very livability of our planet. We can no longer put off an understanding of how the brain and the unconscious mind both contribute to these problems and how they may provide solutions. (2008, p. 11)

Because ICTs correspond to brain and unconscious mind, designers of ICTs should incorporate significant knowledge of neurobiological dynamics. For example, neural binding creates emotional experience. (Lakoff, 2008, p. 27) Dramatic structural circuitry called somatic markers activate convergent pathways, and somatic markers allow the right emotions to go where they should in a story." (Lakoff, 2008, p. 28) Lakoff also says:

Language links words and phrases to structures like these [cognitive frames, narrative, neural binding, event structures, X-schema] via neural circuitry. These circuits, when activated, create an experienced simulation—most likely below the level of consciousness. It is that imaginative simulation experienced inwardly that constitutes "meaning." (2008, p. 236)

It is fairly straightforward to recommend that ICT design be based on principles of neural framing circuitry needed to create frame structures. (Lakoff, 2008, p. 22) These "tend to structure a huge amount of our thought. Each frame has roles (like a cast of characters), relations between the roles, and scenarios played out by those playing the roles." (p. 22) Realizing this dynamic allows for contextualization of e-care software as well as promotion of coherent frameworks in patients; i.e. within the narrative structure of cognitive frames, "appropriate emotions…fit certain kinds of events in the scenarios." Appropriate emotions are coherent emotions within the contextual state.

It may be stipulated that sensory perceptions are "contextual," so ICTs should be designed—using more refined knowledge than relatively simple focus group analysis—to fit a contextual audience. Not only the message, but the epistemology of the medium should be targeted to contextual groups or the context of a personal psyche. If social expectations on the part of the target group are met and meaning discovered, incoherent emotions are less likely to emmerge and coherent psychological states are more likely to ensue. The evidence provided by Reeves and Nass has had a profound effect on the design of "user friendly" PCs because PCs are perceived by users as having personalities. For example, "People prefer computers with personalities similar to their own." (p. 96) Also, "People will perceive a computer that uses dominant text as having a dominant personality, and a computer with submissive text as having a submissive personality." (p. 91) The salient message is that, as far as neural activity goes, "mediated" pictures and sounds produce the same meaningful results that would occur if the people, objects, and places were actually present. (p. 116) Given the relatively simple psychology explored by Reeves and Nass and the profound effect their work had on computer science and markets, it is likely that ICTs design that is sensitive to current knowledge about coherent cognitive frames could contribute to more profound and meaningful media.

The most recent research in neurolinguistics verifies the media equation and explains why the nervous system functions this way. Linguist Charles Fillmore discovered that words are all defined relative to conceptual frames, and scientists have discovered frames by looking for generalizations over groups of related words— metaphorical resonance. (Lakoff, 2008, pp. 22-23) Another way to say this is that the electromagnetic forces that exist at archetypal levels of the unconscious are patterned according to principles of electricity and magnetism and—at conscious levels—are perceived as image patterns that are structured as drama and metaphor. In this context, "metaphorical resonance" is literally a matter of both quantitative and qualitative (contextual) frequency that correlates to the energetic principles of physics.

A paraphrase of this finding is that humans refer their choices and behaviors to dramatic patterns which exist at unconscious levels, and that these stories define morality. Using sophisticated electronic technology, researchers are learning more every day about how the brain works. A salient discovery is that brain function should be studied not solely in terms of location in the brain but in terms of frequency synchronization and plasticity. Researchers have estimated that about 98% of human reason functions at unconscious levels of psyche. Moreover, what we call "reason" incorporates emotion, and is shaped by the vast and invisible realm of functional neural circuitry not accessible to consciousness. Therefore, it can be said that reason is structured according to dramatic frames, metaphors, images, and symbols that are unconscious or archetypal. (Lakoff, 2008, p. 14) Advertisers have been using psychological principles for half a century with extraordinarily predictable results, and governments have just begun to grasp the incredible propagandistic power of psychological design. In-order to foster coherent psychological states, multi-functional coherence as measured by heart rate variability (McCraty & Childre, 2010) provides the more refined ICT framework suggested above. Such cognitive-psychiatric principles of measurable coherence should be used to design ICTs.

Different groups have different—contextual—tastes which, in the advertising industry, are analyzed in focus groups in-order to personify a target group. It can be deduced from Jung's work that the contextual personality of an individual has the same dynamics as the contextual personality of a cultural, ethnic group, or "target" group. Such context is defined by the shared symbolic language, values, and choices of the collective. One group likes reality shows while another watches PBS. One group is Christian, another is Islamic. Once the persona of a contextual group is carefully defined with research, the viewing tastes of the group can be analyzed using Jungian principles of dream analysis within focus groups to address psychic disharmony and to access contextual meaning in the group. This concept can be extended to cultures. Theoretically, the contextual media dream of a culture can be analyzed with ICT algorithms that incorporate dream dynamics to promote coherence as part of their research with focus groups. When a focus group achieves insight, the process leading to the collective insight can be translated and applied to programs and content of a contextual domain in the media.

We know from our longstanding cultural experience and market research that meaningful subliminal messages imbedded in advertisements are relatively predictable in their influence on target groups. Though discovery of meaning is not the objective of advertisers, the nature of such meaningful discovery must become a priority in ICT research. Psychological dynamics have been employed to alter unconscious cognitive frameworks, cultural values, laws, choices, and behaviors. This fact is best illustrated in the Public Relations as conceived by Edward Bernays which changed American culture from a needs-based economy to a want-based economy that has become the "Consumer Culture." (Curtis, a & b) The American context has had obvious influence on the entire Western World context, and it is expanding rapidly to every part of the world. In-order to make the best use of R & D for the emergent ICT industry, our perspective on its vast power to alter cognitive reality must be addressed as a priority. It is only a matter of time before we begin to understand the power of the media—especially the interactive media—as a palpable psychic phenomenon for the discovery of meaning. This understanding will mark a breakthrough in our sense of responsibility for the direct power humans wield with both the causal and non-local energy of their thought and desires. It is within this context that ICT management must pursue research. The optimal e-care is that which heals culture.

Developments in emergent ICT technologies and models in e-Health, e-Social care, and the economics of modern social demands are just the tip of the iceberg. ICTs are the fundamental medium underlying an emergent paradigm shift into a mediated age where Fascism and Socialism are currently at odds. But these alternatives may be outdated phantoms, while other alternatives related to cosmic coherence and sentience may be in the offing. Increasingly, ICTs translate energy and information of psyche-physics into sensory projections that are understandable as "real" and "meaningful" by human beings. In other words, ICTs constitute the language of an emergent worldview that is projected as a sort of Metaverse or mediated dream. This GPS (General Problem Solver) language is analogous to the archetypal language of psyche as defined by Carl Jung. According to Jung, these archetypal energies and information patterns are projected as images from the personal and collective unconscious, (Jacoby, p. 58-59) and Jung based his entire system of dream analysis on the assumption that this archetypal language is interactive (Dream images change according to patient insight as to meaning.) and can be read in the imbedded dramatic symbolism of dream images. This symbolic language—correctly understood—can teach and heal persons and collectives from dimensions of the cognitive unconscious where contextual meaning may be found. (Jacoby; Schafer & Yu) The "media dream" appears to have all the dynamics of dreams as defined by Jung. (Shafer & Yu)

CONTEXTUAL COSMIC SENTIENCE

It only takes a quantum hop to realize that universe is conscious, and that "consciousness" may be better understood in terms of coherent sentience and QED frequencies. Contextual culture is a serious, practical concern of the EU with its many member states. Each culture has its own way of perceiving things—its own sentience. For starters, each cultural persona perceives the world according to its native language and its own contextual personality. It may be stipulated that, like all languages, ICTs have a contextual syntax and symbolism that delimits what can be communicated. This characteristic should be carefully considered when focusing on a target group. As we have seen, context is an important term in Jungian theory. Jung stressed the importance of "context" as it relates to everything knowable about a patient—age, gender, culture, profession, history, language, etc. It is already apparent that cyber-language that allows communication among Asians, Europeans, and Americans has had an impact on world-unification.

The ability to read the contextual language of a patient's dreams with empathy and accuracy leads to meaningful insight and coherence. Everyone has experienced frustration and incoherence resulting from efforts to communicate in an unfamiliar language. Therefore, in-order for ICTs to foster coherence, they must be programmed to understand the contextual languages and unconscious psychological profiles of diverse target personae. In other words, designers of ICTs must now learn the language of dreams and use it to design the images projected from the cognitive unconscious of contextual groups. Unconscious archetypal patterns are projected into dream symbols which tell a contextual story from unconscious dimensions where contextual meaning can be discovered. Like the generative source of dreams, ICT software projects images on the monitor. Using inverse proportion and principles of Fourier transforms, the software can be designed to embed symbolism that evokes insight in contextual groups. Just as the cognitive unconscious employs the language of dreams to evoke insight in the dreamer, ICT software could use images to evoke meaningful insight in target groups. The more successful the design, the more coherent the user response will be, and this coherent energy and information will extend to the media dream and the geo-electromagnetic field.

It may be stipulated that ICTs are central to modern life. As such, they constitute strategic media for the reframing of media dreams. In *Steps to an Ecology of Mind*, Gregory Bateson pointed out that understanding the "territory" depends on some *representation*, and that no matter how carefully it is measured, a map is ultimately a retinal representation—not the territory itself. However, in the same volume, Bateson observes that the usefulness of a map is not necessarily a matter of its literal truthfulness. Rather the usefulness of a map depends on its having a structure analogous (for the purpose at hand) to the "territory." ICTs have the structural-representational capability to simulate the *territory* of a culture's cognitive unconscious. Just as the narrative-metaphorical patterns in a dream can be analyzed to afford insight as to the psychic condition of a patient, the narrative-metaphorical patterns in a culture's media dream can be analyzed to afford meaningful insight as to the psychic condition of a culture. Based on such analysis—as strategic media—ICTs could be developed to help reframe the cognitive unconscious of a culture's people according to non-invasive benign contextual insight.

For the purposes at hand, media dreams—like Jungian dreams—are subject to analysis by-virtue of the analogous narrative-metaphorical structure shared by images in the collective media and images in dreams. In a classical sense (The whole exists within the part; As it is above, so it is below.) Jung understood that the collective psyche (both conscious and unconscious) has recursive relationship with the individual psyche. "Every Collective, every nation, reflects in magnified form the psychic state of its individual components." (Jung, 1933) Jolande Jacoby, the student and colleague of Jung, asks rhetorically, "May one speak of a structure or morphology of the unconscious, and if so, how much do we know about it? Is it possible to obtain definite information about what is 'unknown' to consciousness? The answer is yes." Jacoby answers her own question saying, "Not directly…but only through such effects and indirect manifestations as the symptoms and complexes, images and symbols that we encounter in dreams, fantasies, and visions." (Jacoby,

1973, p. ?ff) Such symbols and complexes, dreams, fantasies, and visions can also be discerned in a culture's media dreams, and they are all processed by the same part of the brain. (Lakoff)

In a footnote, Jacoby adds that, "The parallel with the hypothesis of physics is obvious. We have no direct perceptions of waves and atoms but infer their existence from observed effects." (p. 36) "In *Nature* (p. 215), Jung draws a parallel between 'matter' and 'psyche' and suggests the possibility that they may be two different aspects of the same thing." (Jacoby, p. 62) From a perspective on molecular biology and medicine, Deepak Chopra develops a similar argument in his, *Body, Mind, and Soul*. (Chopra) Furthermore, the theme of the parallels between physics and psyche or myth is observed by many. (Capra, Bohm, Chopra, et al.)

ICT Language Anchors Thought

The position that language anchors thought is longstanding and relevant to research on ICTs as a mediating language. "It was argued cogently by Bhartrihari (6th c.AD) and was the subject of centuries of debate in the Indian linguistic tradition. Related notions in the West, such as the axiom that language has controlling effects upon thought, can be traced to Wilhelm von Humboldt's essay *Über das vergleichende Sprachstudium* ("On the comparative study of languages"), and the notion has been largely assimilated into Western thought." (Psychology Wiki, para. 3)

Paraphrasing information culled from Wikipedia, in linguistics, the Sapir-Whorf hypothesis (SWH) states that there is a systematic relationship between the grammatical categories of the language a person speaks and how that person both understand the world and behaves in it. Arguments relative to the theme are far-ranging, extending from the opposite idea that language has absolutely no influence on thought (Gumperz 1996) to Noam Chomsky's focus on the innateness and universality of language, Steven Pinker's theory that some sort of universal language underlies all language, and George Lakoff's argument that all language is essentially metaphor. For instance, English employs many metaphorical tropes such as, *spend time, waste time,* or *invest time* that equate time with money.

ICTs adhere to the concept of a universal language that underlies all languages. Of particular relevance to this paper is Whorf's observation that, in general, Western languages tend to analyze reality as objects in space wherein *present* and *future* are places and *time* is a path linking them. On the other hand, non-western languages, including many Native American languages, are oriented toward an entirely different worldview—process. Whorf observed that a Hopi speaker would find relativistic physics fundamentally easier to grasp than a speaker of standard average European. ICTs adhere more closely to this idea of language as process, and this warns designers of quality e-care that Western prejudices about time and space may be outdated.

239

ICTs employ the same patterns of energy and information as psyche and they project images according to the same dynamics as dreams. For the purposes at hand, the projected image is the contextual *representation* of the dramatic-metaphorical (archetypal) language of the *territory*. According to Jung, the dream medium is a projection of archetypal energy and information patterns that are generated from the personal and collective unconscious. Like all media, dreams are a language for transmission of energy and information between conscious and unconscious states. Any conversation between two people is a medium for translation of unconscious content into conscious content; what A communicates to B remains unconscious content for B until it is mediated by A and perceived by B.

ICTs the Medium of Dreams

The mediating function provided by ICTs is much like the mediating function provided by dreams. Like the images in dreams, it is the images projected by ICTs that trigger unconscious patterns of percepts and affordances which then generate interpretations and choices. Images provide symbolic clues that contribute to the evolutionary learning process and bring unconscious meaning into a state of consciousness. According to Jung, images are the projections of archetypal "energy" patterns that carry "information" that can be interpreted with reference to their dramatic-metaphorical frameworks. Like dreams, such images constitute a language between conscious and unconscious psychic states.

The manner in which archetypal energy and information can be analyzed by referring to dramatic-metaphorical patterns in the nervous system is discussed at length by George Lakoff. He cites Roger Shank and Robert Abelson in his paraphrase, "Complex narratives—the kinds we find in everyone's life story, as well as in fairy tales, novels, and dramas—are made up of smaller narratives with very simple structures." Lakoff says, "The neural circuitry needed to create frame structures is relatively simple [neural binding circuitry, neural signatures, event structures] and so cognitive frames tend to structure a huge percentage of cognitive function. Sounding remarkably like Jung who observed that dreams have dramatic action that can meaningfully be broken down into the elements of a Greek play (Jacoby, p. 83), Lakoff explains that each frame has roles (like a cast of characters), relations between the roles, and scenarios carried out by those playing the roles." (Lakoff, 2007, p. 22) "There is a protagonist, the person whose point of view is being taken. The events are good and bad things that happen. And there are appropriate emotions that fit certain kinds of events in the scenarios." (Lakoff, 2002, p. 23) Citing Goffman, Dr. Lakoff also observes that words are all defined relative to conceptual frames: "Groups of related words, called 'semantic fields,' are defined with respect to the same frame. Thus words like 'cost,' 'sell,' 'goods,' 'price,' 'buy,' and so on are defined with respect to a single frame," (Lakoff, 2007, p 22) and the roles of Buyer, Seller, Goods, and Money, form a narrative field context for the frame.

In *Moral Politics*, Lakoff explains in detail how "much of moral reasoning is metaphorical reasoning." An example of how narrative-metaphorical resonance can influence morality is discussed by Lakoff in terms of the core metaphor of moral accounting. According to this fundamental metaphor, a syllogism is established: well-being is good; well-being is moral; wealth contributes to well-being; to be wealthy is moral. According to this *Moral Accounting metaphor*, economic words like *owe, debt,* and *pay* are used in a moral context. (Lakoff, 2008, p. 63) The result is a logical framework in which the metaphorical resonance suggests that wealth is better than poverty (good), so being wealthy is moral (good). Lakoff explains:

A conceptual metaphor is a correspondence between concepts across conceptual domains, allowing forms of reasoning and words from one domain (in this case, the economic domain) to be used in the other (in this case, the moral domain)... Thousands of such metaphors contribute to our everyday modes of thought, (and) play an enormous role in characterizing our worldviews. (Lakoff, 2002, p. 63)

Reminiscent of Jungian amplification, Lakoff describes *radial conceptual categories* as the most common form of metaphorical structure. "The radial categories show how the coherent ideologies in each category fit together and what the relationships among them are." (Lakoff, 2002, p. 14)

Like archetypal constructs of energy and information, ICTs complete a feedback loop analogous to Chomske's generative language. ICTs generate energy that is projected as informational images on a computer monitor. At both conscious and unconscious levels, the computer user perceives pixel patterns in terms of symbolic images. The symbols are registered in the nervous system of the user, interpreted, and generate a response. The user response is then interpreted by the ICT software which generates another pixel pattern to which the user responds. This interactive process is registered and preserved in the nervous system and in the software according to very similar dynamics for processing energy and information. Interpretations lead—eventually or spontaneously—to the discovery of meaning (for the user) which resides at archetypal levels of his contextual persona, but the conscious-unconscious process by which that meaningful insight is achieved is preserved both in the nervous system and the software. With the use of imaging technologies such as EEG, ECG, MEG, future Psychecology Games (PEG), and gaze tracking, patterns preserved in the nervous system can be compared with patterns preserved by the software. In this way, patterns tending to coherence can be reinforced and the efficiency of the process improved with appropriate, compensational feedback. Essentially, this is what the Jungian *Amplification Method* does. A computer constitutes an analog of Jungian psyche, and the images on its monitor constitute an analog to dreams. Global Workspace Theory employs the "Theatre Metaphor" to explain the relationship between conscious and unconscious psyche. The lighted stage is consciousness; the audience and backstage constitute a receptive and directive unconscious. (Baars)

- Electrical circuits and programs = conscious-unconscious neurobiological cognitive frameworks
- Pixel patterns on the monitor = projections of the electrical circuits and programs
- Projections = metaphors
- Metaphor = algorithmic recursion of isometric form
- Correspondence = fractal synchronicity
- Computer user (gamer) = dreamer
- Projected images on the monitor = dreamscape
- Consciousness = Computer monitor, the lighted stage of Global Workspace Theory
- Unconscious = audience and backstage of GWT
- Interpretations = percepts (conscious) + affordances (unconscious)
- Choice = conscious + unconscious response to images
- Interactivity of the dreamer with the dream image = Interactivity of the ICT user with the image on the monitor
- Interactive choices create a living feedback loop into the unconscious world of meaning) = responses to symbolic clues that contribute to the learning process and lead to the discovery of meaning

Computer users do not focus their attention on the computer's circuitry, ICTs, or the underlying physics, but on the monitor images that are informed with information patterns based in perceptions of energy fields. Though this fact is self-evident; and, as mentioned above, it has been verified with the research of Reeves & Nass and many others. Metaphorically, a computational process is all energy and information. Like psyche, itself, the energy and information patterns that constitute ICT computations correspond to the patterns of energy and information that constitute neurobiological wetware. They become conscious as they are interpreted by the psyche of a computer user, and the psyche—being integrated—may be quantified according to the dance of Fourier transforms. In the same way, we focus our attention not on the unconscious circuitry and physics of psyche, but on the imagery, symbolic content, and affordances we call *life*. We might ask ourselves, "How real is the metaphor?" Are such processes recursive within the *actual* frequencies of psyche; and, if they are, what constitutes a point of synchronicity among recursions? Extensive HeartMath research has defined coherence as a marker that can be identified using the sign-wave signature of heart rate variability. (McCraty & Childre, 2010)

ICT Drama as Dream

Marketing employs literary-psychological principles to sell products, and no one can deny the success or the effectiveness of advertising. Advertisers research the subliminal workings of a target group, project an image of that identification into the design of an advertisement, predispose the target group to suspend disbelief, and then allow the psychological association to develop between the subject and the product (object). It has been demonstrated that cognitive dynamics are the same whether applied to advertising in games or healing in dreams and video games. As to be expected, the game industry is contemplating the profitability of using advertising in games. Why not contemplate the more profound profitability of healing with games? First, let us consider the nature of the dynamic called drama:

All the world's a stage,
And all the men and women merely players:
They have their exits and their entrances;
And one man in his time plays many parts,
His acts being seven ages. (Shakespeare, *As You Like It*, II, *vii*, 139)

Humans perceive their waking dream in terms of a story—a narrative pattern in which they project their subconscious selves onto an image they perceive as their *real* life. In other words, they project archetypes of the unconscious onto people and events in their reality. As remarked above, they project their subjective identity (the shadow archetype) onto the screen of the waking dream and the totality of the conscious world becomes a stage. The projected self-reflection provided by a role model is one of the more accessible tools with which we design our persona. Both subliminally and consciously, we design our persona after the patterns associated with our role models be they father, mother, or Spider Man. This is part of the dynamic whereby we suspend disbelief and become the persona we perceive as the protagonist in the story. In projections of video game avatars, this psychology is becoming known as the *Imago effect* which is discussed by Brian Keplesky (Keplesky, Brian, 2007a) reporting on a presentation given by Harvey Smith. (Keplesky, Brian, 2007b) It is in this way—perceiving ourselves as separate—that we learn important things like individuality, personal responsibility, the difference between free-will and destiny, the importance of choice, morality, and love. Apparently, such learning constitutes the bennies of suffering experience in the world of form.

Altogether, the four acts of our personal or collective drama (The Ages of Man) have a premise of self-actualization or atonement—the discovery of meaning. According to our greatest teachers and philosophers, knowing one's self—*healing* or making oneself *whole*—is the purpose of the drama of life—the waking dream—in which we play our part in the number of scenes allotted to us. In each of our individual stories, the exposition, backbone, and solution of our drama always relates to a *premise* (Schafer 2007) having to do with self-actualization. We all ask the same questions. Who am I, and why am I here? Where did I come from? Where am I going? During a human lifetime, the answers to these questions reside at subliminal levels of the psyche just waiting to be "realized" or provided with form and pattern according to interpretations of perceived affordances embedded in our unique experience.

Accordingly, we *think* our reality and, doing so, create it. The waking dream, the sleeping dream, and the rhetorical narrative all have the same patterns. This view is critically important relative to quality ICT management because dramatic structure is a recursively isometric form that is a common denominator among the most significant formats of human neurobiological, psychophysiological *reality*. The best advertisements are dreamlike stories implanted with symbols that resonate with archetypal levels of the psyche. Thus it is in game level design of many popular story-based-games that employ the powerful mythic-psychological symbolism and narrative pattern of the Hero's Journey. Because this subliminal pattern in games has such mythic-psychological clout, players enjoy the game without even knowing why. No matter what relative permutations the pattern affords, the theme of self-actualization is intrinsic to narrative structures and Jungian *Individuation* which may be understood as a healing dynamic. (Jung 1933, p. 26)

ICTs and PEGs

The ubiquitous self-actualization questions mentioned above can be researched with simulations of dramatically structured dream images in Drama Based video Games. (Schafer& Yu) The psychological dynamics discussed above are aspects of theoretical PEG design, and they should become dynamics in design of ICTs. PEG can be used in conjunction with an array of brain-scan and biomarker technologies to probe neurobiological patterns, explore cognitive functions, and improve understanding of how humans learn and how they access "meaning." This paper has been addressed to discussion of research on correlated neurobiological and *archetypal* energy patterns and coherence as a healing dynamic that can be programmed with ICT algorithms in- order to enhance quality e-management.

As discussed above, the discovery of psychic meaning constitutes the essence of both learning and healing, and discovery can be measured with degrees of coherence.

An array of experiments verifying this functional dynamic has been done at the Institute of HeartMath using their Em-Wave technology. (2015) The means for using ICT algorithms to research cognitive meaning with PEG has been theorized in a number of publications. (Schafer, Stephen, 2007, 2011, 2012; Schafer & Yu, 2011) The theoretical arguments in these publications—though multi-faceted—are founded on the existence of the unified, energetic, dramatic common denominator among primary cognitive models, the dramatic structure of images, dreams, and the Media-sphere. In brief, the Media-sphere can be understood to have the same dynamics and purposes as cosmic psyche, and research has progressed far enough to make benign use of this dynamic with mediated biofeedback.

Because PEG can simulate all the psychological dynamics of dreams, playing PEG could evoke and measure both conscious and unconscious neurolinguistic patterns associated with human cognition. Using imaging technologies (EEG, ECG, fMRI, MEG, gaze-tracking, and biofeedback), such simulations can be used to probe neurobiological patterns and to correlate them with archetypal patterns related to learning, "meaningful insight", human transformation, and healing—thus bridging the gap between physics and psychology. Interactive player responses to dramatic content in PEG game images can be designed according to Jungian amplification procedures and computationally "remembered", correlated, and articulated in order to induce a *coherent* state in the player, "where our hearts, minds, and bodies are united in a feeling of wholeness." (McCraty & Childre, p. 10) Being in a state of coherence/ Flow enhances "resilience," performance, and learning. "The various concepts and measurements embraced under the term coherence have become central to fields as diverse as quantum physics, cosmology, physiology, and brain and consciousness research." (Ibid) Flow is correlated with insight, learning, and healing, so as a state of *Flow* is achieved while playing PEG, coherent neurobiological pathways in the *contextual* cognitive unconscious of the player can be tracked and reinforced.

So, the true challenge related to development and management of ICTs is not simply to provide information and to move data. The true challenge is to access cognitive meaning, to navigate the media dream, and to foster coherence in the planetary electromagnetic field. In-order to clarify the concept of the media dream and its basis in metaphorical correspondence imbedded in the fractal stories told by images, the following is illustrative.

Jung's entire theory is based on *libido* which he defines as *psychic energy*, and its dynamic function in a unified field of psyche. If ICTs employing the mathematics of recursion can be applied to the programming of Jungian psychic function, they can be projected onto computer monitors. As in dreams, the symbolic "forms" of the personal and collective unconscious can be imbedded in game images to await the conscious/unconscious insights of players. It is with this understanding that the Jungian dynamics of compensational dream analysis may be programmed into ICTs and game mechanics. So too, the mathematics of recursion—perhaps Finite Element Analysis Packages— (Prathap, Gangen, 1993) could be designed and used in the development of game software sufficient to trace the neural pathways of the cognitive unconscious that lead to coherent meaning.

The self-evident cultural influences of advertising, statistics, polls, and propaganda provide sufficient proof of their cultural effect. The subconscious messages of the media are constantly being used to alter personal and cultural values and to change personal and collective choices and actions. It remains only to apply the cognitive framing potentials latent in the media dream to objectives that are more profound and curative than the pursuit of a superficially limited economic delusion at the cost of cultural sanity and environmental catastrophe.

Though it remains to be verified, using the media-dream as a reference point, the contextual premise of a culture can be realized using a process of cognitive re-framing akin to Jung's amplification method. Within the unified field context of Psyche, the narrative dimensions of dream images (dramatic unities, place, time, *dramatis personae*, exposition, *peripety, lysis*, premise, purpose, etc.) also exist in the collective dream field as portrayed in the media-dream. Premise is defined as, "that which a character learns" during the course of a story. (Glassner; Schafer, 2007) For example, referring to the illustration above, a population may understand that the message of the bridge metaphor can be realized not only at physical levels but at psychic levels. Like an individual on the psychiatrist's couch, a contextual collective—with the help of its media—can achieve insight as to the symbolic psychological significance of a crumbling moral infrastructure that needs attention.

ISSUES, CONTROVERSIES, AND PROBLEMS

An emergent epistemology of moral government must be understood in terms of an ontology of coherent sentient energy frequencies in a *Psychecology*. Addressing the Global Crisis will require high frequency creative cooperation. An existing global humanitarian constituency now represents a critical mass of human spirit-energy that agrees as to coherent "Spiritual" values. It is the Heart—distributive & collective—that provides access to the Soul of the planet Earth. The *collective persona must become the collective Soul*. In-order to manifest as a "coherent" Humanitarian Organism, the organism must be *self-conscious* and function as a global cooperative. To do so, the human *True Self*, must coordinate the lower frequency bandwidths of Personality with the higher frequency bandwidths of the Soul—superhuman spiritual sentience. In theological terms, God works through the efforts of humanity. In other words, the source of human creativity consists of higher Order influences that manifest through the human filtering organism. Beyond issues of possession by evil forces, we can speculate that the Divine plan has to do with the ultimate emergence of the *Coherent Planetary Soul* that is the essence of a *Global Culture of Conscience.* Modern science and technology has provided humanity with a new language and science-based worldview with which humanitarians may finally achieve this objective. (Schafer, Stephen Brock, 2018, p. 532)

A conscious understanding of the symbolic message proffered by the world's media dreams will surely lead to psychological-emotional stress and its destructive consequences. But can a whole culture be sick? Can a society lie on the psychiatrist's couch? Can a culture be healed of neurotic or psychotic tendencies? Can a culture's media assist it in understanding the cause of its psychological disharmonies and help to define, disclose, and disarm its psychological defense mechanisms? These questions must be answered with an array of research on the psychological media. We argue that analysis of media dreams can do just that if the mediated dreams are understood as warnings. The average informed individual can sense the covert messages underlying advertisements, but students of symbolism and psychology can provide a detailed exegesis of the psychological-symbolism in advertisements. Barak Goodman in Frontline's *The Persuaders* (2004) explores the psychiatric dynamics underlying the archetypal codes that push the primal psychic buttons of an advertisement's target group. Amateurs of film, drama, and literature understand something about the dynamics of immersion and suspension of disbelief that allows them to project self onto symbolic actors and situations. Students of the media understand the propagandistic methods whereby mediated messages become the atrocities of Rwanda, the final solution of the Nazis, or the eco-systemic fouling of our own nest. The mediated dream is palpable.

But collectively, we seem bemused. Though the psychological dynamics of the modern media should be well-know, few seem to be paying attention. This pervasive apathy relative to media issues and meaning must be due to deeper complications of the psyche. Our inattention, inaction, and willful misdirection must have a psychological explanation—fear, self-loathing, and defense mechanisms must account for our neuroses. At least in the US, this is suggested by the fact that even sitcom hero-projections are often violent, adumbrated, supercilious, narcissistic, and obsessive-compulsive. Where is this trend going? The unwelcome answer is that it's going in the direction of a severely psychotic event. Unless media professionals throughout the world remove the ego-serving hoodwinks, it will be too late. Not much time left.

The controversies and problems related to the theme of the paper are legion, but they can be diminished by opening our minds to a "territory" more vasty than the archaic materialistic model

FUTURE RESEARCH DIRECTIONS

Happily, there may be a solution. It may not work in time, but at least it would be interesting. What if, in this time of fear and loathing, the citizens of the nation were to demand and support a major initiative to study the media *Psyche*cology from the perspective of the media dream? No one can possibly complain about the cost of such an initiative! How much are we paying for wars? How much are we paying for corporate welfare? How much are we paying for the annihilation of our ecosystem? How much are we paying for illegal military black ops? How much are we paying for antiquated systems of education? How much for bailouts of the banks? It boggles the mind! Moreover, none of these costs is redeemable. The costs of war, waste, and deception are permanent and irretrievable. On the other hand, the benefits of right use of the technological media are efficient, synergistic, and economically bullish. Solutions exist. It is the will that is lacking. But perhaps if we begin trying to understand the meaningful messages sent to us from the collective unconscious by way of our media dream, we would experience an epiphany by which contextual personae could atone with the contextual soul.

As it happens, the solution is more specific. There is a particular medium that has the potential to revolutionize education and provide a curriculum for an incipient media age. It has the potential to harness the power of the collective unconscious and to harmonize the collective psyche. What is this panacea? The answer is video games—specifically those called *Psyche*cology video games and Massively Multiplayer Online Games (MMOGs). The media in general and the medium of Video games in particular may conceal the power to mend our cultural bridges.

SUMMARY AND CONCLUSION

We must begin to come to grips with the psychological nature of the electronic media and begin to use benign psychology to reframe the cognitive unconscious. To date, *human consciousness* has had a traumatic influence upon the course of planetary vitality and evolution. What remains unrecognized is that *the unconsciousness of collective humanity* has even more impact. We have the tools to deal with our current crisis of opportunity, but we are not yet making use of them. Just as we have had the solutions to our ecological problems and our energy needs for decades but have ignored them, we ignore the psychological solutions to social pathology proffered by ICTs and the findings of cognitive sciences.

Because they are somewhat rational, humans occupy a dual reality that consists of the known and the unknown, the conscious and the unconscious, the self and the not self, the persona and the shadow. Some say this is a punishment (the fall of man). Others say it is an opportunity for humans to learn about themselves in-order to achieve transcendence. But philosophy and psychology teach that human rationality is only one aspect of their cognitive capacity; and, at subliminal or super-conscious levels, humans are in touch with other dimensions of awareness. However, some form of the media is necessary for any translation of information from one dimension to another—to transform the unknown into the known. On its simplest levels this process is understood as the acquisition of knowledge. On deeper more comprehensive levels the process is understood as the acquisition of various degrees of meaning leading to wisdom which eventually leads to transcendence of the human condition—the realization that the coherent individual is functionally divine.

The ultimate human *premise* is to overcome the illusion of separation. Winning the game of life requires the player to understand and apply the rules. At this particular juncture in human development, the rules of the game seem directly related to the dynamics of dreams. The dreamscape exists within a unified field of psyche, and the human mandate to actualize the self is the premise of the interactive story. Each individual and every human collective shares the evolutionary objective of achieving more light, consciousness, or at-one-ment. Atonement is the objective of the psychological hero's journey. (Campbell, Joseph, 1949) To the degree a player projects his/her self-image on a hero and immerses self in the game, s/he has the potential to learn something about self and to move closer to atonement or self-actualization. S/he has the potential to become more whole—hale and sound. If we look at the definitions of whole and healing, they are essentially the same—difficult to understand. In human terms wholeness is best understood in terms of harmony, love and integrity. Game experiences programmed to Jungian principles and articulated to the dimensions of a unified psyche would have the effect of value-formation and healing.

Presently, we have a window of opportunity with which to address the psychological crisis of the media age while there is still time to study its parameters. If we neglect the opportunity, we may lose track of reality entirely and surrender the planetary psyche to a terminal psychotic episode. Our technological media constitutes our opportunity. Our global media provides insight as to the content of the collective unconscious, and PEG research has the potential to provide meaningful insight and veridical access into both the personal and collective unconscious. This will be the ongoing challenge of a media age with its infinite psychological potential, and its computer scientists will shoulder much of the responsibility for where ICTs and the media dream take us.

REFERENCES

Aiello, Schfanella, & State. (2014). "How Yahoo Research Labs studies culture as a formal computational concept"--reading the source code of social ties. *MIT Technology Review*. Retrieved August 1, 2014 from http://www.technologyreview. com/view/529521/how-yahoo-research-labs-studies-culture-as-a-formal-computational-concept

Armour, J. A. (2003). *Neurocardiology: Anatomical and functional principles*. Boulder Creek, CA: HeartMath Research Center, Institute of Heartmath, Pub. N.

Armour, J. A., & Ardell, J. L. (Eds.). (1994). *Neurocardiology*. New York: Oxford University Press.

Audi, O., Cichy, R., & Pantazis, D. (2014). Where and when the brain recognizes, categorizes an object. *Nature Neuroscience, 26*. Retrieved from http://www. kurzweilai.net/where-and-when-the-brain-recognizes-categorizes-an-object

Baars, B. J. (1997). In the theatre of consciousness: Global workspace theory, a rigorous scientific theory of consciousness. *Journal of Consciousness Studies, 4*, 292–309.

Barrios-Choplin, McCraty, & Cryer. (1997). An inner quality approach to reducing stress and improving physical and emotional wellbeing at work. In US Naval Postgraduate School of Systems Management & Institute of Heartmath. John Wiley & Sons, Ltd.

Bateson, G. (1972). *Steps to An Ecology of Mind: Collected Essays in Anthropology, Psychiatry, Evolution, and Epistemology*. University Of Chicago Press.

Boyd, F. (2015). Immersive media: to the holodeck and beyond. *Knowledge Transfer Network*. Retrieved May 6, 2015 from http://www.ktn-uk.co.uk/immersive-media-to-the-holodeck-and-beyond/

Bradley, R. T. (2006). The psychophysiology of entrepreneurial intuition: a quantum holographic theory. *Institute of Whole Social Science & Institute of Heartmath: Proceedings of the Third AGSE International Entrepreneurship Research Exchange*.

Campbell, J. (1949). The hero with a thousand faces. Bollingen/Princeton University Press.

Cherry, K. (2015a). What is Flow? *AboutEducation*. Retrieved November 6, 2015 from http://psychology.about.com/od/PositivePsychology/a/flow.htm

Cherry, K. (2015b). What are peak experiences? *About Education*. Retrieved November 12, 2015 from http://psychology.about.com/od/humanist-personality/f/peak-experiences.htm

Childre, D., & Rozman, D. (2005). *Transforming Stress: The HeartMath Solution to Relieving Worry, Fatigue, and Tension*. Oakland, CA: New Harbinger Publications.

Chomsky, N. (1957). *Syntactic structures*. The Hague: Mouton.

Chopra, D. (1995). *Body, mind & soul*. PBS Home Video.

Creating massive virtual worlds for training. (2015). Halldale Group. Retrieved August 26, 2015 from http://halldale.com/news/defence/simthetiq-releases-122000-km2-correlated-vbs3-openflight-training-environment#.Veh2xdJRGUl

Curtis, A. (2002). The century of self. *BBC*. Retrieved from http://topdocumentaryfilms.com/the-century-of-the-self/

Dionisio, J. D. N., Burns, W. G., III, & Gilbert, R. (2013). 3D Virtual Worlds and the Metaverse: Current Status and Future Possibilities. *Computer Science Faculty Works*. Retrieved from http://digitalcommons.lmu.edu/cs_fac/8

Dooley, R. (2015a). The TMI Effect for Pictures Can Reduce Your Sales. *Neuromarketing*. Retrieved November14, 2015 from http://www.neurosciencemarketing.com/blog/articles/tmi-effect-pictures.htm

Dooley, R. (2015b). The Brainfluence podcast, episode #81: The brain lady, a.k.a. Susan Weinschenk. *Neuromarketing*. Retrieved November 6, 2015 from http://www.rogerdooley.com/wp-content/uploads/2015/10/EP081-BrainfluencePodcastTranscript.pdf

EmWave Technology. (2015). *Institute of HeartMath*. Retrieved November 14, 2015 from http://www.heartmath.com/emwave-technology/

Europe's Information Society. (2011). ICT for Better Healthcare in Europe. *Europa*. Retrieved April 27, 2011 from http://ec.europa.eu/information_society/activities/health/index_en.htm

Foster, D. (1985). *The philosophical scientists*. New York: Dorset Press.

Freedberg, S. J., Jr. (2015). Marines explore augmented reality. *Breaking Defense.* Retrieved September 1, 2015 from http://breakingdefense.com/2015/09/marines-explore-augmented-reality-training/

Frysinger, R. C., & Harper, R. M. (1990). Cardiac and respiratory correlations with unit discharge in epileptic humantemporal lobe. *Epilepsia, 31*(2), 162–171. doi:10.1111/j.1528-1167.1990.tb06301.x PMID:2318169

Galeon, D. (2016). An AI was taught to hunt & kill humans in a video game. *Futurism.* Retrieved 7/11/2017 from http://futurism.com/scientists-taught-an-ai-to-hunt-and-kill-humans-in-a-video-game/

Geere, D. (2015). A robot just passed the self-awareness test. *Techradar.* Retrieved July 16, 2015 from http://www.techradar.com/news/world-of-tech/uh-oh-this-robot-just-passed-the-self-awareness-test-1299362

Gillin, Lapira, McCraty, Bradley, Atkinson, Simpson, & Scicluna (n.d.). Before cognition: the active contribution of the heart/ANS to intuitive decision making as measured in repeat entrepreneurs in the Cambridge TECHNOPOL. *Heartmath Institute Research Library.* Retrieved November 6, 2015 from https://www.heartmath.org/assets/uploads/2015/01/language-of-entrepreneurship.pdf

Ginsberg, J. P., Berry, M. E., & Powell, D. A. (2010). Cardiac Coherence and PTSD in Combat Veterans. Alternative Therapies in Health and Medicine, 16(4).

Glassner, A. (2004). *Interactive storytelling.* Natick, MA: A.K. Peters.

Goodman, B., Dretzen, R., Rushkoff, D., Soenens, M., & Fanning, D. (2004). *The Persuaders. Frontline. WGBH Educational Foundation distributed by PBS Home Video, a department of the Public Broadcasting Service.*

Grammar, T. (2007). In *Wikipedia.* Retrieved April 27 from http://en.wikipedia.org/wiki/Minimalist_Program

Greenyear, F. (2015). Simthetiq Releases 122,000 km2 Correlated VBS3 & Openflight Training Environment. *Halldale Group.* retrieved November 14, 2015 from http://halldale.com/news/defence/simthetiq-releases-122000-km2-correlated-vbs3-openflight-training-environment#.VkYlJ9JdHnO

Hall, M. P. (2003). *The secret teachings of all ages.* New York: Jeremy P. Tarcher/Penguin.

Hameroff, S., & Penrose, S. R. (2014). Discovery of quantum vibrations in "microtubules" corroborates theory of consciousness. *PhysOrg*. Retrieved January 16, 2014 from http://phys.org/news/2014-01--discovery-quantum-vibrations--microtubules-corroborates.html

Hardesty, L. (2015). System automatically converts 2-D video to 3-D: Exploiting video game software yields broadcast quality 3-D video of soccer game in real time. *MIT News*. Retrieved November 4, 2015 from http://news.mit.edu/2015/software-converts-2-d-3-d-video-1104#.VjsetvPiDfc.linkedin

How Yahoo Research Labs studies culture as a formal computational concept. (2014). *MIT Technology Review*. Retrieved January 25, 2015 from http://www.technologyreview.com/view/529521/how-yahoo-research-labs-studies-culture

Hull, R. F. C. (1974). *Dreams*. New York: Princeton University Press.

Institute of Heartmath. (2007). New research project: global coherence monitoring system. *IHM Summer 2007 Newsletter*. Retrieved May 1, 2009 from http://www.heartmath.org/templates/ihm/e-newsletteer/2007/Summer-2007/summer_2007_newsletter.htm

Jacobi, J. (1973). *The psychology of CG Jung*. London: Yale University Press.

Jung, C. G. (1933). *Modern man in search of a soul*. Harcourt Brace & Company.

Kaplesky, B. (2007b). *The imago effect—notes on presentation by Harvey Smith of Midway Games*. Retrieved November 14, 2015 from http://www.secretlair.com/index.php?/clickableculture/entry/notes_the_imago_effect_avatar_psychology/

Karavides, M. K., Leehrer, P. M., & Vaschillo, V. (2007). Preliminary reports of an open label study of heartrate variability biofeedback for treatment of major depression. *Applied Psychophysiology and Biofeedback*, *32*(1), 19–30. doi:10.100710484-006-9029-z PMID:17333315

Keplesky, B. (2007a). The Imago Effect: Avatar Psychology. *Behind the Door SXSW07*. Retrieved November 14, 2015 from https://doornumber3.wordpress.com/2007/03/14/the-imago-effect-avatar-psychology/

Khodarahimi, S. (2009). Dreams in Jungian psychology: The use of dreams as an instrument for research diagnosis and treatment of social phobia. *The Malaysian Journal of Medical Sciences: MJMS*, *16*(4), 42–49. PMID:22135511

Kirk, T. (2014). Superconducting spintronics pave way for next-generation computing. *PhysOrg*. Retrieved January 15, 2014 from http://phys.org/news/2014-01-superconducting-spintronics-pave-next-generation.html

Knight, W. (2015). A new tool for analyzing academic papers uses cutting-edge AI to find meaning in billions of words. *MIT Technology Review*. Retrieved from http://www.technologyreview.com/news/542981/academic-search-engine-grasps-for-meaning/

Knox, Lentini, & Alton. (2012). Effects of game-based relaxation training on attention problems in anxious children. *Priory.com.*

Kosslyn, S. M. (1994). *Image and Brain*. Massachusetts Institute of Technology.

Kowal, E. (2015). *Computer simulations improve lethality*. Retrieved May 19, 2015 from http://htl.li/N8e9W

Lakoff, G. (2002). *Moral politics*. Chicago: University of Chicago Press. doi:10.7208/chicago/9780226471006.001.0001

Lakoff, G. (2008). *The political mind*. Viking Penguin.

Lakoff, George, & Narayanan. (2010). Toward a computational model of narrative. *International Computer Science Institute and University of California at Berkeley*. Retrieved from http://www1.icsi.berkeley.edu/~snarayan/narrative-aaai-fs2010.pdf

Lee, D. (2015). Facebook set to share AI advances. *BBC News*. Retrieved November 5, 2015 from http://www.bbc.com/news/technology-34717958?post_id=10206805820649209_10208064398872878

Lehrer, P., Vaschillo, E., Lu, S. E., Eckberg, D., Vaschillo, B., Scardella, A., & Habib, R. (2006). Heart rate variability biofeedback: Effects of age on heart rate variability, baroreflex gain, and athsma. *Chest, 129*(2), 278–284. doi:10.1378/chest.129.2.278 PMID:16478842

Lindmark, S., Wiklund, U., Bjerle, P., & Eriksson, J. W. (2003). Does the autonomic nervous system play a role in the development of insulin resistance? A study on heartrate variability in first degree relatives of Type 2 diabetes patients and control subjects. *Diabetic Medicine, 20*(5), 399–405. doi:10.1046/j.1464-5491.2003.00920.x PMID:12752490

Ludlow, P. (2007). Noam Chomsky (1928). In Encyclopedia of the Philosophy of Science. Routledge.

Luskin, R., & Newell, Q. (2002). A controlled pilot study of stress management training of elderly patients with congestive heart failure. *Preventive Cardiology, 5*(4), 168–172, 176. doi:10.1111/j.1520.037X.2002.01029.x PMID:12417824

McCraty, R. (2002a). Heart rhythm coherence: And emerging area of biofeedback. *Biofeedback, 30*(1), 17–19.

McCraty, R. (2002b). Influence of cardiac afferent influence on heart-brain synchronization and cognitive performance. *International Journal of Psychophysiology, 45*(1-2), 72–73.

McCraty, R. (2005). *Enhancing emotional, social, and academic learning with heart rhythm coherence feedback*. Heartmath Research Center, Institute of Heartmath.

McCraty, R., Atkinson, M., Stolc, V., Alabdulgader, A. A., Vainoras, A., & Ragulskis, M. (2017). Synchronization of human autonomic nervous system rhythms with geomagnetic activity in human subjects. *IEJRPH*. Retrieved from http://www.mdpi.com/1660-4601/14/7/770/htm

McCraty, R., & Childre, D. (2010). Coherence: bridging personal, social, and global health. *Alternative Therapies, 16*(4). Retrieved November 6, 2015 from https://www.heartmath.org/assets/uploads/2015/01/coherence-bridging-personal-social-global-health.pdf

McCraty, R., & Tomasino, D. (2006). Coherence-building techniques and heart rhythm coherence feedback: New tools for stress reduction, disease prevention, and rehabilitation. In E. Molinari, A. Compare, & G. Parati (Eds.), *Clinical Psychology and Heart Disease*. Milan, Italy: Springer-Verlag. doi:10.1007/978-88-470-0378-1_26

Morris, S. M. (2010). Achieving collective coherence: Group effects on heart rate variability coherence and heart rhythm synchronization. Alternative Therapies, 16(4).

Orme-Johnson, D. W. (n.d.). Maharishi Effect. *Global Good News*. Retrieved November 12, 2015 from maharishi-programmes.globalgoodnews.com/maharishi-effect

Parkin, S. (2015). Virtual reality startups look back to the future. *MIT Technology Review*. Retrieved March 7, 2014 from https://www.linkedin.com/grp/post/1039687-6003159104225366019

Particle based simulations. (2014). Particle based simulations (physX flex). *NVIDIA*. Retrieved December 9, 2014 from https://www.youtube.com/watch?v=1o0Nuq71gI4&feature=share

Postman, N. (1985). *Amusing ourselves to death*. Viking Penguin Inc.

Postman, N. (1992). *Technopoly: the Surrender of Culture to Technology*. New York: Vintage.

Prathap, G. (1993). *The finite element method (FEM).* Retrieved from http://www. nal.res.in/oldhome/gages/fepace.htm

Reeves, B., & Nass, C. (1996). The media equation. Cambridge University Press.

Rein, A. (1995). The physiological and psychological effects of compassion & anger. *Journal of Advancement in Medicine, 8*(2).

Saffell, N. (2015). *On the origin of robot species: robots building robots by "natural selection".* University of Cambridge. Retrieved August 12, 2015 from http://www. cam.ac.uk/research/news/on-the-origin-of-robot-species?sthash.zMSyp5OS.mjjo

Sapir-Whorf Hypothesis. (2007). In *Wikipedia.* retrieved April 27, 2011 from http:// en.wikipedia.org/wiki/Sapir-Whorf_hypothesis

Schafer, S. (2007). Premise: The key to interactive storytelling. *Game Career Guide.* Retrieved April, 3, 2007 from http://www.gamecareerguide.com/features/357/ premise_the_key_to_interactive_.php?page=1

Schafer, S. (2011). Articulating the paradigm shift: Serious games for psychological healing of the collective persona. In *Business Social Networking: Organizational, Managerial, and Technological Dimensions.* IGI Global. Retrieved from http://www. igi-global.com/book/handbook-research-serious-games-educational/5

Schafer, S. (2012). Optimizing Cognitive Coherence, Learning, and Psychological Healing with Drama-based Games. In *Video Game Play and Consciousness.* Nova Science Publishers. Retrieved from http://www.facebook.com/insights/?sk =po_261980910540561#!/pages/Video-Game-Play-and-Consciousness/2619809 10540561?sk=wall

Schafer, S. (Ed.). (2017). *Exploring the collective unconscious in a digital age.* Hershey, PA: IGIG Global.

Schafer, S., & Yu, G. (2011). *Meaningful video games: drama-based video games as transformational experience.* Hershey, PA: IGI Global. doi:10.4018/978-1-60960-567-4.ch019

Schafer, S. B. (2018). *Generating a superconductive culture of conscience.* Beau Bassin, Mauritius: LAP LAMBERT Academic Publishing.

Simonite, T. (2015). A better way to design brain inspired chips. *MIT Technology Review.* Retrieved May 6, 2015 from http://www.technologyreview.com/ news/537211/a-better-way-to-build-brain-inspired-chips/

The curious evolution of artificial life. (2014). When it comes to research into Artificial Life, commercial projects have begun to outpace academic ones. *MIT Technology Review*. Retrieved July 30, 2014 from https://www.linkedin.com/grp/post/1039687-5900533809526378496

The emerging science of human-data interaction. (2015). *MIT Technology Review*. Retrieved January 11, 2015 from http://www.technologyreview.com/view/533901/the-emerging-science-of-human-data-interaction

The emerging science of human-data interaction—simulation of living systems. (2014). *MIT Technology Review*. Retrieved July 31, 2014 from https://www.linkedin.com/grp/post/1039687-5900533809526378496

Trafton, A. (2014). New brain-scanning technique allows scientists to see when and where the brain processes visual information. *Medical Press*. Retrieved January 27, 2014 from http://medicalxpress.com/news/2014-01-brain-scanning-technique-scientists-brain-visual.html

Urban, T. (2015). AI revolution—road to superintelligence. *But Wait Why*. Retrieved November 5, 2015 from http://www.technologyreview.com/news/525301/virtual-reality-startups-look-back-to-the-future/

Yohn, D. L. (2015). The Secret Behind Retail Customer Experience Success is Brain Science. *Neuromarketing*. Retrieved November 20, 2015 from http://www.neurosciencemarketing.com/blog/articles/retail-customer-experience.htm

Zaltman, G., & Zaltman, L. (2008). *Marketing Metaphoria*. Harvard Business Press.

Zucker, T. L., Samuelson, K. W., Muench, F., Greenberg, M. A., & Gevirtz, R. N. (2009). The effects of respiratory sinus arrhythmia biofeedback on heart rate variability and posttraumatic stress disorder symptoms: A pilot study. *Applied Psychophysiology and Biofeedback*, *34*(2), 135–143. doi:10.100710484-009-9085-2 PMID:19396540

ADDITIONAL READING

Bardy, B., & Stoffregen, T. (2004). *Multi-sensory enactive interfaces and the global array: what is an illusion?* http://www.interdisciplines.org/enaction/papers/3

Bell, J. S. (1988). Nonlocality in physics and psychology: an interview with John Stewart bell, in Psychological Perspectives.

Bohm, D. (1987). Hidden variables and the implicate order. In B. J. Hiley & F. David Peat (Eds.), *Quantum Implications*. London: Routledge & Kegan Paul.

Briggs, J. P., & Peat, D. D. (1984). *Looking glass universe*. New York: Simon & Schuster.

Broodryk, C. W. (2006). The moving image: contemporary film analysis and analytical psychology. *Submitted in fulfillment of the requirements of the degree Magister Artium in the Department of Drama, Faculty of Humanities*, University of Pretoria. http://upetd.up.ac.za/thesis/available/etd-08212007-125813.unrestricted/00dissertation.pdf

Campbell, J. (1973). *The hero with a thousand faces*. Princeton: Bollingen.

Capra, F. (2000). *Tha tao of physics*. Boston: Shambhala.

Chalmers, D. (1996). *The conscious mind*. New York: Oxford University Press.

Chomsky, N. (1957). *Syntactic structures*. The Hague, Paris: Mouton.

Coles, R. (Ed.). (1997). *Carl Gustav Jung: selected writings*. New York: Princeton University Press and Random House.

Dainton, B. (2003). *Stream of Consciousness: Unity and continuity in Conscious Experience*. London: Routledge, International Library of Philosophy; http://psyche.cs.monash.edu.au/symposia/dainton/prec.html

Davies, P. (1988). *The cosmic blueprint*. New York: Simon & Schuster.

Dunniway, T. (2000). Using The Hero's Journey in Games. *Gamasutra*, http://www.gamasutra.com/view/feature/3118/using_the_heros_journey_in_games.php

Eddington, S. A. (1935). *The nature of the physical world*. Cambridge University Press.

Freeman, D. (2002). Four Ways to Use Symbols to Add Emotional Depth to Games. *Gamasutra*, http://www.gamasutra.com/view/feature/2974/four_ways_to_use_symbols_to_add_.php

Freeman, D. (2004). *Creating emotion in games*. Boston: New Riders Publishing. doi:10.1145/1027154.1027179

Fromm, E. (1951). *The forgotten language*. New York: Grove Press.

Garrett, J. (2007). *Aristotle on Metaphor: The Poetics, Chapter 21, 1457b1-30*. Retrieved Nov. 3, 2015 from http://people.wku.edu/jan.garrett/401s07/arismeta.htm

Gibson, J. J. (1979). *The Ecological Approach to visual Perception*. New Jersey, USA: Lawrence Erlbaum Associates.

Glassner, A. (2004). *Interactive storytelling*. Natick, Massachusetts: A.K. Peters.

Glassner, A. (2004). *Interactive storytelling*. Natick, Massachusetts: A.K. Peters.

Grasse, R. (1996). *The waking dream*. Wheaton, Illinois: Quest Books.

Grasse, R. (1996). *The waking dream*. Wheaton, Ill: Theosophical Publishing House.

Grof, S. (1985). *The Adventure of self-Discovery*. Albany, N.Y.: State University of New York Press.

Hameroff, S. (2008). *The 'conscious pilot': Synchronized dendritic webs move through brain neurocomputational networks to mediate consciousness. Center for Consciousness Studies, Toward a Science of Consciousness 2008*. University of Arizona.

Harnad, S. (2007). *Symbol Grounding Problem*. Scholarpedia http://www. scholarpedia.org/artcile/Symbol_Grounding_Problem

Isbister, K. Better Game Characters by Design. Morgan Kaufmann Publisher. San Francisco, 2006. (ISBN 10: 0-12-369535-X)

Jacobi, J. (1974). *Complex, archetype, symbol in the psychology of C. G. Jung*. Princeton: Bollingen.

Jahn, R. G., & Dunne, B. J. (1987). *Margins of Reality: The Role of Consciousness in the Physical world*. New York: Harcourt Brace Dovanovich.

Jenkins, H. (2005). *Game Design as Narrative Architecture*. http://web.mit.edu/21fms/www/faculaty/henry3/games&narrative.html

Jenkins, H. (2005). Game Design as Narrative Architecture. *Publications*, http://homes.lmc.gatech.edu/~bogost/courses/spring07/lcc3710/readings/jenkins_game-design.pdf

Jung, C. G. (1933). *Modern man in search of a soul*. San Diego, New York, London: Harcourt Brace & Company.

Jung, C. G. (1974). *Dreams*. Princeton University Press.

Koriatt, A., & Goldsmith, M. (1996). Memory metaphors and the laboratory/real-life controversy: Correspondence versus storehouse views of memory. *Behavioral and Brain Sciences*, 19(2), 167–228. http://www.bbsonline.org/Preprints/OldArchive/bbs.koriat.html. doi:10.1017/S0140525X00042114

Ludlow, P. (2007). Noam Chomsky (1928-). Draft: forthcoming in Routledge Encyclopedia of the Philosophy of Science, Sahotra Sarkar and Melinda Fagan (eds).

Martin, J. W., & Ostwalt, C. E. (Eds.). (1995). *Screening the sacred: religion, myth and ideology in popular American film*. Boulder: Westview Press.

Meehan, D. B. (2003). *Phenomenal Space and the Unity of conscious Experience*. http://psyche.cs.monash.edu.au/symposia/dainton/meehan.html

Noë, A., & Thompson, E. (2004). Are there Neural correlates of consciousness? *Journal of Consciousness Studies*, *11*(1), 3–28.

Noë, I. (2004). Experience without the head. Draft: to appear in Perceptual Experience, Tamar Szabo Gendler & John Hawthorne (eds)

Norman, D. A. (1999). Affordances, Conventions and Design. In Interactions, 6 (3) p. 38-41 doi:10.1145/301153.301168

Pearce, J. C. (1971). *The Crack in The Cosmic Egg*. New York: Julian Press.

Peat, F. D. (1987). *Synchronicity: The Bridge between Mind and Matter*. New York: Bantam books.

Pert, C. B. (2003). *Molecules of emotion*. New York: Scribner.

Pinker, S. (1997). *How the mind works*. New York: W.W. Norton.

Postman, N. (1984). *Amusing ourselves to death*. New York: Penguin Books.

Prathap, G. (1993). *The finite element method (FEM)*. Kluwer. Reviewed in *The FEPACS Saga: from concepts to commercial products*. http://www.nal.res.in/oldhome/gages/fepace.htm

Pribram, Karl (1969). The neurophysiology of remembering. *Scientific American* 220 p, 75.

Pribram, K. (1977). *Languages of the Brain. Monterey*. Calif: Wadsworth Publishing.

Sasse, D. B. (2008) *A framework for psychophysiological data acquisition in digital games*. Retrieved: June 5, 2008 from http://www.gamecareerguide.com/features/542/masters_thesis_a_framework_for_.php

Satinover, J. (2001). *The quantum brain*. New York: John Wiley & Sons.

Seielstad, G. A. (1983). *Cosmic Ecology*. Berkeley: University of California Press.

Sharma, H., & Clark, C. (1998). *Contemporary Ayurveda*. Philadelphia: Churchill Livingstone.

Strassman, R. M.D. (2001). DMT the spirit molecule. Rochester, Vermont: Park Street Press.

Talbot, M. (1991). *The holographic universe*. New York: Harper.

Vallor, S. (2006). An enactive-phenomenological approach to veridical perception. *Journal of Consciousness Studies*, *13*(4), 39–60. http://www.ingentaconnect.com/content/imp/jcs/2006/00000013/00000004/art00004

Wallace, Robert Keith (1986). *The Physiology of consciousness*. A joint publication of Institute of science, technology and public policy & Maharishi international university press.

Wolf, F. A. (1987). The Physics of dream consciousness: Is the lucid dream a parallel universe? *Second lucid dreaming symposium proceedings*. Lucidity Letter 6, no. 2, p. 133)

Zohar, D. (1990). *The quantum self*. New York: William Morrow and Company.

Zohar, D., & Marshall, I. (1994). *The quantum society*. New York: William Morrow and Company.

KEY TERMS AND DEFINITIONS

Contextuality: Jung's principle of compensation demands that dream interpretation must incorporate significant familiarity and understanding of the individual or patient who is doing the dreaming. In order for ICT software to provide authentic compensation, the game must be specifically programmed to the psychological profile or "context" of the player.

Media Dream: The symbolic, semiotic, metaphorical map projected by a culture's visual media—particularly film, television, the internet, and video games—that afford insight as to psychic harmony or imbalance of a culture.

Media Sphere: Has been defined by the author as the collective ecology of the world's media including newspapers, journals, television, radio, books, novels, advertising, press releases, publicity, and the blogosphere; any and all media both broadcast and published.

Psychological Immersion: As applied in the dramatic arts, psychological immersion is known as suspension of disbelief. In current cognitive research, it applies mostly to the psychic function called emotion and is defined mostly in terms of feeling associations. The author uses the term relative to the infinite field of the unconscious—including elements of all the Jungian functions—not just the emotions. Precisely, immersion is the process of being submerged in the cognitive unconscious but retaining a degree of consciousness as one does in lucid dreaming states.

ENDNOTES

¹ Many of the world's healing philosophies and practices such as Ayurveda and Homeopathy are based on sophisticated reading of symptoms that are understood to correspond with unconscious (multi-functional) bio-disharmony. Based on complex understandings of correspondence, these healing methodologies have been practiced for thousands of years. In the case of Homeopathy that was discovered in the 19th century, the "doctrine of signatures" (likes cure likes) dates back to Celtic healing principles which claimed that illnesses could be cured with plants that cause the same symptoms as an ailing body.

² The Jungian contextual personality has been effectively programmed and employed for decades in Myers-Briggs profiles that can be effectively analyzed using questionnaires with as few as thirty questions.

Conclusion

CRITICAL BALANCES BETWEEN HEALTHCARE INNOVATION, QUALITY, AND INFORMATION PRIVACY

Throughout the book *Emerging Trends and Innovations in Privacy and Health Information Management* the various chapters discuss some of the ongoing changes in the context of health conceptions and healthcare systems. The implications and readjustments associated to the introduction of increasingly advanced scientific knowledge and technical innovations and devices, both in the way health information is mined, stored and screened, as well as in the treatment and prevention of diseases, are debated under differentiated theoretical and disciplinary frameworks. Issues of efficacy and functionality, but also of ethical concerns and quality, namely of the health professionals' practice, permeate the various contributions and put in the forefront of the debate the need to profound and understanding the impacts of the ongoing changes in the conception of health and healthcare themselves. In fact, renewed analytical challenges emerge from the ongoing transformation from a pathogenesis to a "salutogenesis" (Antonovsky, 1979) point of view, and the introduction of a more "technical" construction and delivery of healthcare.

In this concluding part, the discussion about the main structuring analytical pillars of the book are pursued – health conception; innovation, technology and healthcare quality; science, politics and moral; ethical concerns and health information management – under the thesis that even in an increasingly technical healthcare delivery and management moral conceptions continue to pervade the debates and the expectations or resistances of the individuals towards healthcare innovation. Under this scope, a deeper debate is required on the relationship between science, moral and politics, putting in the forefront the rationales in confrontation and on the ways information can be managed in the interconnection between ethical concerns and the economic and managerial pressures of healthcare systems today.

To this extent the chapter is structured in two parts. The first one - Understand health and healthcare today: background issues – and the second - Emerging trends and critical debates in healthcare innovation and privacy. Beginning with a discussion around the transmutation of the conception of health and healthcare, under the influence of technological discoveries, its possibilities and impacts (namely in the increasing of medicalization), the chapter proceeds with the debate concerning the ethical questions associated with health information mining, screening and storage, namely privacy and security issues.

UNDERSTANDING HEALTH AND HEALTHCARE TODAY: BACKGROUND ISSUES

Health, as a construct, as an objective and as a product, reflects the prerogatives and circumstances of a given time and context. Therefore its definition and the practices it encompasses depend not only on the scientific and technical knowledge available in a given time-space but also on how it is understood and appropriated politically and culturally. The boundaries of what is considered to be "good health" or "being healthy" vary according to the perceptions and values of a given historical epoch and the expectations, intervention possibilities, and ways of comparison. Thus, the conception of health, and in contrast that of illness have a dimension of relativity that is particularly important, though not sufficient, for the understanding of what can be framed in a notion of well-being.

In fact the thresholds of a particular sense of well-being, both objective and subjective, are defined either by the levels of scientific knowledge, gained and integrated or not into the practices (of citizens and health professionals), or by cultural, moral or religious issues that influence the conceptions of what can be classified as "pathological" and, as such, justify actions for its eradication and/or control (medically, socially or politically). The boundaries between what is known and what is believed, or accepted, are in fact complex and porous. For example, at one time masturbation was classified as a mental disorder, with physical implications associated with malnutrition. "Patients", under this conception, were subjected to diets, electric shocks or even the removal of the genital organs in more extreme cases. Inherent to an explication seemingly "scientific", a moral and normalizing view of what was considered to be a *"counter natural"* and sinful practice was present. A view effectively rooted in a religious morality of guilt (namely associated to pleasure) and punishment. Although this radical dimension of what can be considered abnormal is now being overcome, different rationalities - cultural, moral or religious (and even in some cases aesthetic or prophylactic) - continue to be invoked to justify male or female genital mutilation[1] in various countries and cultures. The definition of what falls within the notions of health and illness, or of normal or abnormal, is not therefore a linear and close debate. The current example of the albino children in Africa, persecuted and often murdered for superstitious reasons (because they are believed to possess magical powers or are a living proof of curses and bad omens) is paradigmatic. The complexity and multidimensionality of the dimensions that this debate entails require thus a constant and attentive consideration of the angle of vision that is being adopted and of the possible combination of universal principles and contextualized concretizations.

Health and Illness: Between Science, Moral, and Norm

Since ancient times the control of the disease and of the threats (individual and collective) that it can behave is a concern of humanity. The ways of doing so vary however over time. From the magical-religious conceptions to the rationalist approaches, the search for a certain state of health and harmony has been populating peoples' concerns.

The sorcerer, in certain tribes, would have the function of expelling, through rituals of spirit's summoning and sacrifices, the demons that prevent the connection of the person in the macrocosm of a Nature personalized. Such conceptions start from the assumption that the "disease" is a manifestation of forces external to the body and that in the "flesh" is objectified the curse or the sin.

Religious or moral grounds are also manifest in some conceptions of health and illness. For example, for the Hebrews the disease translates a manifestation of God's wrath against the imperfection of the human being. An imperfection associated with the disrespect for the divine law and the submission to the human will and sinful instincts (3), and objectified as a disease in the body, envelope of this imperfection. Leprosy is, in this context, the most visible dimension of the manifestation of the discontentment of God. This also explains in some way the legitimacy of the social exclusion of lepers, not only by the contagious dimension of the disease, but also by the seal of sin that their body translate[2]. The healing of lepers by Christ, often referred to in the New Testament as "proof" of a divine progeny, is thus not only the cure of a disease, but also the forgiveness of the sins that justify it.

Nevertheless, some rules of a religious nature also seem to be anchored, although not justified in this way, in "good reasons". For example, some of the religious precepts of Judaism preserved to date, such as dietary norms, in addition to maintaining the cohesion of the group and its differentiation through shared symbolic rules, have an intrinsic rationality, namely related to the prevention of certain diseases. Thus, even if infectious diseases were still unknown, and as such the scientific explanation could not be pointed out, what is certain is that the prohibition of mollusk intake, for example, prevents certain diseases such as oyster-transmitted hepatitis; or that the ban on slaughter of animals by a person with skin diseases can prevent the contamination of the meat.

The relationship between sickness and sin remained in the Middle Age in Europe through the influence of Christianity. The *contra naturam vivere* was identified and fought as the cause of all evils, including physical ones, associating thus health and disease with a moral issue. Although this religious and moralizing reading has been preserved (with distinct contours in different contexts and religions) up to the present time, with the advent of modernity a more rational and empirical understanding of the states of health and illness overlaps.

With the development of chemistry, for example, the comprehension of disease as a result of chemical processes related to the functioning of the organism, as Paracelsius (1493-1541) asserts, allows to find a rational explanation for the states of organic imbalance that were previously difficult to understand, justifying also chemical treatments. Likewise, advances in anatomic knowledge, and particularly in pathological anatomy, allow to associate disease, no longer to fluid imbalance as Hippocrates of Cos (460-377 BC) believed (4), but to the malfunction of the body and its various components. As René Leriche (1879-1955) refers, health "«is life lived in the silence of the organs» [73, 6.16-1]. Conversely, «disease is what irritates men in the normal course of their lives and work, and above all, what makes them suffer» [73, 6.22-3]" (cited in Canguilhem, 1989 [1943], p. 91).

Hence it is no longer pain or functional incapacity and social infirmity which makes disease, but rather anatomical alteration or physiological disturbance. Disease plays its tricks at the tissue level, and in this sense, there can be sickness without a sick person (Canguilhem, 1989 [1943], p. 92).

This "ontologization" of the disease contributed in fact to a taxonomic identification of symptoms and, as such, to a negative definition of health. This would be the state corresponding to the absence of disease symptoms. The symptom is, in this perspective, the language of the body, the expression of a message only intelligible by the mastery of the signs that constitute it.

Medical expertise and the objectification of its language thus reflect the emergence of the modern clinic, and with it, a whole set of expectations associated with the liberation of physical "demons", objectified in a symptomatology, and the search for harmony and well-being. The doctor is thus the new shaman. With his "powers" he manages to free the subjects from physical and psychological maltreatment, thus transforming their existence and their connection with the collective. All this in a transformed and rationally organized context for the pursuit of the new objectives of healing, treatment and empirical collection of evidence. Hospitals acquire different objectives and structures than they did in the Middle Age. They are no longer sites for the charitable collection of the sick and excluded, and become places of healing and learning. They are thus organized and structured around medical expertise and reference frameworks that allow: patient separation and classification, systematic information gathering based on increasingly deep and reliable technical expertise, and the assumption of a more objective language in describing the symptoms. A language that in fact delimits an increasingly specialized intervention space.

Medical knowledge and practice are thus guided and legitimized by the constant search for effective control over death and disease. With the so-called Pasteurian revolution at the end of the nineteenth century, an essential advance in the treatment and differential understanding of health and disease is assured. It opens the possibility of preventive medicine anchored in a deeper understanding of the etiology and evolution of diseases. The discovery of microorganisms allows the development of sera and vaccines and, consequently, the eradication or control of diseases (smallpox was eradicated, according to WHO data, in 1977). Alexander Fleming's (accidental) discovery of penicillin in 1928 opens up new possibilities for successful treatments with the antibiotic revolution.

At the same time, epidemiological studies, allowing a better understanding of the contextual factors that explain the prevalence and risk factors in the emergence and spread of some diseases, are developed mainly from the study of John Snow (1813-1858) about cholera in London. The search for indicators and regularities was also aided by statistical advances (2). Noteworthy, in this context, are the pioneering studies conducted in the seventeenth century by William Petty (1623-1687) and John Graunt (1620-1674). Graunt produced those that are considered the first studies on vital statistics by comparing mortality rates between different groups and correlating sex and place of residence. Similarly, in the nineteenth century, Louis René Villermé (1782-1863) conducted a study focusing on the levels of mortality in different districts of Paris (*Tableau de l'État Physique et Moral des Ouvriers*), having concluded that low income levels were correlated with high mortality rates.

The pioneering use of health statistics seems, however, to be due to the physician William Farr (1807-1883) as part of his duties at the General Register Office of England. The Annual Reports highlighted inequalities in health and disease levels across regions. In this context, the Report (1842) produced by Edwin Chadwick (1800-1890) became famous. It describes the living and sanitary conditions of the proletarians of industrialized Britain, which led to the promulgation of the Public Health Act in 1848. The relationship between epidemiological studies and influence on political decisions thus begins to acquire visibility. The same thing happened in the US through Lemuel Shattuck's Report of the Sanitary Commission of Massachusetts (1850).

Although epidemiological studies do seek to emphasize supra-individual explanatory factors capable of influencing public policies and interventions, advances in knowledge about anatomy, physiology and microbiology have contributed to the affirmation of a purely biomedical health concept. It is, moreover, a paradigm that continues to support a large part of the innovations in health technologies today, especially in the areas of diagnosis and monitoring of health status.

The mobile of health professionals is oriented to the preservation of life in the best possible conditions, focusing on the well-being of the patient and on their choices, as priorities and guiding principles. Even if some voices currently raise suspicions about the prioritization by health professionals of economic interests, relegating to the background the essential interest of patients (the case of aesthetic interventions is one of the most pointed examples), the deontological principle of medical practice, embodied in the Oath of Hippocrates, remains untouchable. Even if permeated by renewed ethical dilemmas fostered by ongoing scientific and technological advances. That way, it is understandable the continuity and priority in the valuation of a biological view about health issues. For example, the biostatistical conception of Cristopher Boorse (1977), with great impact on the medical field, highlights a negative definition of health. In Boorse's conception, health would be conceived as an objectively apprehensible state - "value-free as a statement of biological function" - of absence of disease. By releasing a substantive understanding based on value judgments, the notion of "normality" must be defined, from the perspective of the author, statistically and functionally, based only on biological data and pathological indicators. Data that, in fact, health professionals are prepared to identify, diagnose and treat.

The definition of health advocated by the WHO, on April 7, 1948 (since then the World Health Day), seeks to overcome this biomedical paradigm and highlight the various dimensions (biological, psychological and social in the broad sense) that are articulated to the production of a state of "complete well-being". However this notion of "completeness" has, on the backside of the medal, the "non-concretization", either because of the difficulty of determining what fits into a goal of wellbeing (which necessarily involves subjective dimensions and value judgments), or because the constant search of complete satisfaction that is, as such, unattainable, or still, due to the operational difficulties of applicability by the allocation of the necessary and adequate means to its accomplishment. To this extent, the criticisms of idealism (which are not unrelated to the attempt to overcome the horrors of World War II) and the inoperability of such a goal not only failed to overcome the concentration on a biomedical perspective of health but also contributed to its prevalence, and actually to its deepening, namely through the current use of technological innovations and devices.

268

The Normative Focus

In the Preamble of the Constitution of the World Health Organization the States recognize health as a universal public good and their multidimensionality and complexity are evidenced in favor of an intention of well-being, harmony and happiness:

The States parties to this Constitution declare, in conformity with the Charter of the United Nations, that the following principles are basic to the happiness, harmonious relations and security of all peoples: Health is a state of complete physical, mental and social well-being and not merely the absence of disease or infirmity. The enjoyment of the highest attainable standard of health is one of the fundamental rights of every human being without distinction of race, religion, political belief, economic or social condition. The health of all peoples is fundamental to the attainment of peace and security and is dependent upon the fullest co-operation of individuals and States.

In the same way, Marc Lalonde, Minister of Supply and Services of Canada, also defends, in 1974, in the so called Lalonde Report - A New Perspective on the Health of Canadians – that the field of health is multidimensional and encompasses human biology (genetic inheritance and biological processes, including aging factors); the environment (soil, water, air, housing, workplace); the lifestyle (smoking or quitting smoking, drinking or not, practice of physical exercise or not) and the organization of health care (medical care, outpatient services, hospitals and medication).

Thus, a positive definition of health, both as a product and as a process, emerges as well as the need to integrate it into a broader development logic, referring to a political consideration of the means and ends to be considered. Health, as a fundamental human right, involves a set of arguments and political prioritization. The means allocated for the realization or not of the possibilities of treatment and prevention actually depend not only on the scientific and technological developments in the medical, epidemiological and pharmaceutical fields, but also on the political priorities defined by both the State and health organizations. The Ottawa Charter for Health Promotion (1986) states that,

To reach a state of complete physical mental and social well-being, an individual or group must be able to identify and to realise aspirations, to satisfy needs, and to change or cope with the environment. Health is, therefore, seen as a resource for everyday life, not the objective of living. Health is a positive concept emphasizing social and personal resources, as well as physical capacities. Therefore, health promotion is not just the responsibility of the health sector, but goes beyond healthy lifestyles to well-being.

In the same line of reasoning the Declaration of Alma-Ata (1978) - adopted at the International Conference on Primary Health Care in Almaty (formerly Alma-Ata), Kazakhstan (formerly Kazakh Soviet Socialist Republic) - expressed the need for urgent political action to minimize the enormous inequalities in the world concerning health, as well as the need for health professionals and development workers to promote actions aiming to protect health for all. To this end, health actions should be: practical, achievable and socially acceptable; accessible to all; implemented in participatory and cooperative way, and financially sustainable.

Health and Development

The importance of socio-economic conditions in the construction of well-being (in itself a concept with a strong material component) and health is not a new subject. Several authors have demonstrated, in the context of epidemiological studies, that adverse (material, sanitary and economic) living conditions have negative impacts on the health status, mortality and morbidity of populations. These conclusions have contributed in a way to the determination of policies and measures that aim, under different orientations in various times and contexts, to question that connection, either by priority intervening in health and hygiene care, or to promote progressive changes in the socioeconomic contexts and labor markets. The demand for integrated and non-sectoral actions is nowadays affirmed with particular incidence.

In the 1980s, the philosopher Lennart Nordenfelt, especially in the works Causes of Death (1983) and On the Nature of Health (1987) defends a perspective of health as "the ability to achieve vital goals", that is, the conditions for a happy and prosperous life in the long term - such as Aristotelian eudaimonia – or, as he has more recently stated (1995) in line with the notion of "decency" advocated by the ILO (International Labor Organization), the "minimally decent life", more than mere survival.

Similarly, the notion of vital inequalities is explored by the Swedish sociologist and Professor of Cambridge University, Göran Therborn, in Inequalities of the World: New Theoretical Frameworks, Multiple Empirical Approaches (2006). What the author calls the Killing Fields of Inequality (2012) relates to the increase in one of the three types of inequality he points out: vital inequalities ("inequalities in health outcomes and life expectancies"), alongside economic and existential inequalities. As stated by Therborn,

Hard evidence is accumulating that health and longevity are distributed with a clearly discernible social regularity. Children in poor countries and poor classes die more often before the age of 1, and between the age of 1 and 5, than children in

rich countries and rich classes. Low-status people in Britain die more often before retirement age than high-status people. Vital inequality, which can be measured relatively easily through life-expectancy and survival rates, destroys millions of human lives in the world every year. (https://www.opendemocracy.net/article/the-killing-fields-of-inequality)

If we take into account, for example, data revealed by the United Nations (FAO, 2010, 2012; UNAIDS, 2010; UNICEF, 2006, 2007), it can be seen that approximately 925 million people worldwide do not feed enough to be considered healthy. This means that one in seven people on the planet starves. Starving is the first on the list of the top 10 health risks. Indeed, the number of hungry people has increased in recent decades compared to the percentage of the world's population. More than half of the world's hungry people, about 578 million people, are living in Asia and the Pacific. Africa fits more than a quarter of the world's hungry population, killing more people annually than AIDS, malaria and tuberculosis combined. Only among children under the age of five, a third of deaths in developing countries are linked to malnutrition.

In addition, according to the projection of statistical data, it is assumed that by 2050 irregular climate change will lead more than 24 million children to hunger, of which almost half live in sub-Saharan Africa. Such numbers are even more dramatic if we consider that hunger is currently the only major solvable problem facing the world. Given the definition of human development of the United Nations Human Development Program (2010), in addition to the level of income, people should be able to "live a long and healthy life, obtain education and knowledge and enjoy a standard of decent life". The search for solutions to current problems should seek to create access to resources and solutions that allow each person the freedom, through their knowledge and skills, to concretize as fully as possible their human potential. This challenge, coupled with the pressing scarcity of natural and social resources, requires creative and effective solutions that respond to local needs, counteracting measures that are too centralized and far from the real challenges. Effectivelly, studies in India conducted by Drèze and Sen (1997) have shown that increasing economic growth does not necessarily and automatically improve quality of life in such important dimensions as health or education, nor does it imply intervention and suppression of the causes of inequalities.

Also climate change is a new uncertainty to consider. Climate change occurs due to two main causes: natural causes (variations in the sun's brightness and the parameters that define the Earth's orbit around the sun) and anthropogenic causes, such as changes in atmospheric composition due to the burning of fossil fuels and changes in land use, in particular deforestation. It is also known today that the impacts of climate change are having adverse effects on the ecological, social and economic systems of the European Union (EU). Numerous initiatives and studies have been carried out in Europe with the aim of producing a sound knowledge base on the impacts of climate change. From these studies and from the scientific literature, the concept of adaptation emerges as a "multiscale multi-sectoral decision-making problem, characterized by enormous uncertainty about the precise impacts of climate change" (BASE Project, p.1). This uncertainty hampers political decision-making and conditions the success of the measures envisaged. Some of the critical elements that cause these effects are the dispersion and insufficiency of integrated knowledge and gaps in research on human responses to climate change and adaptation policies, for example.

In the mid-twentieth century, in the context of development economics, the term "sustained" arises associated with the need to critically revise the development process based on unlimited economic growth, which in itself would ensure the generation of welfare benefits and the gradual improvement of situations of poverty. However, especially with the great economic crisis of the 1970s, exacerbated by the peak of oil, there are evidences about the inadequacies of this linear model of development and the discussion about its "unsustainability" for the maintenance of life on Earth erupts. In 1987 the celebrated Brundtland Report inaugurated the concept of sustainable development, bringing to the discussion the environmental dimension of sustainability, as opposed to the strictly economics view that did not pay attention to the scarcity of natural resources, rather considering them as mere externalities that had nothing to do with economic equations. In this way, it is taken into account that the needs of the present generations cannot compromise the satisfaction of the needs of the generations of the future. At the 1992 Earth Summit in Rio de Janeiro, the environmental component of sustainability is valued (Roque Amaro, 2009; Schmidt, & Valente, 2004).

Ten years later, at Rio + 10, in 2002, Johannesburg, the concept is reformulated now proposing a greater integration of three societal goals: economic growth; environmental preservation and social cohesion. With this new framework, it is maintained that sustainable development would able to harmonize social justice and equity of access for all with the satisfaction of their basic needs and development opportunities. A notion and a practice that allow to meet the needs of future generations through preservation of natural resources, without neglecting economic growth. More recently, in relation to COP21 (Conference of the Parties) in Paris, it was rectified the new Sustainable Development Objectives and concluded a historic global agreement to address the effects of climate change. However, there are 17 targets to be met, and given the slow pace of ownership of top-down measures by the general population and the rapid pace of geopolitical and economic transformations and unexpected events, such initiatives may incur in exercises that are unable to overcome a mere rhetorical exercise (Schmidt, & Valente, 2004).

Today, the systemic dimension of the multiple crises of the world is even more evident. Given this scenario of intricate relationships between the causes and effects of the climatic, ecological, social, cultural and economic aspects of the various problems, it is increasingly pressing to develop strategic visions and holistic and integrated actions that are able to reconcile the multiple dimensions of human life and all the systems in which it operates.

In this sense, the sociologist Roque Amaro (2011) proposes a more complete perspective of sustainability, since it integrates more dimensions and assumes the need to build on the experience accumulated from organizations and initiatives of solidarity economy. If on the one hand, initiatives should contribute to the construction of sustainability in a broad sense in the world, on the other hand, they should also be able to face the challenges to their internal sustainability (organizational, institutional) and ensure their viability and durable sustainability, so that they can generate lasting systemic changes. In general, it is accepted that Development will only be Sustainable if it guarantees the "Sustainability of Life (including Humanity)" (idem, p.165), through a so called Integrated Sustainability.

In general, the assumptions presented previously have to do with aspects related to culture, social macro systems, and the environment. However, there are other scales and dimensions that guide individuals, groups, organizations, and ecosystems' behavior, etc. Authors who have worked on the Integral perspective (Brown, 2005; O'Brien, & Hochachka, nd; Hargens-Esbjörn, 2009) propose an understanding of reality by means of more systemic analyzes, from the point of view of four dimensions (crossed as a quadrant) that they consider fundamental to evaluate any element or system: individual, collective, exterior and interior (Brown, 2005). Thus individual subjective questions of morality, ethics, and spirituality are as important as the more material issues of behavior. Collective issues such as cultural identity, communication and education are as important as the use and development of technology, the design of the financial-economic system, as well as the production and consumption structures (energy, food, construction, etc.).

One of the most subtle and often ignored dimensions in the equation of building solutions to sustainability has been pointed out by several authors (Macy, 2014). Hopkins (2008), in naming the principles of the transition process to a post-carbon society admits three fundamental tools: the hands, the head, and the heart. In the author's view, generating positive visions for the future that increase the empowerment of communities (through the generation of new stories, new visions of the future); the promotion of inclusion and responsiveness within the community; sharing and networking; and the self-organization and decentralization of decision-making processes, as the basic principles for building community resilience, must also recognize the need for personal and inner transition. That is, recognize and understand the psychological dimension of change.

Other fields beyond the medical domain must therefore be aggregated to achieve a more integrated health perspective. Thus, its implementation would not only be linked to the practice of health professionals, but also to the intervention of other professionals guided by other rationalities (political, social and managerial) beyond medical and scientific rationality. The connections between these different rationalities are not always linear and can produce blockages and contradictions. The case of the "social discharge from hospital" in several European countries is a paradigmatic example. From a clinical point of view, the patient is ready to leave the hospital context and release the bed, but can only do so if the social conditions for their departure are ensured in conditions of dignity and safety (housing or institution of care; and family or community support). In this way medical power is associated with social power in determining what lies behind health care. Medical rationality, which evaluates the state of health recovery, is associated with the rationality of hospital management and the costs associated with the occupation (unnecessary from the medical point of view) of a bed, and the socio-political rationality that evaluates the possibilities of preserving the health, understood in a broad sense, after leaving the hospital.

The application of technological innovations and advanced biological research in the field of healthcare makes it possible to ensure, with greater speed and less recovery time in the hospital context, the essential purpose of curing and restoring the functional balance of the organism, or even to prevent diseases. Thus it contributes potentially to a better health realization from a biomedical perspective. There is still however a long way to go in articulating medical technologies and social-medical technologies, for example at post-operative care at home. Although there are already a number of advances, as some chapters of the book point out, in terms of support, via technology, to dependent patients at home, people with disabilities or caregivers, the accessibility to such technologies is still limited, either by the costs involved or by the difficulty of making these supports operational for all those who need them. Technological development and innovation in the health field can effectively contribute to a more appropriate combination of the aforementioned rationalities, thus towards a more integrated notion of health: the rationality of health professionals (achievement of well-being, control and overcoming symptoms, healing and follow-up); the rationality of health managers (the liberation of hospitals from large population inflows, often with small malaria, and the faster evacuation of hospital beds, reducing costs) and the rationality of social professionals (ensuring adequate care outside the hospital context).

Medicalisation: The Pervers Effect?

The breadth of the WHO health concept (also visible in the Lalonde Report) has been effectively permeated by criticism over the years. Some of philosophical and technical nature - health would be an ideal, a judgement of value and, as such, unattainable - others of sociopolitical nature. In this perspective, under the pretext of preserving and defending the health of populations, public authorities can now intervene in the lives of citizens, normatively imposing an ideal of well-being guided by moralizing presuppositions of what is appropriate or inadequate in behavioral terms. The establishment of criteria for the homogenization of behaviors can lead to a reduction in the margins of autonomy of people and to a kind of precautionary and hygienist authoritarianism.

Medical discourse can thus become a juridical discourse. This ensures a dual legitimation of practices and behaviors: the legitimacy of legal imposition stems from medical-scientific reasons; the legitimacy of some medical impositions stems from the need to comply with a legal determination. In the first case, we have, for example, the prohibition, under individual and public health protection assumptions, of smoking in public places (in fact an increasingly wide prohibition, initially in enclosed spaces and currently, in some countries, extended to open spaces). In the second case, we have, for example, the vaccination programs (which are now heavily controversial as highlighted in the preface to this book) or health tests for the performance of certain occupational functions (e.g., tuberculosis, tetanus, among others).

At the same time, the constant search for a full state of well-being can contribute, paradoxically, to the growing dependence on medical and pharmacological care. Several authors emphasize, especially since the 1960s, this dimension. For example, Foucault's perspectives on the discipline of bodies and the resulting bio-power are well known.

In the seventies of the twentieth century, Michel Foucault developed the concept of biopolitics to designate how power in the eighteenth and nineteenth centuries was transformed into a "discipline" of individuals and the population. In other words, "to designate what brings life and its mechanisms into the realm of explicit calculations and makes power-knowledge an agent of transformation of human life" (Foucault, 1976, p. 188).

In this way, the human being and his behaviors, added to the concepts and principles of "normal" and "pathological", constitute an object of political action and new socioeconomic strategies, giving rise to a normalizing "biopower" related to public health, hygiene, food, sexuality and birth. This type of power manages, models and orders the forces of life, controls and medicalizes populations, under the argument of favoring their growth and well-being. As Foucault (1976) states, the first pole of life management

Was centered on the body as a machine: its training, the enhancement of its skills, the extortion of its forces, the parallel growth of its usefulness and docility, its integration into effective and economic control systems, all this was ensured by processes of power that characterize the disciplines: anatomy-politics of the human body. The second, which formed a little later in the middle of the eighteenth century, was centered on the body of the species, on the body traversed by the mechanics of the living and supporting biological processes: proliferation, births and mortality, the level of health, the duration of life, longevity with all the conditions that may make it vary; its appropriation operates through a series of interventions and regulatory controls: a biopolitics of the population. (p. 183).

Likewise, biopolitics has constituted itself as an indispensable element of the capitalist system through the controlled inscription of "bodies" in the productive system and of populations in economic processes. At the end of the seventies, Foucault emphasized the transformation of the subjects into economic agents, submitted to processes of appreciation and amplification of skills and abilities in the face of increasingly competitive global markets. The functionality of "bodies" and comportments, according to economic-political criteria of productivity, would, in the view of the author, be a central element for the development of Fordist societies. In reference to neoliberalism, Michel Foucault introduces an element that is essential for the understanding of contemporary politics: the fusion between *homo oeconomicus* and the perspectives of "human capital". This way he affirms that *homo oeconomicus* is not only, in the present contexts, a producer-consumer, but also a constructor of itself and of his framing as ethical, social and economic being (Revel, 2005).

The notion of biopolitics seems to be a pertinent concept, as pointed out by several authors (Agamben, 1995, 1998; Negri, & Hart, 2002; Cocco, & Negri, 2005; Messu, 2008) for the understanding of contemporary politics. Lives, assumed as political categories, become increasingly exposed and managed. It is enough to think of measures for dependent populations, insertion and activation programs, unemployment management, among others. The insertion or activation policies associated with employment derive from this logic of public action, seeking to inscribe individual temporalities in collective, normalized and institutionalized temporal frameworks. A "de-socialized" subject, for example for a long period of unemployment in which he manages his own time is, by public action, intimated to submit to a set of tests that have as essential presupposition the regulation of the gaps between individual and collective, inscribing it in social times, valued, legitimized and institutionally recognized: periodic presentations in the services; vocational training; obligation of community services, etc.

The so-called "medicalization" corresponds, in particular according to Conrad's (2004, 2007) perspective, to broadening the scope of medicine to various spheres of human life, which produces numerous impacts (Illich, 1975; Maturo, 2012). The last two chapters of the book seek to accurately reflect on some of these impacts.

On the one hand, the "medical gaze" placed on certain problems and phenomena allows to dilute prejudices and stigmas around certain behaviors, no longer classified as vices, dysfunctions (so responsibility of the individual), or metaphysical possessions, but as diseases. This is the case of alcoholism, erectile dysfunction, epilepsy, drug addiction, attention deficit hyperactivity disorder, among others.

Still, and in counterpoint, new stigmas can be generated by transforming human differences into pathologies and contributing to the conception that there is a standard of normality and excellence, a filter for the hygienist evaluation and monitoring of individual behaviors and options. This way, the possibility of medicalization of affections and behaviors is accentuated, adjusting them to rules of normality, which is not only expected but desirable. It is enough to remember the strong consumption of stimulants to be able to work more hours or the behavioral controllers of the children with a diagnosis of hyperactivity and attention deficit. Indeed the deficit of attention is often paradoxically enhanced by the digital and multi-stimulant contexts in which we live.

Another element to be considered in this context is patient safety in the face of exacerbated drug use (Bernstein, & La Valle, 2015) and medical interventions. Some of the nefarious effects are known. For example aesthetic interventions performed at progressively earlier ages in an attempt to adapt to a pattern of preconceived beauty, sold as the key to happiness and social valorization.

In addition, the evolution and sophistication of current diagnostic and treatment techniques, notably through the use of technological innovation, allows detecting minor functional abnormalities or anticipate diseases that are still asymptomatic, often leading to unnecessary treatments "just to be safe". At this level, there are for example controversial debates about the surgical interventions for the removal of breasts by the simple detection of genetic markers that can produce eventually cancers in a diffuse future time. This increases the belief of control over death by benefiting from advances in medical care and research (for example in the field of genetics).

It should be noted that often the process of medicalization is initiated not by the medical class but by certain social movements that stress the importance of classifying certain situations or problems as illness before the doctors themselves do it. This was the case for movements in favor of classifying alcoholism as a disease. The health problem is thus constructed socially and politically before being constructed scientifically. The reverse is also true. For example with regard to mental disorders and disability. Anti-psychiatry movements challenge the classification and diagnosis of certain behaviors as mental illness. The same way, the movements of disabled people challenge the classification of "abnormality" associated with the conception of disability as a disease. Irving Kenneth Zola's book Missing Pieces: The Chronicle of Living With Disability (1982) is at this level particularly relevant.

Medicalization is also evident in determining choices and lifestyles. The consumption of drugs and the increasing use of all kinds of treatments and exams is magnifying exponentially at the present time. According to OECD data (2017), antidepressant use had risen, in just four years, 46% in Germany and 20% in Portugal and Spain. In the U.S. 11% of Americans over the age of 12 take an antidepressant.

Citizens today become consumers of health products and perform their own self-diagnosis (digital technologies enhance this possibility). In addition, the evaluation of quality health care is increasingly associated with the prescription of exams and medications. If this does not occur in an appointment, the patient considers that he/she were not properly attended and that the health problem was devalued by health professionals.

The cross-fertilization of these various conditions, coupled with the pressure of the pharmaceutical industry and biotechnology companies, leads to what might be called currently of "over-medicalization", often calling into question the "harm principle" that guides practice clinic. H. Gilbert Welch, a professor at the Dartmouth School of Medicine, reports in the book Less Medicine, More Health: 7 Assumptions That Drive Too Much Medical Care (2016), overdiagnosis practices and the transformation of citizens into "guinea pigs" and their subjection to treatments that are often unnecessary or inadvisable.

Avoiding death and suffering become the essential motivations that justify uncritical acceptance and the pursuit by citizens of treatments and drugs. In the background, they seek happiness, in fact unattainable, as Freud, in the work Civilization and Its Discontents (1930) argued, in a civilization that encourages high performance and hedonism as essential pillars of collective life.

Pain and Suffering: Ethical Issues

Medicine treats pain, can it treat suffering? The distinction between suffering (of the soul) and pain (of the body) is at this point of the reflection essential. Suffering engages a representation; pain is a perception, an experience. Pain can be protective (alarm of the body), suffering can be redemptive (Christianity) or destructive (of the image of oneself). It is essentially a mode of being in the world (Scheler, 1936).

"Who increases knowledge, increases pain", predicted Ecclesiastes (1:18). All the ethical reflection in philosophy will resume this formula to try to deduce the practical principles of a "good life". This will lead the defense of ethics as contrasted as those of Spinoza and Schopenhauer. Yet, with science - as we understand it today - particularly the science of the brain, our knowledge of the physiological mechanisms of pain offers the possibility of alleviating its perceptual and functional manifestations. In other words, a thorough knowledge of our bodily and cerebral "machinery" - to adopt Descartes' lexicon - does not lead to an increase of our pain (except, perhaps, for the researcher or for the one who tries to acquire knowledge). On the strictly empirical level, that of medical practice and the relationship between the doctor and his patient, the increase of medical knowledge results in a gain that can be described at least in terms of comfort. Would the prediction of Qoheleth (The Preacher) prove erroneous? Better, would neuroscience make vain philosophical speculation and the quest for ethics? A positive answer would simply forget that the biblical statement deals with the reflective consciousness which, by definition, has always material to operate. And, in fact, the technical means of reducing physical pain have by no means reduced to nothing the reflection on the suffering inherent to the human condition, the one that the Toranic maxim deals with.

Max Weber in his famous conference Wissenschaft als Beruf, pronounced for the first time in 1917 in Munich, returns to this question in order to clarify in what sense the social sciences can make use of the notion of "progress", and of scientific "progress" in particular. As the author states, the physician has technically the means to prolong the life of the dying person, even if she implores to dye. And she implores to dye, because, for her, life has no more value, it is no longer worth living. As we would say today, life no longer confers the dignity that is attached to a sense of human life. The means available to physicians to technically master life, dispel, or at least imply, that it is solved the question of the meaning and dignity of the life in their hands. They dismiss it or presuppose it because their goal is to implement the technical "progress" that is available to them. In doing so, the question of the meaning or dignity of life remains outside the logic of scientific "progress".

It is therefore necessary to distinguish the logic of scientific "progress", internal to the scientific discipline that carries it, from its interpretation or its valorization as a "progress" of the human condition as an inescapable step towards an assured "better being". And even if the progress to a "better being" is not achieved, the historical "progress" in the conditions of existence can and must be recognized. Nevertheless, the life that is worth living is each time to be interpreted, to be mastered, both individually and collectively, drawing on the representations and values that are shared. That is why it will be in the field of professional ethics and moral prescription that the doctor will have to interrupt his technical gesture to preserve the dignity of the life entrusted to him. It can do so because morality proposes to give meaning to life and human dignity, and therefore to the pain and suffering endured.

Pain and suffering are thus longstanding philosophical, existential and ethical questions. Various attitudes have been adopted over times that sway between acceptance and escape. Stoicism, Epicureanism, Christianity, etc., all practical or moral philosophies sought to define the right attitude that men had to adopt in the face of pain and suffering. Both in front of the one they know themselves and the one they perceive in others. Each time, the attitude to be adopted sought its foundation in the understanding of the meaning and the value that should be given to them. In sum, it was about coping with only mental convictions. Contemporary medicine based on the knowledge of the physiochemical mechanisms of pain has substantially renewed the way in which these questions can be apprehended, without ever answering them absolutely.

Indeed, by adopting the vision of Cartesian dualism, distinguishing the spirit of the body, but seeking their point of communication, we have been able to attribute the pain to the body and the suffering to the spirit. The pain could thus appear as a signal of the body when it knew some disturbance, when its organic unit was to be disturbed. The pain, as Darwin will say, is the alarm of the body. By reserving suffering in the mind, we assure only just a "conscience", a double psychic, the pain of the body. Suffering is an affection of the mind that has an intention that transcends bodily pain. Jean-Paul Sartre will say in *L'Être et le Néant* how, when "I have a headache", an intentional affectivity goes to my pain to "suffer" it. That is, to flee, to accept, even to value the suffering. In this sense we can say with Max Scheler (1936) that suffering is a mode of being specific to the world. For him, suffering calls for sacrifice. It claims that we renounce some particular property to preserve the general good of our person. In a way, restore our psychic balance. Thus suffering leads to rethink our being in the world and, probably, if we remove the direct causes, social, historical, accidental, to find the tragic dimension of our human condition, our *fatum*. We understand why the *"visage"*, especially when it expresses suffering, may have become in Levinas the metaphor of the human condition. I can experience and suffer myself from the suffering of others. We also understand why, over time, our sensitivity to suffering has been able to increase to the point of chasing all forms of cruelty and to find ourselves today in a position to blur the distinction between man and the sentient animal.

Under this scope, it may be questioned if contemporary medicine liberating the pain from the body does not dispossess the individual of his suffering. Not, first of all, the mystical suffering that borders on holiness - in the absence of preserving health - but the suffering that awakens as much to the world around us as to the relationship with the other or the affirmation of his existence. This may lead either to victim's complaint or to the heroic action. The eradication of the pain of the body may remove the sacrifice but it does not remove what pain can engage in terms of reflexivity. Alzheimer's disease, which does not give rise to many approaches in terms of pain, remains fully understood in terms of suffering. The one that we think we can impute to the sick person and the one expressed by those with who she is still in contact. In the latter, suffering expresses the loss of the other who is no longer the same, an another who has already disappeared, an another who is radically different. In short, the other which must be sacrificed, according to Scheler's perspective.

The Subjective Focus of Health

As it was already underlined the narrative associated with the conception of healthcare is currently under transformation. Not only in terms of the relationship between health professionals and patients - the autonomy of the individual in the active choice of health care and in the appreciation of the results to see materialized - but also in the way health services themselves are structured and articulated. Today the person is not only responsible for maintaining positive lifestyle choices across life, but also for preserving and controlling their own health. To this extent the responsibility for healthier options became a sort of public moral, guiding the rudder of personal and collective options.

The importance and the role of the patient in the healthcare system are thus reconfigured under a principle of healthfulness. The person is no longer only the object of action of health professionals, but also a consumer of healthcare, determining how and where to be cared for. Under this scope, the subjective or personalized dimension of health constitutes as a central element of the ongoing paradigmatic shift.

The definition of health by the symptomatological prism is considered very limited today. New conceptions in the understanding of health, advocated for example by Kleinman, Eisenberg, and Good (1978), make it possible to distinguish between "disease" and "illness". This involves not only the physical manifestation of the disease but also the subjective experience and the meanings attributed by the person experiencing it, as well as the "cultural construction of clinical reality".

In fact, understanding health and illness as subjective experiences, such as Sigerist (1941), Knottnerus (1983), Illich (1975), among others, allows to comprehend well-being as achievement and as perception. In the conception of Canguilhem (1978), for example, the pathological implies *pathos*, that is, a feeling of suffering and impotence. Medicine must therefore work with the complete individual and not only with their organs and how they function. The "subjective body" and its language, of pain or pleasure, cannot, from the author's perspective, be ignored. Thus, health is, for Canguilhem, a vulgar concept, in the sense of common and accessible to all, and not a scientific notion.

Similarly, the epidemiologist André Knottnerus (1983) puts the focus on the patient's self-perception in the definition of what fits the notion of well-being. Likewise, physical health is associated with social determinants that must be taken into account in the preparation of medical diagnoses, adopting a personalized and integral perspective.

Indeed, several authors have sought to justify the importance not of a "state" of "complete well-being", but rather of resilience and adaptability to ever-changing and largely adverse circumstances. More than a state, health would be a process in which the capacity for adaptation of the human being to cope with life's own anxieties and inadequacies is essential (Huber, 2014). The resilience and "sense of coherence" that some people demonstrate - and that is associated with the concept of salutogenesis worked by Aaron Antonovsky (1979)[3], allows to understand how certain people resist to serious and potentially pathogenic factors. This way it is possible to conceive illness and health, not as opposites, but as extremes on a continuum.

Critical Shifts in Healthcare Conception: Clash of Rationalities and Ethical Conflicts

Around the world there are conflicts in the hospital setting about how to direct care to certain patients. In the name of personal convictions some patients refuse to be lavished the professional gesture provided. A clear conflict arises between the medical rationality that governs the organization of care and the existential rationality that guides the patient. This conflict involves value systems. On the one hand, the one adopted by the medical profession which is agreed to find the origin in the Oath of Hippocrates. It is a system built, unified, generalized and used as a basis for professional ethics. On the other hand, the one conveyed - so to speak - by the patient. It varies from one patient to another. It is not always formulated or stated by the patient and is often expressed through reactions to the hospital's ways of doing things. But it is the source of an ethical conflict that engages both parties.

A paradigmatic case stands out about clash between different rationalities. It has often been the subject of public debate, sometimes of cartoons, but it clearly lays the foundation on which the antagonism of the ethics that put doctors and patients in conflict. As Max Weber had quite rightly explained, it is the caricatural traits of a social phenomenon that best enable to identify the ideal type and thus to gain access to its objective understanding. This paradigmatic case is one that sees a patient, in the name of his religious beliefs, refuse to be examined and treated by a doctor who is not of the same sex.

The story circulated in all media: a man arrives in the middle of the night in the hospital with a high fever. The medical team is solely female. The man, a deeply believing Muslim, refuses to allow care by female doctors. When a male caregiver arrives to take service in the early morning, the man was already in an advanced state of sepsis. He dies in the day. Taking care of him earlier in the night may have saved him. All hospital departments, in one way or another, have had to face this type of situation, which sometimes puts them in a position not to be able to fulfill their primary mission. The refusal of blood transfusions by Jehovah's Witnesses, the refusal to be "touched" by male doctors by Muslim women or their husbands, the refusal to leave their clothes, etc., all these refusal in the name of religious convictions forced the hospital, that is to say the professional medical and nursing bodies, the administration and, beyond, the political guardianship, to clarify the rule that was to prevail. It should be noted that the same difficulty could have arisen within the medical and nursing teams themselves when staff members asserted their religious beliefs so as not to comply with the behavioral rules adopted by the service in which they work. For example, in Great Britain, in 2008, a woman, a radiologist and a Muslim doctor, had to give up her job because she refused to apply the hygiene rule adopted by all health care institutions that asked staff to keep bare arms below the elbow. She emphasized the imperative of modesty and veiling of the body demanded by the Koran.

As we can see, the hospital has become a place where conflicts between the ethics of conviction and the ethics of responsibility are concentrated, to use the conceptions of Max Weber. But, unlike what Weber envisioned, the conflict here does not lead to a simple alternative: either conviction or responsibility. Here, at least on the side of the hospital, responsibility and conviction must seek to coexist. Although they are presented as antagonistic.

Let us first consider the person who proclaims religious convictions. The Muslim believer, for example, is required to show modesty (Hayâ). This is, first of all, a moral virtue that must guide the believer in his relationship with God, but also in his relationship with others and in his relationship with himself. So there is a public morality that emerges and prescribes particular veil parts of the body. Islamic legal traditions will vary as to which parts of the body of the man and woman should be kept veiled, under what circumstances, in what places, and so on. And of course, according to the traditional rule followed, the unveiling of the body can be admitted under certain conditions, tolerated under others or radically proscribed. Obviously, the doctrinaire background is inherited from Genesis, the biblical text that makes the vision of the human body the expressive manifestation of sin. The religions of the Book will draw different lessons. The Koranic religion will draw its social morality. From there, the refusals encountered in the confines of the hospital to offer his body to the sight, the touch, manipulations of doctors and caregivers because it entails a break in the observance of the imperative of modesty.

On the side of the hospital and the nursing staff, they have become accustomed to obey an imperative of efficiency in order to achieve the primary objective of their mission, namely the Hippocratic objective of restoration and preservation of the well-being of the person. To do this, they are required to implement the knowledge and technical actions that form their knowledge and medical skills. This implies that a type of behavioral rationality can be identified and that it depends, of course, on the degree of knowledge and experience attained by medical practice. It has therefore varied over time. In other words, the medical ethics imposed on the hospital is that of the appropriate behavior, the appropriate gesture, which promotes the well-being of the patient who suffers. It is an ethics of action that is finalized and adjusted to the sensitive affects of which the patient testifies. In other words, a pragmatic ethic of responsibility, of what one must be able to account for. No wonder that a logic of effective action is widely needed in the hospital compound and that it takes on the appearance of ever greater submission to the technoscientific imperatives that dominate today largely the medical act. This is to the point where, when they are strongly subject to a managerial rationality of actions, we will be able to blame them for not knowing how to integrate the "human factor". It is therefore that the newly adopted codes of ethics in hospitals have hastened to reaffirm, without abandoning the Hippocratic objective.

If on the philosophical frame, that of the ethical debate precisely, these two ethics can be analyzed and compared from the point of view of the principles that they implement: ethics of the belief founded on the creed in revealed principles. on the one hand; and on the other, ethics of responsibility based on know-how articulated on universal principles relating to human dignity. On the social and political level, their assessment will also be made with regard to the values that dominate in each society. But we belong to societies that are largely secularized, who put human rights at the heart of their public morals, who always intend to master nature - human nature in particular - and who believe profoundly in the efficiency of their science and their techniques. This is the collective morality of today's secularized and developed societies. This is why a precedence of this collective morality will prevail and take precedence over what will appear as a morality only individual.

And, it is probably to limit the social effects of the confrontation of these two morals, to avoid that the fundamental principles of the collective morality are reduced in their effective application, that a compromise will be sought and will take the form of professional ethics and charters circumscribed to the sphere of action that is the hospital. The order of values that controls the normative analysis - Weber spoke in the same sense of "dogmatic" analysis - and which is adopted in our societies - opposed to theocratic societies - no longer operates empirically. Empirically, that is to say for any individual forming the social collective, it is his "personal" system of values that is essential. He can adopt the values of collective morality or subordinate them to those of his religious belief, that is, to the revealed values of his dogma. This in some cases leads him to reject the values of the collective in which he finds himself, since he does not recognize the same dogma. Conflict is therefore inevitable and the risk is that of mutual rejection and / or coercive imposition. In both cases, the empirical conflict remains since its normative source remains. It lies in the impossibility of fully satisfying the primary imperatives of each value system. It is ultimately in order to avoid these consequences that the hospital institution and the whole of society behind it engage in ethical compromise solutions.

The ethical conflict that is expressed in the hospital is therefore never a simple hospital conflict, that is to say a conflict born of the fact that the hospital norm, the ethics that apply to it, would come up against the norms and the heterogeneous values provided by the patient. The conflict is not - or can not be reduced to - a border conflict as if the hospital could function as a closed, extraterritorial space, which would follow its own law. A space in which the "law" of the hospital would have full authority. Although tendentially, it is what directs the action of the hospital, we must however hold it as a social space deeply penetrated, crossed, agitated, by conflicts of values that flourish in the rest of society. And these are somehow imported by all the social agents we meet there, that is to say the patients, these people who consult and come to be treated, and the hospital agents: doctors, personal caregivers, managers, etc. Everyone, indeed, joins the hospital with his stock of personal convictions that will de facto vary axiologically. They also vary on an axis that can be limited by: in one pole, the common values socially shared, those which are first in the type of society in which we live, in the other pole, the most important values, those who are part of his intimate beliefs, his adhesions and personal elections, in short, his good life options.

Our democratic societies "ideally" distribute these values between those which, on the one hand, underlie a "public space", common, axiologically defined by the principles of democracy and formally guaranteed by rights, and, on the other hand, the values which are left to the discretion of each individual and constitute the pragmatic content of his liberties. This distribution, however, always causes in practice conflicts of interpretation. Hence the codes, regulations and other legal mechanisms for managing disagreements that arise. These devices anticipate in a way the "response" to bring to the conflicts. This works very well in a stabilized society, where the differences are appreciated and sanctioned to the height of their importance. It works less well in a society subject to mutation and agitated by contrary normative movements. Hence the permanent exercise of codification that one meets there, sometimes disordered but supposed to bring the discordant facts in the right considered fundamental: the constitutional right. Our societies are experiencing large-scale mutations of all kinds, particularly mutations affecting their populations: environmental, professional, cultural, etc. Mutations which are upsetting not only the relationship we have with each other, but also the role and place that we hold in this society and therefore the social status that we think we have. For this reason, the elaboration of new rules - new rules of living together as it is said -, the adoption of ethical charters and monitoring committees and the application of these charters, become important activities in the political and social regulation of our societies. This general regulation activity is also found in the hospital.

But, as this is also a space which, by definition, is governed by a particular ethical imperative, the Hippocratic imperative, a sort of transcendent law peculiar to the medical sphere, the social conflict when it is transported in calls for a social name of a singular nature. A social name which surpasses the values invoked in the rest of society, those guaranteed by constitutional law, has its own reason. To put it another way, when a conflict concerns the values that structure the hospital activity because an individual, a group, an organized community, contest its application, this conflict tends to blow up the balance that could have to settle between public values and private values, even between collective ethics and singular deontological imperative.

This is why, after some time when the rigid application of the ethical imperative led to questions about the respect of collective values, there was a relaxation in the way of finding a response to the conflicts that arose. Indeed, refusing to hear the request to satisfy the rule of "modesty" expressed by the Muslim patient - a personal rule, private since only related to a religious belief - may lead to a renunciation of care by the patient and in a life-saving emergency, an act of non-assistance to a person in danger. Such an act becomes reprehensible in court because it derogates from the fundamental values of "fraternity" / "solidarity" and "equality" of citizens. But, as it may be the same if we meet the demand (case of the Muslim nurse mentioned above), it is the application of collective ethical values and the hospital ethics itself that has become necessary to rethink.

A more precise and detailed code of ethics will emerge in most countries claiming the values of democracy. It aims to provide the framework within which ethical conflicts in the hospital must now be answered. Roughly speaking, it is considered that in the event of a life-threatening emergency, it is the Hippocratic imperative that prevails and must be imposed on the patient. When such a prognosis is not engaged, the hospital undertakes to seek, within the limits of its means, to meet the particular request of the patient. In other words, the private ethics of the patient obliges the public institution (in the sense that it addresses the community). It is true, only within the limits of its possibilities, which can be restricted. This leads, of course, to new conflicts, but these are no longer fundamentally ethical, they are more related to the service relationship and its satisfaction.

As we can see, the secularization of our societies has given religious beliefs and the values associated with them an elective status for the citizen and not, that of shared evidence, of what must be accepted by all. Our democratic societies have instituted, in the strong sense of the term, the break. Churches have long struggled to accept it. But this will be done in different ways depending on the nations. In any case, the confusion of politics and religion no longer exists. Most often, ethical conflicts of religious origin have ceased to be collective conflicts and have found their answers in the private sphere of choices and personal options. Yet today we are witnessing a kind of return of the pendulum. The ethical conflicts that erupt often put to evil the public / private partition, they crack the consensus on the supreme values of democracy historically built in the West. They produce this effect because they carry a religious belief that refuses the division of areas of competence between religion and politics. As regards Islam, which we have mentioned here, it appears with great vivacity nowadays, probably under the impulse of the forces of radicalization of the interpretation of the dogma, whereas during a good part of the twentieth century this one had proved compatible with the secularization of societies, including in the Middle East and the Maghreb. But, constituted religions are not the only ones involved. There is also a general movement in our societies which, without first challenging the democratic division of the spheres of competence, aspires, however, that its personal expectations are met at best and finds that the collective rule in the rigidity of its application too much of the expression of choices and personal values.

To put it another way, the secularization of our societies by sending back to the individual the affirmation of religious values has strengthened the power of the latter to assert the choice of his values - what has been called also the individuation of society. In doing so, common or commonly accepted collective values, such as freedom of expression, of claim, of behavior in the public space, etc., were recomposed from individuals and no longer from an abstract collective, almost transcendental, and perceived very far apart, if not in contradiction with individual aspirations. In this sense, it can be said that it is the fundamental ethical principles of our democratic societies which, by promoting the affirmation of individual values, have provoked the conflicts that come to question them. We understand why it is on the double register of the confirmation of transcendent public values and the recognition of the variety of individual values that embody them empirically, that re-adjustments are now taking place through codes of ethics and other normative regulations. This, both in the hospital and in many sectors of civil society.

EMERGING TRENDS AND CRITICAL DEBATES IN HEALTHCARE INNOVATION AND PRIVACY

Guided by the desirability of a "complete state of well-being", advances in scientific and technical knowledge have largely enabled, in countries with higher levels of development, to control infectious diseases, minimize or delay the impacts of disabling illness, and reduce the consequences of invasive surgical interventions. It is now possible, thanks to technological innovation in health and the emergency of a new paradigm in terms of care, to ensure an ever greater precision and mastery of the medical act. Currently, the development by researchers around the world of precision tools and anticipation of diseases allow results unimaginable just a decade ago. The ultra-rapid sequencing of DNA - which 30 years ago was a kind of "fairy tale" in the words of Razelle Kurzrock -, the cellular reprogramming and tissue engineering, the "4.0 surgery" (or "cognitive surgery"), the precision medicine, the miniaturized devices for continuous monitoring of health conditions, the advances in home automation, among others, are just examples of processes capable of producing systemic and disruptive innovations in the field of medical care.

The so-called precision medicine, for example, enables currently treatment protocols to be adapted to the molecular specificities of each individual and to predict the risk of emergence of certain diseases, such as cancer, even without visible manifestations of the disease. The All of Us Research Program - inserted in the Precision Medicine Initiative (PMI) and promoted by the National Institutes of Health - is a good example of the alliance between science, politics and technological innovation to assure individualized health care. The Program intends to gain "better insights into the biological, environmental, and behavioral influences on these diseases to make a difference for the millions of people who suffer from them", assuming that precision medicine is "a revolutionary approach for disease prevention and

288

treatment that takes into account individual differences in lifestyle, environment, and biology" (https://allofus.nih.gov/about/about-all-us-research-program). For this purpose DNA and other health information from a million people were collected and stored for use in research. These biospecimens are preserved in the biobank at the Mayo Clinic (Rochester, Minnesota) and combined with other lifestyle and health information provided by participants. In Europe it is the United Kingdom who leads these big studies. The biobank is situated in the industrial area of Stockport and stores biological samples of five hundred thousand British volunteers aged between 40 and 69 years.

Research in the field of precision medicine is currently oriented towards personalized therapy in cases of more resistant cancers. The case of success in the recovery of metastatic breast cancer from Judy Perkins in the USA is particularly well known. After tumor DNA sequencing by a team at the National Cancer Institute headed by Steven Rosenberg, it was possible to identify the patient's own tumor-infiltrating immune cells. These cells were then replicated and injected into the patient, leading to complete eradication of the tumor.

The relevance of precision medicine is therefore unequivocal, pointing to future research prospects that may prove both very stimulating and very disturbing. Stimulant, because they allow scientific advances of great impact, as well as relevant practical effects like decrease the hospital costs, the consequences of inadequate treatments adapting them case by case (theranostics), and the quick recovery of the patients. Disturbing for the possibilities it opens for example to the modification of genes in embryos. Biological repair - now possible - opens the door to an unprecedented revolution in the field of disease prevention and treatment. The mankind ancestral dream of living longer and better seems ever closer, but the fears of manipulation and eugenics do not cease to emerge clearly.

Innovation in Healthcare: Critical Issues

Any innovation produces, inherently, fear and withdrawal. Especially when associated with possible implications in life and in the sense of human, as in the case of health innovations. It is enough to remember the negative social reactions to the first in vitro fertilization in 1978. However, after the birth of Louise Joy Brown, in vitro fertilization and other reproductive technologies have been used to raise thousands of children around the world. The initial fear of "custom-ordering babies" has been gradually diluted. Similarly, the fears associated with the production of the early death of comatose patients for organ transplantation in the course of the first heart transplant in 1967 - by the team of the South African surgeon Christiaan Barnard

- became gradually incongruous. The repetition of the surgeries and the obtained successes contributed to pacify the fears.

Innovating, despite the polysemy of the concept, always implies modifying something - services, processes or products - either by introducing a new way of thinking and doing, or by incremental readjustment of procedures or instruments. It presupposes, therefore, to embark on untrodden paths and accept the risks that this decision entails.

Joseph Alois Schumpeter (1911), a major reference in this field, focuses on the notion of "creative destruction" to exemplify the changes brought about by the introduction of an innovation in business cycles. In other words, he focuses on the capacity for progression of the capitalist system, through the constant revolution of the economic structure. The Schumpeterian concept of innovation refers thus to different ways of carrying out a particular activity, the introduction of a new good or a new quality of a good, a new production method (thus defining the opening of a new market), the conquest of a new source of supply of raw materials, or the emergence of a new structure of organization.

In fact, there are several perspectives on how to conceive innovation. From broader understandings associated mainly with incremental changes, to disruptive processes capable of structurally transforming processes, organizations and ways of life. Similarly, the notion of innovation may entail a more restrictive view associated with the technical and technological dimension, or a broader view that allows to aggregate technical-scientific innovation and social innovation (Moulaert, 2009, 2005; Oosterlynck, van den Broek, Albrechts, Moulaert, & Verhetsel, 2010).

With regard to innovations in the field of health care, many authors focus on the introduction of new knowledge and technology in the field of diagnostic, surgical, treatment, prevention and monitoring of disease and health (Thakur, Hsu, & Fontenot, 2012). Organizations, in turn, foster or encourage these changes, adapting, quickly or progressively, to the uncertainties arising from them and making the best use of them for the accomplishment of their mission. It therefore acquires particular relevance the impact of innovations on the various stakeholders and how they are appropriated or not as useful and relevant. An innovation does indeed involve not only novelty but the application of it and the production of associated value. In services aimed at people the appreciation of the impacts of innovations on value production - not merely economic but also scientific, social and relational - is particularly important.

The notion of "value" is associated, in this case, with a global welfare concept that the introduction of innovation, whether of product or of process, may entail. The fundamental debate is associated, in this perspective, with the "value" conception and with the identification and assessment of the value produced, particularly with regard to the thresholds and the balances between "value creation" and "value appropriation" (Santos, 2009). The relevance and weight of each of these axes actually determines the type and the legitimacy of a given initiative. In other words, the choice of a particular model of action and the coherence between objectives and effective practices must be recognized and valued by health professionals and health consumers as appropriate, in line with the organizational mission. Bell, Masaoka, and Zimmerman (2010, p.41) identified seven criteria to evaluate the value produced by innovation in a given organization: a) alignment with the core-mission; b) excellence in execution; c) scale or volume; d) depth, by analyzing the relevance or importance recognized by the beneficiaries to a particular action or process regardless of scale, and evaluate their level of participation since the conception to the evaluation; e) filling an important gap; f) community-building and g) leverage. The respect for human beings and their choices, the respect for environment and the good use of the material and immaterial resources is also, or must be, an important indicator of the value created with innovative procedures and instruments. In other words the primary focus is to increase the potential and possibilities of the various stakeholders, making them indispensable and integral parts of the praised initiatives. For example, the use of mobile devices to promote telemedicine increases the possibilities to an easier and more efficient access to health information, conscious choices of treatments and health monitoring. Quality of health care can, this way, be deepened and diffused.

Innovations in healthcare, whether in the process, or in the instruments and techniques, should always be guided by the structuring principle of not causing harm and helping health professionals to best perform their mission, preferably more efficiently, more effectively and more sustainably (in terms of patient sequelae and cost of services). Safety and trust in healthcare lies, among other factors, in the development of prior tests and demonstrated results, as well as in detailed information on the level of reliability of a certain treatment, which may still be experimental, or on treatments with best-outcomes or more adapted to the concrete situation of the patient.

Of course, resistance to innovation does not come only from the recipients of the actions. The hospital environment itself, with all the internal and external influences that cross it, may be more open or closed to changes, especially from an administrative perspective and not so much from the one of health professionals and medical care. The adoption by the health manager of a more commercial orientation will potentiate the discovery and acceptance of distinctive and customer focused factors, so it will generate processes of collecting pertinent information about "target" publics, their needs and expectations and the results that can be provided. Critics of this approach accuse it of turning health services into companies, often for profit, which justifies denying treatment to patients who cannot afford it, or encourages treatments or examinations that might be unnecessary. Proponents of this more managerial perspective of the hospital organization emphasize above all the possibility of a more strategic and accountable fulfillment of their mission, creating customer-value. Of course this also presupposes a particular organizational culture, a certain notion of service and the non-questioning of the basic principles of the relationship between health professionals and clients. A relationship that, in fact, as numerous studies show, is one of the central pillars for the quality of health care,

Better doctor–patient communication (e.g. more question-asking, more information giving, shared decision-making and more empathic behaviour) seems to have a positive influence on the consultation, and represents an important determinant of accessibility in health care (Stewart, 1995; Kaplan, Greenfield, & Ware, 1989; Willems, De Maesschalck, Deveugele, Derese, & De Maeseneer, 2005). The quality of information exchanged during the consultation and understanding between doctors and patients may be key to the delivery of high quality counseling. (Schieber, Delpierre, Lepage, Afrite, Chantal, Cases, *et al.*, 2014, p. 707).

Public health policies themselves also tend to increasingly emphasize this dimension of "partnership" between health professionals and patients in prescribing and applying care. A perspective that is not free from risks and paradoxes. In order to know consciously, it is necessary to know and understand adequately the information available, both about the disease and about the treatment and possible consequences of its adoption or rejection. Adequate and accessible access to this information is also an opportunity generated by information technologies applied to health.

Similarly, the appropriation of certain innovations depends on their usefulness and ease of use or the level of novelty and relevance attributed to them, for example in terms of distinctive advantage and the level of adaptations they require.

Studies indicate that besides relative advantage, perceived complexity and compatibility of the new technology also influence its adoption decision. For example, although electronic medical records (EMRs) have been around since the early 1960s, until recently they were not adopted extensively by the majority of healthcare management organizations (Walker, 2006) because of the complexity of maintaining the electronic medical records of the patients. (Thakur, Hsu, & Fontenot, 2012, p. 564).

Healthcare Strategic Assets: Information management, Commitment, and Reflectivity

In fact, one of the most important elements for the efficacy and safety of treatments in health contexts is related to the speed of access and reliability of the information collected about a given patient and their clinical history. The use of information register and secure sharing technologies is essential for the good fulfillment of the mission of health professionals and managers of health organizations. This is because it allows not only the reduction of inadequate and often dangerous treatments for patients (e.g. non-disclosure of intolerance or pharmacological interactions), but also important savings in time and budget resources. Avoiding a repeat of an earlier examination or subjecting the patient to unnecessary testing, ensuring effective sharing of information between health professionals and between services, helps to preserve not only the patient's well-being, but also to identify more easily the origin of a possible error and contribute to the greater economic rationality of the health system. The use of information logging technologies can facilitate this process and support the medical decision or strategic decisions of hospital managers (where to allocate resources, what to transform, how best to articulate the services, etc.), as well as contribute to the transformation of organizational culture. Health information management thus becomes currently a key strategic resource for health organizations (Inamdar, Kaplan, & Bower, 2002).

The dimension of the relationship between managers and other staff is also very relevant. The commitment-based strategy and the clear sharing of information and operational decision-making appear to be not only more productive and effective (Khatri, Baveja, Boren, & Mammo, 2006), but also more potential for intangible gains (e.g. at the level of the relationship between professionals and between professionals and patients) essential to a greater humanization and quality of the services provided. Among others, the study of Ekedahl and Wengstrom (2008) found that organizations that promote positive relationships in the workplace and that establish a relational and sharing culture have more successful performances and effects on better organizational learning.

In healthcare organizations, sometimes the manager is also someone of the clinical staff who helps to keep the focus on the organization's essential mission. Bottom-up management with information flows from a lower level to a top level is however essential, as is the role of the patient in defining and evaluating the services provided and the expectations they have in terms of their quality.

Peter Drucker (1985), a relevant name in organizational management studies, stresses that organizations' success relates to their strategic ability to identify opportunities and align with the needs and characteristics of audiences, professionals and new knowledge and instruments.

Health organizations also need coping strategies to enhance the quality and effectiveness of services. What is assured namely by the support of the organization to its staff and by the apprenticeship from mistakes and omissions. Mistakes that in the case of the healthcare sector can be dramatic and painful. It is enough to recall the consequences of contaminated blood transfusions, surgeries performed on the wrong part of the body or the wrong side of the brain, accidentally turned off vital signs machines, incorrectly given anesthesia, misinterpretation of vital signs, inadequate removal of injured from accident sites causing trauma irrecoverable, among many others.

Despite technical advances in diagnosing and recording information, the number of recorded medical errors leading to the death of patients, whether through negligent practices or incorrect decisions, has been increasing. The U.S. Institute of Medicine's To Err Is Human report reported, in 1999, approximately 98,000 patient deaths from medical errors. In 2010, the Office of Inspector General for the Department of Health and Human Services registered 180,000; a number that has been increasing exponentially in the last decade. Of course, these numbers may be due mainly to the improvement of recording techniques of occurrences and the greater ability of families to face the powerful class of health professionals increasingly subject to lawsuits. However, these data suggest the need for further reflection.

Studying errors and learning how to avoid or minimize them contributes to advancing health care and changing standards of care. Increased regulation and standardized practices have contributed to the transformation of care protocols, which now allow better protection of patients, health professionals themselves and health organizations. Many of these standard practices stem from learning from mistakes made and are now assumed to be normal and necessary, and mostly based on scientific evidence. For example, the prevention of wrong-site surgery has become one of the norms inscribed in the Joint Commission for Accreditation of Healthcare Organizations (JCAHO) in U.S. Preoperative procedures are standardized and guidelines that oblige the marking of the surgical site, with the participation of the patient, and double-check information by all the members of the surgical team. Other examples of apprenticeship after dramatic medical errors and the advancements of medical knowledge are: postoperative sponge and instrument counting; medical forms that include information about allergies; breast self-examination, and mammograms as a standard of care (and even a health policy measure in some countries, encouraging examinations for all women over the age of 45); procedures associated with trauma care, standardized in the Advanced Trauma Life Support; among many others.

A carefully collecting and sharing of information about patients is a central element of surgical success, as well as the establishment of medical routines. For example, time-outs before each surgery to check patient's identification and clinical history, equipment, professionals engaged and the roles of each one in the surgery, anticipated risk events, etc.

The origin of the errors may be related, either with negligence and insufficient knowledge, or with errors of the health system itself or the instruments used. Technical-scientific advancement and the introduction of advanced technological innovation can help to minimize some of the most frequent errors, however the risk inherent in any treatment or surgery can never be totally eliminated.

It is possible only to underline some essential strategies to increase the quality of health services, such as: better communication between health professionals (for example in shift changes and emergency services), can be emphasized alongside technological advances; better communication between physician and patients that enables the collection of more complete information about the clinical history and about elements that can affect decision making; increased levels of hospital hygiene and infection control; improvement in the training of new professionals subjecting them to pressure tests and the resolution of unexpected situations; reserving the most complex surgeries for the most experienced surgeons so as not to turn patients into guinea pigs and learning objects (advancement in robotic models of human simulation for surgery training is a good way to associate learning and protection); the request for a second opinion in more complex diagnostic cases, among other aspects.

A relevant and complex issue in the field of health care mistakes lies in the responsibility of medical personnel. While on the one hand it is important in terms of preserving trust in health professionals that certain errors are recognized and punished, on the other hand, it is necessary to consider the complex question of the intentionality of the act and the risk that always persists in any treatment process. In this case, it is necessary to distinguish between gross errors or omissions and negligent and careless practices, from the normal consequences of the decision made on the basis of the best available scientific and technical knowledge. Decision-making (often in a minimal time span) calls for this expertise gained from experience and available knowledge for the best possible decision-making. However, the human factor is always there even with the most sophisticated instruments and the most standardized procedures. The decision is always human and in unexpected situations a prudential judgment is in the background of the action. It is enough to recall the "Sully" case. Chesley "Sully" Sullenberger was the captain of US Airways Flight 1549 taking off from LaGuardia Airport (New York City), on January 15, 2009. Loss of power in both engines due to a large flock of birds forced to a quick decision. Assuming that it was not possible to reach either LaGuardia or Teterboro airport, the captain made the decision of landing on the Hudson River and saved all 155 people on board.

It was a decision-making marked by rationality and based on acquired knowledge, experience (derived from other similar situations) and ability to control emotions. This knowledge to act, that in situations of crisis and uncertainty is affirmed, although starting from an identified risk situation, thus minimally controlled, does not fail to produce unexpected and often dramatic results. A drama that, in the case of health services, can produce irreparable damage to the life of a human being, which subjects health professionals to high levels of stress and controlled distress.

What we might call "knowing how to act" must therefore include the following analytical dimensions of structuring action itself: a) the unavoidable presence of a component of order and uniformity, manifested in shared medical language and organizational and deontological orientations; b) the plurality of principles and rationalities coexisting in the same context, together with a tacit dimension of "between us" essential for the proper functioning of health services; c) the contingency and unpredictability at the heart of the action, resulting from the profound daily variability of situations, accompanied by an "inspired" component of the practice, thus a strong presence of "sensorial gestures" (feeling, intuiting, perceiving) and singularity, used by professionals in the development of the practice and difficult to translate in terms that others (professionals or not) can recognize and understand.

In fact, the indetermination and contingency of the practices of health professionals, despite an increasing routinization and parameterization of procedures, are not negligible. It is therefore central to the understanding of the architecture of the decisions of these professionals to consider that not only their knowledge and techniques intervene, but also their complicity with chance, emotion, *kaïros* (that is, the acuity of the right moment to act), the inescapable force of circumstances and the tactical dimension of practice. Therefore, the intrinsic and extrinsic paradoxes of decision and priorities, and the confluence or co-possibility of heterogeneous elements in the construction of situations. This is because the "matter" for the production of the action - the patient and the manifestation of the disease - has largely unknown contours and the elaboration of a diagnosis and the resulting treatment has a strong dimension of trial and error. A dimension that even the most advanced diagnostic techniques cannot override.

The inescapability of acting, most often under the pressure of the moment, for example in emergency services, emphasizes the importance of reflective capacity as constitutive of the action itself. Using a prudential rationality, health professionals construct the deliberative situation with other professionals, with the patients and with the families under assumptions of reasonability and admissibility. The situational character of the exchange of arguments does not imply, however, a radical relativity of the procedures of action. As the notions of reasonableness and admissibility presuppose, the argumentative dynamics, although situationally constructed, must be susceptible of being registered in a public space, that is, taking into account criteria shared and recognized by all those who do not directly construct the situation (team, community, etc.). Saying it differently, construct an argument that articulates the general and the particular, the one and the multiple, in a daily dynamics of de-composition, re-composition and inter-composition of the practices and of their modalities of justification. These are essential elements not only to explain to patients or families the unexpected results of a certain treatment that was deemed appropriate or an unsuccessful surgical intervention. Likewise, this ability to translate medical arguments externally is fundamental in internal investigation processes or in legal proceedings.

At the heart of the analysis is the power to act, that is, the explication of the capacity to justify the how and why one acts in a certain way and the core of values and principles inherent to this process of explanation and justification of the action. The hospital space, as demonstrated by Anselm Strauss's sociological studies, especially in the classic works Boys in White (1961), Psychiatric Ideologies and Institutions (1964) and Chronic Illness and the Quality of Life (1975), this one in partnership with Barner Glaser, is permeated by tacit logics and shared languages, grounded in the context, and often incomprehensible to the outside. The cohesion generated in this way is also a mechanism of management of the unforeseen with several implications in terms of speed and effectiveness in the answers.

This way, a rational (dynamic and flexible) conception of rationality stands out, which can be called "prudential", by reference to the Aristotelian concept of *phronèsis,* that is, a practical judgment in situation. This takes place, and at the same time triggers, the reorientation of discourse and practices. The conversation between the one and the multiple, and the composition that results from it, presupposes a continuous movement of re-composition and argumentative deconstruction, in view of the coherent coordination of the action with other agents. As Donald Schön (1994) puts it, a "coherent and uniform improvisation" presupposes a common *"canevas"*, a repertoire to be mobilized at the right moment, which may even lead to a re-adaptation of the practice in a new direction. Using the metaphor of the jazz music mentioned above,

When good jazz musicians begin to improvise as a group, they also demonstrate that they "feel" their instrument and that they adjust to the music as it emerges. By listening themselves and listening to others, they feel where the music is heading and adjust their performance accordingly. They can do this primarily because, in their collective creation effort, they use a common basis - rhythm, melody and harmony are familiar to each musician - which allows to predict in part the following of the passage (p. 83).

The dynamics and attunement of this process of articulation with other professionals and other rationalities is, in fact, an important component of the "competence in act" of health professionals and of the consecration of reflexivity in the daily practice of professional practice.

Reflectivity assumes itself as a product and a producer of dialogue with situations and contexts. One of the key aspects in this perspective is the evidence that practice is rooted in an "experiential" core of the subject's relationship with his / her knowledge and learning, in the course of a dynamic theoretical-practical "dialogue" with the situation, the *loci* of action and the agents that they frame. It is a kind of "logic of concert", that is, the sharing of a common sense, a shared repertoire to be mobilized at the appropriate time and place, and allowing the mutual justification and adaptation of professional acts and decisions. We can therefore distinguish three dimensions of reflectivity associated with action: a) reflexivity in action, that is, the construction of the current practice by mechanisms of appreciation, adaptation and feedback, in order to increase the adequacy between purposes, processes and results; b) reflexivity by action, that is, knowledge and elements derived from action that will become readjustments in the forms of intervention and treatment protocols for example. The reflexivity by action allows the mobilization and the conjugation of previous knowledge and experiences, in consonance with the specificity of the situation constructed and under construction, thus building a renewed corpus of knowledge and abilities; c) reflexivity for action, that is, the strategic preparation of action. In our analysis, we understand the notion of strategy as a translator of the exercise of a competent rationality in the combination of different logics and principles taking into account the aim to be reached and the overcoming (not denial) of contingency. A dose of freedom and interactive construction is therefore inherent to possible determinisms.

The use of technologies by health professionals seeks not only to increase the accuracy of the medical act but also to reduce as much as possible the circumstantial components. However, as it has already been said, the human dimension associated with unpredictability persists and resists to various types of control. The relationship between health professionals and patients, for example, involves the combination of different knowledge and a repertoire of expectations, representations and analogies, anchored in the "familiarity" constitutive of trustworthiness. The critical detachment, which many people call "the coldness of healthcare professionals" as if an emotional barrier had been built, is therefore crucial. Reflection, for action and in action contribute, as Schön (1994) points out, to the correction of this "excess of knowledge", that is, the "familiarity" with contexts and situations (only apparently) similar and iterative.

In this perspective, reflectivity is a circular process of mutual influence between situational and contextual data, values, theories, convictions and experiences, of the various actors in the interaction situation and that allows reassessing the way in which situations are understood considering also the way others understand them and according to the evidence of their value. Reflectivity implies, therefore, not only personal and professional characteristics, but also the knowledge of the context and relational spaces, by the assumption of an open, critical and predictive posture, as well as the relevant mobilization of their knowledge and the elements of "return of experience" into processes of continuous adjustment and learning.

In this way, reflexivity is diatopic insofar as it involves, on the one hand, ethical parameters - the principles "beyond" the act and the consideration and respect for the values of the other, placing trust in the argument and the acquired knowledge - and bon the other hand by expressive parameters - an argumentative construction adapted to the situation and to the public visibility of the arguments, that is, the "good reasons for ..." (Boudon, 2003). The "expressive" axis emphasizes both the pertinent construction of the argument itself, that is, the way in which the different arguments and premises are articulated, or the uniqueness arising from the association, concerning a concrete situation, of general principles (namely of deontological character) and the professional's ability to interpret, innovate and adapt (O'Sullivan, 2011).

The term responsibility comes from the Latin *respondere* (answer). Thus responsibility would be the quality of the one who "responds by his own actions or those of others", and of those who must respect "their commitments" (Michaelis Dictionary). It is, therefore, a concept anchored in action and in close connection with the contexts. In this perspective, its substantiality results, on the one hand, from the existence of other living beings in articulation in the different shared contexts and, on the other hand, from the role played by different segments of society (citizens, public organizations, companies, State, communities) considering the articulation between multiple factors of economic, political and cultural order.

Thus, responsibility lies at the heart of the sense of humanity and citizenship. It is the existence and consciousness of the Other, "infinite in his finitude" according to Lévinas (1993). As human beings and as citizens we are responsible for our acts and omissions. A responsibility that is even greater today, given the fading of certainties and the affirmation of the plurality of values and behaviors admissible.

The notion of social responsibility thus becomes the true balance between the right to freedom of choice and the duty to consider the consequences of these same choices, towards other human beings, towards nature and towards the cosmos. The concept is, however, ambiguous, acquiring differentiated connotations depending on the prism of analysis, the domain of application and the underlying ideological perspective.

The presuppositions of order, stability and prediction of regulatory mechanisms were, in modern societies, conditions for technological development and foundations of progress that was considered linear and virtuous, and which was at the same time the product and producer of the same order.

The knowledge of the world, based on this normative conception, was based on the Cartesian perspective of reducing complexity through the divisibility and classification of the real into progressively simpler elements. Thus, from the simplicity and regularity of the laws of nature, we sought the predictability and control of phenomena, with the purpose not only of understanding the real, but especially of transforming it into principles of (presumably) universal order. The Newtonian laws accurately translate the simplism of a mechanistic reading of the world, with causality as principle. The social sciences themselves have appropriated and adapted such a paradigm, classified, consequently, as dominant, to the understanding of society and of social dynamics and structures. In this perspective, it was considered that society itself could be explained and regulated, based on the same factualist, mechanistic and organicist principles (as Comte, Durkheim or Parsons theorized), proper to natural phenomena. Therefore, with potential for predictability and generalizing explanation.

This thought classified by Ortega y Gasset (1987, p. 39), as "orthopedic thinking", has reduced the understanding of the problems and the concrete questions that are posed to humanity, to the logic and concepts that have emptied it of content. In this respect we can highlight, for example, the effects of the institutionalization and professionalisation of the production of knowledge, namely in the Academy. It ends up, in the limit, reducing science to the answers to the problems which it itself articulates, in a largely self-legitimating sterile spiral.

Indeed, this model of thinking embodies a rationality that has contributed to the affirmation and consolidation of potentially disaggregating paradigms of progress and development because they are dissociated from self-monitoring and from self-criticism of the boundaries between power and duty. The effects of a socially autistic model of economic and technological growth, for example, on the environment, are not, according to the "orthopedic paradigm", thought to be harmful, but as a "small" price to pay for development, understood in the strict sense, that tends to generate the own mechanisms (economic, social and political) that allow reproducing it.

However, in the last three decades, the first signs of questioning about the reducibility of such a model of thought and the incongruity of the assumptions that support it begin to emerge. First of all, Truth, associated with a scientific discourse in some unquestionable way, becomes relativized by processes of refutation and argumentation in pluralistic, conflicting and unpredictable societies (Popper, 2000). In this sense, concepts and guarantees of objectivity, predictability, causality and order, as well as the plausibility of unique and universal languages are questioned. In this way, other truths emerge as legitimate and appealing science to achieve the "second rupture with common sense", returning to society, the so-called "profane space", the scientific discoveries and achievements. The forms of understanding of the real which the "dominant paradigm" has provided and which emerge as the diffuse, uncertain, and sometimes even contested traits of a new form of intelligibility, objectivity and practice.

In this context, Giddens (2000) highlights the concepts of "end of nature" and "end of tradition" as the basis for understanding this new paradigm of knowledge, based on a renewed perspective of participation and social responsibility. The "end of nature" translates, in the view of the author, a mutation in the relation human being-nature. From a concern with the action of nature on his life, man begins to worry, today, with his actions on the nature and the impacts of this action on the future. In this perspective, the principles of "prudence", the sustainable use of natural resources and the "respect" for the preservation of life in its various manifestations are evidenced. These principles are based on an "imperative of responsibility" as a safeguard of the future or, in a "future oriented ethics", as defined by Jonas (1995), in his reference work published in Germany in 1979.

The "end of tradition", in turn, corresponds to an understanding of events, all, not as the product of predetermined forces, but as something built and rebuilt permanently, under a logic of "active trust", of freedom, of will and of individualism. Contemporary societies are characterized by "manufactured risks" (Giddens, 2000), that is, the risks arising from a set of processes that seek to build human progress and development in contexts of uncertainty, unpredictability and co-responsibility for future. Risks that are manufactured and expand in almost all dimensions of human life. In this context, self-affirmation in today's societies also reveals its less positive side: fragility tends to constitute itself as a living brand; freedom, at the same time as it is desired, becomes a difficult burden to manage; autonomy, which necessarily entails ties of aggregation to others, tends to become a kind of over-individualization, by defect or excess, of "over-accountability of self," as Ehrenberg (2000) wrote. In this context, a new sense of responsibility seems unavoidable, appealing to each and everyone's capacity for a multidimensional and always incomplete and uncertain understanding of the role and the respective impacts on the construction of the future or alternative futures.

The conception of today's societies as risk societies (and at risk) implies, as Mattedi and Butzke (2001) point out, in overcoming the modern dichotomy that allowed the separation of nature and society. According to this conception, society would be produced independently of nature, using it only as a resource for the service of developmental logic. The understanding of modern society as a "risk society", according to Beck (1992), however, highlights the need to reflect deeply on the relations between the knowledge society, nature, social, economic and political.

In a context of "reflective modernity," as Beck, Giddens and Lash (1995) read, the notion of progress and the knowledge that underlies it, in fact, acquires renewed and more complex contours. Indeed, if the modern "risk societies" conceptualized by Beck (1992) include a set of impacts and contingent factors resulting, in a first line, from a globalized process of accelerated modernization, and the consequent production of pluri-insecurities, the current societies, marked by increased uncertainty and complexity, increase this effect and constitute not only as societies of risk, but also as societies at risk. In fact, a new conception of risk, with a greater degree of unpredictability, puts the use and reliability of knowledge, in particular scientific knowledge and the technical applications resulting from it, in a new light.

More information about phenomena and possible impacts (in terms of education, health, environment or socio-economic integration) creates new mechanisms of insecurity and re-dimension the notion of responsibility, both citizens and judged by the ability to anticipate risks and control them (Beck, Giddens, & Lash, 1995). The very mechanisms of control, intensified given the difficulty in accurately determining the risk thresholds, themselves become sources of new insecurities, in a sort of spiral of continuous reproduction of causes and effects. The political and social alert surrounding the pandemics of the last decade and the mass vaccination programs resulting therefrom are an example of this. The relationship with opposing temporalities is, at this level, obvious and poses important political challenges. On the one hand, there is a need to act in the present, under a logic of urgency and in a context of proximity in order to safeguard the possibility of future (considering the knowledge we have about the eventuality and effects of various natural and military disasters). On the other hand, it is necessary to orient the action in the long term in face of the urgency of global transformations and of civilizational changes at the global and local scale.

In this context, a new framework of social responsibility acquires relevance. In view of the increase and complexity of the risks, the increase of social inequalities and new dynamics of exclusion, cause and consequence of (which eventually leads to) the breakdown of traditional mechanisms of integration and social participation such as salaried work. In this sense, it is increasingly advocated a greater political, social and educational commitment to the construction of a global ethic. Here, it is a question of assuming a morality of responsibility which, at the root, constitutes the imperative of responding to its actions. As Etchegoyen (1995, p. 31) states, the morality of responsibility translates "the complex synthesis of a global requirement and specific situations". Responsibility must therefore underlie a project of society based on sharing, prudence and respect. These principles derive from a knowledge anchored not only in science, but also in the social experience of different groups. In short, we seek a knowledge that is transmuted into wisdom. A general understanding is sought that the community, the historical patrimony and the polis constitute themselves as "common goods".

Healthcare Information Management: Confidence and Accountability

Additionally, we must considerer that each innovation and change is accompanied, to different degrees, by a set of benefits, but also by risks and constraints, forcing a serious reflection on the balance between them and the ethical and sociopolitical implications entailed.

It is important to ensure the distinction between the knowledge produced by science and its application. Science is guided by a presupposition of increasing knowledge, knowing more and better to better respond to a given question. Intrinsically, it is morally neutral. It is not a method of deciding what priorities to take, the acceptable or unacceptable risks, or the benefits or harms of certain technical applications. These considerations call for a different kind of rationality than scientific rationality. Although science often serves to give them legitimacy.

Innovation fear is understandable, but it is diluted along with continued application of innovations and proof of results. In fact, many of the resistance to innovations in the field of treatment and prevention of disease stem not from the potentially associated technical risks, but of moral dimensions. For example, although transplants of various organs, such as kidneys and corneas, have been performed at the time, heart transplantation has proved to be much more controversial. The argument that the heart was not an organ equivalent to the others was centered on the belief, of mystical and religious roots, that it housed the soul and was the stronghold of the noblest sentiments of the human being. To transplant it would correspond to an attack on the "essentiality" of the human being. Thus, arguments of a moral nature often tend to be involved in medical-scientific processes. The same is true today of many of the arguments invoked for example concerning precision medicine.

The continuity of the research on human genome editing is inevitable and the enabling technology is rapidly evolving. The Human Genome Project took 13 years (1990-2003) to sequence a genome. Today it is possible to do it in one day and with relatively low costs. Modification of embryos seems to be the next step. The report of the US National Academy of Sciences, Engineering and Medicine - Human Genome Editing: Science, Ethics, and Governance (2017) - stresses the importance of further deepening clinical trials, while maintaining some constraints and reserves: promotion of well-being as a principle; transparency of information accessible and understandable to stakeholders; due care supported by sufficient and robust evidence; responsible science; respect for persons, their dignity and personal choices; fairness and equity in risks and benefits, and transnational cooperation and respect of different cultural contexts (NAS, 2017, pp. 11-12).

Often associated with human genetic engineering, the human enhancement technologies are a group of techniques that aim, above all, by the association of nanotechnology, biotechnology, information technology and cognitive science, to improve human performance and capacities (enhanced memory, enhanced communication, enhanced senses, multi-dimensional thinking, extending the body, machine thinking). They go beyond strict concern about the treatment of diseases and disabilities. These developments lie at the basis, for example, of the controversial transhumanist movement, which focuses on the development of human potentialities, eliminating natural limits and constraints that hinder the maximum physical and mental expansion of the human being (Hughes, 2004; Bailey, 2004). According to the National Intelligence Council's Global Trends 2030 report (2012), "human augmentation could allow civilian and military people to work more effectively, and in environments that were previously inaccessible (...)", superhuman "abilities, enhancing strength and speed, as well as providing functions not previously available" (p.100). However,

Owing to the high cost of human augmentation, it probably will be available in 15-20 years only to those who are able to pay for it. Such a situation may lead to a two-tiered society of an enhanced and non-enhanced persons and may require regulation. In addition, the technology must be sufficiently robust to prevent hacking and interference of human augmentation. Advances in synergistic and enabling technologies are necessary for improved practicality of human augmentation technologies (NIC, 2012, p.100).

A new dimension of individual responsibility and fulfillment of desires or expectations for greater well-being therefore find in technological innovations in health an important field of action.

The definition of norms and directives of data protection is very relevant and contributes to create a climate of accountability and confidence on healthcare systems and professionals. Patients trust that the personal information they share with health professionals is confidential, and even deontological and legally privileged. They assume an assumption of confidence. Confidence in health professionals, confidence in the results of science and medical treatments, confidence in the responsible use of data and information collected (Checkland, Marshall, & Harrison, 2004; McKinlay, Marceau, 2002; Porter, Morphet, Missen, & Raymond, 2013; Zheng, 2014).

Some studies, however, show a progressive loss of confidence in health professionals today (Davies, 1999; Donaldson, 2001; McKinlay, & Marceau, 2002; Zheng, 2015). For example, a study by Hui Zheng in the U.S. referring to the last three decades revealed an increase in distrust in these professionals. A mistrust not so much associated with their scientific authority ("obedience to doctors 'instructions"), but with their professional ethics and power ("trusting physicians' standards of practice") (Zheng, 2015, p.702).

Particularly, confidence in medicine is most directly affected by the performance of this institution. Declining confidence in medicine may be related to specific trends in medical institutions, such as the erosion of physicians' power. Pescosolido et al. (2001) found that the lack of confidence in medicine is associated with negative sentiments toward physicians. Negative attitudes towards physicians have become more widely endorsed over time, possibly in response to the penetration of managed care and the changing landscape of health insurance. In the past half-century, physicians have become increasingly specialized as a result of "the burst of new knowledge flowing from the dramatic rise and productivity of biomedical research since World War II, the array of technology deriving from those advances, and a widespread desire among physicians for related expertise" (Barondess, 2000:1300). (Zheng, 2015, p. 702).

The loss of confidence in health professionals and institutions in recent years is closely related, as has already been mentioned, to the mediatization of errors, scandals and reprehensible practices. For example, the high death rates from pediatric cardiac surgery in Bristol Royal Infirmary in UK; the errors in the screening of blood products in France and Portugal; the omissions in the rapid control and information about the bovine spongiform encephalopathy; the removal, in the Alder Hey hospital (Liverpool) of organs at post mortem examination from children without their parent's consent, among others.

Accountability and regulation concerns increase in this context, generating paradoxical effects of increasing security, but also greater risk and error intolerance (Checkland, Marshall, Harrison, 2004). On the other hand, the effects that these issues may have on the self-confidence and practice of health professionals deserve greater consideration in terms of training and hospital management (Connick, Connick, Klotsas, Petroula, Tsagkaraki, & Gkrania-Klotsas, 2009; Porter, Morphet, Missen, & Raymond, 2013).

Regulation (particularly associated with data protection) contributes to the increase of confidence in health systems and establishes thresholds of accountability. However, the overemphasis on the dimension of confidence and its regulation can lead, as

Harrison and Smith (2004) show, to a loss of flexibility in professional practice and gesture and to obscure the essential uncertainty associated with diagnoses and treatments. Paradoxically, this obscuration can generate unrealistic expectations in patients who, when not met, lead to new regulations and attempts at control. It is therefore important to maintain, as the authors say, the trust between professionals and patients. So it is impossible to regulate everything and control all the margins of uncertainty and the moral dilemmas that pervade the practice. In fact,

There is some evidence in practice that concentrating upon measures to increase confidence does have dysfunctional consequences. The most obvious of these is the potential for the distortion that occurs when particular performance targets are privileged above all else, with the consequent de-prioritisation of aspects of practice that are not being measured. (Checkland, Marshall, & Harrison, 2004, p. 132)

The Ethos of Confidence

Confidence is, by definition, the ex-ante and ex-post product of a risk control relationship. In this way, she always admits a relative dose of uncertainty and unpredictability. This is why, as Niklas Luhmann (1979) affirms, trust is only fully achieved in a familiar world, that is, a world that re-inscribes events within a framework with known and relatively predictable thresholds. The social, moral and psychological "tranquility" of social individuals derives from the quietude they experience, a feeling of confidence they feel in the continuity of objects, behaviors and social activities. The security environment that derives from this "routine" quietness embodies the promise of the perpetuation of the world and its order. This means that the production of "social tranquility" focuses precisely on the creation of common routines that mark both the scope of its possible actions and the interpretation of the actions of others.

Trust has thus become established as the essential ballast of life in society. It is this that allows us to leave the house every day and get closer to others and institutions without fear of being destroyed by this "openness", this "availability" to interact with it, this ethos of confidence. The ethos of confidence is also at the root of the governance of the complex and unpredictable societies of modernity, as well as the development of the modern economy, as Peyrefitte (1995) and Fukuyama (1996) rightly pointed out, or the management of organizations. There is no trust without reliability, and trust oblige. In order for trust in others, and vice versa, to exist, everyone must be "trustworthy": true to their commitments, duties and mutual expectations. The Lockean notion of *fides* allows the association of one human being with another, that is to say, the duty to respect the mutual commitment and virtue resulting from the fulfillment of that duty. Although this is beyond social obligation, because it is above all a duty of the man as man, it is also a duty which obviously finds its translation in the social behaviors. A kind of "tacit agreement" in which, like the Garfinkel formula, each person engages in an unspoken conjuncture of "good faith" and according to a common definition of the situation and shared knowledge.

Modern confidence is also "tooled confidence", to use the expression of Mangematin and Thuderoz (1997). It calls for devices (contracts, legal codes, etc.) in order to model and frame the social relations of trust. It also serves as a basis for various conventions, often supported by "tacit mental devices", symbolic or imaginary, such as the recognition of shared roles and values associated with honor, loyalty or solidarity. We must recall, for example, the faith in the word given as a source of legal commitment and social obligation to do.

It thus appears that confidence is assumed, in modern societies, as the base of normality, of the expected. "All is well," is to say that things seem to be what they should be. Logic closely associated with the luhmannian notion of familiarity. From a modern perspective, trust is only possible in a world that has become familiar, such as the hospital or health care. Familiarity, anchored in a historical and experiential perspective (one that allows for the development of mutual expectations), is even turned into a precondition for trust.

People's appeal to healthcare services is based on this "familiarity" assumption of what is expected of a healthcare service: being "well" treated and produce life, not harm. A familiarity anchored in the confidence that the people who treat them will have the best knowledge and experience possible and that the information they will provide will be treated with discretion, privacy and security. Questions today particularly pertinent given the amount of information available and the ease of its recording and sharing.

Health Data Protection: Accountability and Privacy

There is now an international consensus on patients' rights to the privacy and confidentiality of information transmitted in the therapeutic relationship, as well as informed consent on the possibilities and consequences associated with a given treatment (WHO, 2015). For example, the right not to be over-medicated or subject to unnecessary treatment or testing. In sum, it is the duty of professionals to fulfill a "moral ideal" associated with the organization's mission and the deontological rules of its own practice which, as Brown and Moore (2001) refer, are at the heart of accountability processes.

Accountability is, in fact, a concept of relational nature, which must be analyzed within the framework of relationships that organizations establish with agents to whom they are accountable, and from which they seek to construct shared meanings and meanings (Christensen and Ebrahim, 2006; Ebrahim, 2003). In defining accountability Kearns (1994) focus on the importance of the relationship with stakeholders, that is, the means by which it seeks to manage and respond to its diverse expectations and needs., building a model of mutual accountability.

Crack (2013) refers to these processes by grouping them into two perspectives. The first is centered on the demonstration of sound financial management and in accordance with the legal presuppositions that regulate the performance of social organizations. For this reason, accountability mechanisms focus on the management of resources and the results obtained in the short term and are essentially oriented to respond to the interests and expectations of the agents who finance and supervise these organizations. The second perspective stems from the need to meet the expectations of the people who support the organization's raison d'être and therefore presents a holistic perspective of accountability processes in relation to all social actors, with a particular focus on the people and communities they serve. It is inspired by the notions of people-centered development, empowerment of communities and participatory decision-making, and presupposes a reflexive and critical practice of mutual and continuous learning. It focuses, therefore, on creating moral and socially binding expectations among stakeholders around common values and goals rather than economic and legal incentives. In this way, the parties involved take responsibility and mobilize to act in accordance with the shared objectives. In this model, the sanctions for the violation of the expectations among the stakeholders are of a social and relational nature, but also of an economic or legal nature (Brown, Moore and Honan, 2004).

The right to privacy, in particular, advocates that patients have the right to reject interference in their bodies and to make their own choices. For this purpose, the information must be accurate and scientifically reliable, as well as its intelligibility, ie adequacy to its educational level, culture and cognitive ability.

Confidentiality relates to the duty of health professionals to keep patient information confidential. It is a fundamental deontological principle of medical practice, also recognized by law as privileged communication and, as such, protected and safe. Safety refers to the processes used to protect the privacy of health information and to ensure the attended confidence between health professionals and patients. The use of electronic medical records, for example, facilitated the sharing of information and processes between professionals and between services, but on the other hand, it has complicated the process of information security, requiring constant attention to possible attacks on software and dynamics for permanent updating. A system that becomes more complex as more data is collected and more processes expand, for example using mobile health devices. The level of electronic security, however, allows higher levels of security of the information collected than paper records. First of all because it fits the "digital footprint". It is possible to know when, who and where given information was accessed. However, it is also easier to violate and change the registered information.

The patient-consumer is at the center of the paradigm shift in health as it has already been pointed out, so the safety assurances of health information management are a relevant factor to emphasize as the mechanism that produces trust in healthcare system. Nevertheless, complex aspects such as those related to the ownership of information and the decision on what to reveal and what to keep secret acquire particular complexity, generating a new professional field in health institutions - information managers - in order to proactively anticipate problems in the protection of information and to determine the way of access to it by different professionals, with different objectives (even outside the hospital scope such as insurers or community agents), and the patient and the family. In this context a particularly pertinent aspect relates for example to the level of information protection after the death of the patient. The fundamental principle is that the owner of the substantive information is the patient and therefore has the right to consult and clarify the dimensions that may constitute it as not very precise, as well as determine when and if they can be revealed. Health services are the owners of the physical registry and therefore must ensure their privacy, confidentiality, security, integrity and availability. The ethic of privacy is therefore not centered on the decisions made by health professionals based on the information they have access to, but rather on the possibility for people to control information about them and determine the limits for their disclosure or noninterference. The clarification of the rules of the game and the processes for its implementation (for example by the use of more advanced technological processes) goes beyond the dimension of ethics in favor of a technical and even conceptual dimension (the discussion about identity, the notion of public and private, intimacy, autonomy, cooperation, among others). The relationship between what can be done (viability and legality) and what must be done (ethics) should thus be balanced and continually revised. That is why it is vital to accelerate research on the subject of privacy and data security and invest in prospective analysis.

The necessary reorganization of technology in continuity, currently demanded by the health services, advocates rethinking the subjects, the team relationship, the ways of working and the organization of the practices. In fact, in the face of a paradigm shift in health care by the introduction of diagnostic and treatment technologies that often go beyond physical interaction between health professionals and patients (through the use of surgical robotics or telemedicine), the subject of health practice it also broadens, extending beyond the traditional offer of health services, sanitary and preventive campaigns in the community or programs of epidemiological surveillance, for the development of techniques of anticipation and treatment of asymptomatic diseases and for the technological education of medical personnel. In this context, Emerson Mehry (2002) refers to the "technological valises" of current health practices and the profound way in which they have impacted on care itself.

Likewise, a more holistic conception of health and its respective social, economic, cultural and ecological constraints requires a greater planning of health care and policies thought of a broader focus. New professionals therefore come into the field of health care (engineers, development agents, environmentalists, lawyers and the community itself) and not just doctors and nurses.

This also implies a change in the training of health professionals themselves. Not only more technological, but also more focused on ways to react to unexpected situations and humanization as a fundamental element of a quality service. A quality that will always be associated not only with the results of the treatments, the surgical interventions and the postoperative follow-up, but also with the accessibility to the care and the form of treatment. Empathy is in this domain the element to be preserved in increasingly digitized contexts.

CONCLUDING REMARKS

As noted throughout the book, the scientific and technical achievements of modern science and its contribution to the promotion of well-being and quality of life, particularly in the fields of health and economic and social development, are now relatively consensual. However, on the other hand, the awareness of the paradoxes inherent in some of these achievements, because of the perverse and unexpected effects they can produce in different dimensions of individual and collective life, is intensely emphasized in today's contexts.

It is enough to recall the often ambiguous and contradictory discussions about the limits and possibilities of research on the human genome, stem cells, or the production of transgenics. Such discussions often go beyond the scientific sphere to fit into political and geo-strategic decisions, or into reactive and "precautionary" movements fueled by the more or less conscious or implicit fear of a "brave new world" in which freedom is progressively suppressed in favor of the mass programming and production of human life itself. Nevertheless, whether a paradigm of dissociation between science and morals is advocated or the reverse perspective is considered, it is currently consensual that the information about the effects of the application of certain technical-scientific knowledge makes it responsible, which forces a critical relations between scientific freedom and the autotelic justification of knowledge production, its applicability and the ethical responsibility of the agents involved in the construction and monitoring of the increasingly diffuse sources of knowledge and action.

The greater social regulation of science (beginning especially in the health sciences), through legislation, ethics commissions or systems for detecting academic fraud, stems from the effect associated with increasingly blurred boundaries between what might be called "ontological"and operational utility of scientific knowledge (Israel & Hay, 2006).

Indeed, as Homan (1991) suggests, the need for ethical regulation of research stems, to a large extent, from the often dilemmatic relationship between distinct expectations in terms of scientific results and the effects they may produce. So-called scientific policies emerge in this context to promote not only the management of science, but also to define thresholds of action and introduce priority criteria that are supposedly translators of the values of a given society in a given space-time. Under such assumptions, legitimated in principles of protection of society itself against the possible abuses of scientists, technicians and professionals, both in the form and content of what is investigated and disseminated, the regulatory policies of scientific research emerge and impose limits to discoveries and the way they are conducted. These limits should be subject to a wider critical discussion. A discussion that is currently considered to be promoted not only within the scientific community itself, but also, increasingly, in the societal context. The *Commission Mondiale d'Éthique des Connaissances Scientifiques et des Technologies* (COMEST), founded by UNESCO in 1998, set out principles to guide scientific and technological decision-making, not by economic assumptions but by ethical criteria. In this context, the Commission (UNESCO, 2005) points out the precautionary principle as a central axis in a time of risk and uncertainty management, where prevention is increasingly difficult.

The production of answers, which are intended to be alternative and effective, to the current social and economic needs, finds in the paradigm of innovation, technological and social, its full realization. Assuming itself politically as an essential orientation for the pursuit of goals of progress and competitiveness, the rhetoric of innovation emerges, in the current scientific, technological and social context, as the fundamental factor for the production of results with greater impact and greater potential of competitiveness in national and international contexts. In this sense, it is simultaneously a condition for the production of new knowledge (for example, for the development of technology) and a product of them. In this context, the debate about scientific responsibility does not arise in an abstract way, nor does it relate to the products derived from science and technology, but rather to their applicability and the desired effects, thus with an evident political dimension. Social responsibility, in this context, is related, on the one hand to the production of value deriving from action in specific contexts and, on the other, with the stimulus to dynamics of accountability and political and organizational governance that do not disregard people over efficiency. In this sense, the so-called responsible innovation (Grunwald, 2011; Siune et al., 2009) reflects the idea that innovation cannot be uncritically and self-imposed (innovating for innovation), but it must conform to the expectations of populations, services and a better society. It is, in essence, a committed innovation, a social practice that is not confused with science, but which maintains a synergistic coexistence relationship with it (Almeida, & Albuquerque, 2018).

The critical appropriation of knowledge, in the sense of social emancipation and the affirmation, of solidarity and responsibility, of a project and of a collective action, constitutes the central axis of construction of the individual as a political subject. A subject capable of thinking and influencing the course of History, building a dimension of autonomy, which necessarily implies the ability to balance individual projects and options, with choices and determinations thought and concretized collectively. The possibility of accessing knowledge and especially of understanding and mobilizing it, in order to transform oneself and the contexts (organizational, professional or community) is therefore a relevant factor of social change, inherent to a multidimensional conception of health, and building an emancipatory critical consciousness. It advocates a sense of justice and sustainability that transcends the private and immediate sphere for the benefit of a new being simultaneously local / global and individual / collective. In other words, it is urgent to think about the thresholds of the public and private space in today's global, technological and multicultural societies. Decisions have cross-impact and unpredictable impacts. Additionaly, under this new conditions (which can be both empowering and limiting) effective participation of all citizens in decisions about their own health is expected. Therefore, the meaning of democracy and the rights and duties that it behaves (or should behave) is today, in fact, the central axis of an inescapable global social and political debate capable of re-dimensioning the concept of citizenship and health, opening it to broad education, pluralism, solidarity, emancipation and ethical, environmental and socially sustainable responsibility.

In fact, understanding current societies and the challenges they face presupposes that we take into account a set of frameworks of change that allow to delineate a framework reading of current phenomena and contexts, simultaneously complex, transdisciplinary and dynamic. An interpretative framework that takes into account, namely: the uncertainty as a structuring factor of individual and collective experiences; the redesign of the concept of risk and responsibility and, in the first line, the renewed processes of access and use of knowledge and information.

In this context, the definition of roles, which fit each and every one of the citizens and the presuppositions and limits of their respective spheres of action, constitute the "Ariadne thread" of a complex debate about the democratic sense and the values to preserve in the present time. The reinterpretation of the concept of social responsibility associated, on the one hand, with an increasing awareness and knowledge of the impacts of the actions and, on the other hand, a lesser control of the course of these same actions, poses renewed questions about how to construct a substantial dynamics of responsibility in plural contexts. In other words, the central question is how to ensure the necessary balance between individual and collective or between freedom, pluralism and order on the basis of a renewed democratic project. Even if these are substantive issues, these debates are no longer considered relevant factors in the field of health care today, as it was possible to emphasize throughout the book.

Understanding currently for example what can be conceived as "common good" becomes a central point for the reconstitution of the meaning of political, social and civic citizenship in different parts of the world. The rupture with the principles of predictability of modern societies and the emergence of new forms of risk puts in the forefront of the debate the need to find alternative rationalities for the joint experience that go through the revaluation of interactive processes, the valuation of people and their potential (by overcoming the mere functional dimension), the proximity and revaluation of the living place, the creativity and entrepreneurship, in short, the affirmation of specificities and the respect for singularities, without neglecting the global and structural framework of the issues we currently face. This is today one of the most pressing debates for the resizing of public policies in general and of health policies in particular.

Cristina Albuquerque
University of Coimbra, Portugal

REFERENCES

Agamben, G. (1995). *Moyens sans fins. Notes sur la politique*. Paris: Rivages.

Agamben, G. (1998). *Homo Sacer: Sovereign Power and Bare Life*. Stanford University Press.

Almeida, F., & Albuquerque, C. P. (2018). Ciência e Responsabilidade Social. In Ética Aplicada: Investigação Científica (pp. 321-342). Lisboa: Edições 70/Livraria Almedina (publicação simultânea em Portugal e no Brasil).

Antonovsky, A. (1979). *Health, stress and coping*. San Francisco: Jossey-Bass.

Bailey, R. (2004). Transhumanism: The most dangerous idea? *Reason*.

Beck, U. (1992). *Risk Society: Towards a New Modernity*. New Delhi: Sage.

Beck, U., Giddens, A., & Lash, S. (1995). *Modernização Reflexiva. Política, Tradição e Estética na ordem social moderna*. São Paulo: Editora UNESP.

Bell, J., Masaoka, J., & Zimmerman, S. (2010). *Nonprofit Sustainability. Making strategic decisions for financial viability*. San Francisco: Jossey-Bass Books.

Bernstein, J., & La Valle, R. (2015). Because of Science You Also Die. *International Journal of Health Policy and Management*, *4*(9), 615–616. doi:10.15171/ijhpm.2015.102 PMID:26340492

Boorse, C. (1977). Health as a theoretical concept. *Philosophy of Science*, *44*(4), 542–573. doi:10.1086/288768

Boudon, R. (2003). *Raison, Bonnes raisons*. Paris: PUF.

Bragazzi, N. L., & Del Puente, G. (2013). Why P6 medicine needs clinical psychology and a trans-cultural approach. *Health Psychology Review*, *1*(e5), 21–22. PMID:26973894

Brown, L., & Moore, M. (2001). Accountability, Strategy, and International Non-Governmental Organizations. *Nonprofit and Voluntary Sector Quarterly*, *30*(3), 569–587. doi:10.1177/0899764001303012

Brown, L., Moore, M., & Honan, J. (2004). Building Strategic Accountability Systems for International NGOs. *Accounting Forum*, *1*(2), 31–43.

Canguilhem, G. (1989). *The normal and the pathological*. Cambridge, MA: The MIT Press, Zone Books. (Original work published 1943)

Checkland, K., Marshall, M., & Harrison, S. (2004). Re-thinking accountability: Trust versus confidence in medical practice. *Quality & Safety in Health Care*, *13*(2), 130–135. doi:10.1136/qshc.2003.009720 PMID:15069221

Christensen, R., & Ebrahim, A. (2006). How does Accountability Affect Mission? The Case of a Nonprofit Serving Immigrants and Refugees. *Nonprofit Management & Leadership*, *17*(2), 195–209. doi:10.1002/nml.143

Cocco, G., & Negri, A. (2005). *Glob(Al). Biopoder e lutas em uma américa latina globalizada*. Rio de Janeiro: Record.

Conrad, P. (2007). *The medicalization of society: on the transformation of human conditions into treatable disorders*. Baltimore, MD: The Johns Hopkins University Press.

Conrad, P., & Leiter, V. (2004). Medicalization, Markets and Consumers. *Journal of Health and Social Behavior*, *45*, 158–176. PMID:15779472

Crack, A. (2013). Language, listening and learning: Critically reflective accountability for INGOs. *International Review of Administrative Sciences*, *79*(4), 809–828. doi:10.1177/0020852313500599

Davies, H. (1999). Falling public trust in health services: Implications for accountability. *Journal of Health Services Research & Policy*, *4*(4), 193–194. doi:10.1177/135581969900400401 PMID:10623032

Donaldson, L. J. (2001). Professional accountability in a changing world. *Postgraduate Medical Journal*, *77*(904), 65–67. doi:10.1136/pmj.77.904.65 PMID:11161069

Drèze, J., & Sen, A. (Eds.). (1997). *Indian Development: Selected Regional Perspectives*. New Delhi: Oxford University Press. doi:10.1093/acprof:oso/9780198292043.001.0001

Drucker, P. (1985). *Innovation and Entrepreneurship*. Harper & Row Publish, Inc.

Ebrahim, A. (2003). Making Sense of Accountability: Conceptual Perspectives for Northern and Southern Nonprofits. *Nonprofit Management & Leadership*, *14*(2), 191–212. doi:10.1002/nml.29

Ehrenberg, A. (2000). *La fatigue d'être soi. Dépression et Société*. Paris: Odile Jacob.

Ekedahl, M., & Wengstrom, Y. (2008). Coping processes in a multidisciplinary healthcare team— A comparison of nurses in cancer care and hospital chaplains. *European Journal of Cancer Care*, *17*(1), 42–48. doi:10.1111/j.1365-2354.2007.00801.x PMID:18181890

Etchegoyen, A. (1995). *A era dos responsáveis*. Linda-a-Velha: Diffel.

FAO. (2010). *The State of Food Insecurity in the World. Addressing food insecurity in protracted crises*. Rome: FAO UN.

FAO. (2012). *The State of World Fisheries and Aquaculture*. Rome: FAO UN.

Foucault, M. (1976). Histoire de la sexualité: Vol. 1. *La volonté de savoir*. Paris: Gallimard.

Fukuyama, F. (1996). *Confiança, Valores sociais & criação de prosperidade.* Lisboa: Gradiva.

Giddens, A. (2000). *Conversas com Anthony Giddens: O sentido da Modernidade.* Rio de Janeiro: FGV.

Grunwald, A. (2011). Responsible Innovation: Bringing together Technology Assessment, Applied Ethics, and STS research. *Enterprise and Work Innovation Studies, 7,* 9–31.

Hargens-Esbjörn, S. (2009). *An overview of integral theory – An all-inclusive framework for the 21st century.* Integral Institute, Resource Paper. Disponível em: http://integraleurope.org/wp-content/uploads/2013/05/IT_3-2-2009.pdf

Harrison, S., & Smith, C. (2004). Trust and moral motivation: Redundant resources in health and social care? *Policy and Politics, 2*(3), 371–386. doi:10.1332/0305573041223726

Holmgren, D., & Mollison, B. (1978). *Permaculture one. A perennial agriculture for human settlements.* Melbourne: Transworld.

Homan, R. (1991). *The Ethics of Social Research.* Londres: Longman.

Hood, L., & Auffray, C. (2013). Participatory medicine: A driving force for revolutionizing healthcare. *Genome Medicine, 4*(110). PMID:24360023

Hopkins, R. (2008). *The Transition Handbook. From the oil dependency to local resilience.* Chelsea Green Publishing.

Hughes, J. (2004). *Citizen Cyborg: Why Democratic Societies Must Respond to the Redesigned Human of the Future.* Westview Press.

Huxley, J. S. (1957). *(Transhumanisme) New Bottles for New Wine.* Londres: Chatto & Windus.

Illich, I. (1975). The medicalization of life. *Journal of Medical Ethics, I*(2), 73–77. doi:10.1136/jme.1.2.73 PMID:809583

Inamdar, N., Kaplan, R. S., & Bower, M. (2002). Applying the balanced scorecard in healthcare provider organizations. *Journal of Healthcare Management, 47*(3), 179–195. doi:10.1097/00115514-200205000-00008 PMID:12055900

Israel, M., & Hay, I. (2006). *Research Ethics for Social Scientists.* Londres: Sage. doi:10.4135/9781849209779

Jonas, H. (1995). *El principio de responsabilidad. Ensayo de una ética para la civilización tecnológica.* Barcelona: Editorial Herder. (Original work published 1979)

Kearns, K. (1994). The Strategic Management of Accountability in Nonprofit Organizations: An Analytical Framework. *Public Administration Review, 54*(2), 185–192. doi:10.2307/976528

Khatri, N., Baveja, A., Boren, S. A., & Mammo, A. (2006). Medical errors and quality of care: From control to commitment. *California Management Review, 48*(3), 115–141. doi:10.2307/41166353

Kleinman, A., Eisenberg, L., & Good, B. (1978). Culture, illness, and care: Clinical lessons from anthropologic and cross-cultural research. *Annals of Internal Medicine, 88*(2), 251–258. doi:10.7326/0003-4819-88-2-251 PMID:626456

Levinas, E. (1993). *Entre nous. Essais sur le penser-à-l'autre.* Paris: Grasset.

Macy, J. (2014). *Coming back to life. The Updated Guide to the Work That Reconnects.* New Society Publishers.

Mangematin, V., & Thuderoz, C. (2003). *Des mondes de confiance. Un concept à l'épreuve de la réalité sociale.* Paris: CNRS-Éditions.

Mattedi, A., & Butzke, I. (2001). A relação entre o social e o natural nas abordagens de hazards e de desastres. *Ambiente & Sociedade, 9*(9), 93–114. doi:10.1590/S1414-753X2001000900006

Maturo, A. (2012). Medicalization: Current concept and future directions in bionic society. *Mens Sana Monographs, 10*(1), 122–133. doi:10.4103/0973-1229.91587 PMID:22654387

McKinlay, J. B., & Marceau, L. D. (2002). The end of the golden age of doctoring. *International Journal of Health Services, 32*(2), 379–416. doi:10.2190/JL1D-21BG-PK2N-J0KD PMID:12067037

Mehry, E. (2002). *Saúde: A cartografia do Trabalho vivo.* São Paulo: Editora Hucitec.

Messu, M. (2008). Le temps social fractal. In V. Châtel (Ed.), *Les Temps des Politiques Sociales* (pp. 49–71). Fribourg: Academic Press.

Moulaert, F. (2009). Social Innovation: Institutionally Embedded, Territorially (Re) Produced. In D. MacCallum, F. Moulaert, J. Hilier, & S. Haddock (Eds.), *Social Innovation and Territorial Development.* Ashgate.

Moulaert, F., Martinelli, F., Swyngedouw, E., & Gonzalez, S. (2005). Towards Alternative Model(s) of Local Innovation. *Urban Studies*, *42*(11), 969-90.

NAS - National Academies of Sciences, Engineering, and Medicine. (2017). *Human Genome Editing: Science, Ethics, and Governance*. Washington, DC: The National Academies Press. doi:10.17226/24623

Negri, A., & Hart, M. (2002). *Império*. Barcelona: Paidós.

NIC. (2012). *Global Trends 2030: Alternative Worlds*. National Intelligence Council.

Niklas, L. (1979). *Trust and Power*. John Wiley & Sons, Ltd.

O'Brien, K., & Hochachka, G. (n.d.). Integral adaptation to climate change. *Journal of Integral Theory and Practice*, *5*(1), 89–102.

O'Sullivan, T. (2011). *Decision making in Social Work*. New York: Palgrave-Macmillan. doi:10.1007/978-1-137-28540-9

OECD. (2017). *Health at a Glance 2017: OECD Indicators*. Paris: OECD Publishing; doi:10.1787/health_glance-2017-

Oosterlynck, S., van den Broek, J., Albrechts, L., Moulaert, F., & Verhetsel, A. (2010). *Bridging the Gap between Planning and Implementation: Turning Transformative Visions into Strategic Projects*. Routledge.

Ortega, Y., & Gasset, J. (1987). *El tema de nuestro tiempo*. Madrid: Alianza Editorial.

Peyrefitte, A. (1995). *La société de confiance. Essai sur les origines et la nature du développement*. Paris: Éditions Odile Jacob.

Popper, K. (2000). *Conjecturas e refutações*. Coimbra: Almedina.

Porter, J., Morphet, J., Missen, K., & Raymond, A. (2013). Preparation for high-acuity clinical placement: Confidence levels of final-year nursing students. *Advances in Medical Education and Practice*, *4*, 83–89. doi:10.2147/AMEP.S42157 PMID:23900655

Revel, J. (2005). *Michel Foucault: Expériences de la pensée*. Paris: Bordas.

Roque Amaro, R. (2009). A Economia Solidária da Macaronésia – Um Novo Conceito. *Revista de Economia Solidária*, *1*, 11–29.

Roque Amaro, R. (2011). Projeto ECOS. *Revista de Economia Solidária*, *3*, 157–171.

Santos, F. (2009). *A positive theory of social entrepreneurship*. Working paper, INSEAD, Faculty & Research.

318

Scheler, M. (1936). *Le sens de la souffrance*. Paris: Aubier.

Schieber, A. C., Delpierre, C., Lepage, B., Afrite, A., Chantal, J. P., & Lombrail, P. (2014). Do gender differences affect the doctor–patient interaction during consultations in general practice? Results from the INTERMEDE study. *Family Practice*, *31*(6), 706–713. doi:10.1093/fampra/cmu057 PMID:25214508

Schmidt, L., & Valente, S. (2004). Factos e opiniões: uma abordagem transnacional ao desenvolvimento sustentável. In L. Lima, M. Cabral, M. & Vala, J. (Eds.), Atitudes Sociais dos Portugueses – Ambiente e desenvolvimento. Lisboa: Imprensa de Ciências Sociais.

Schön, D. (1994). *Le Praticien Réflexif. À la recherche du savoir caché dans l'agir professionnel*. Montréal: Les Éditions Logiques Inc. (Original publication 1983)

Shumpeter, J. (1911). *The theory of Economic Development*. Boston: Harvard University Press.

Siune, K. (2009). *Challenging Futures of Science in Society. Report of the MASIS Expert Group*. European Commission.

Thakur, R., Hsu, S., & Fontenot, G. (2012). Innovation in healthcare: Issues and future trends. *Journal of Business Research*, *65*(4), 562–569. doi:10.1016/j.jbusres.2011.02.022

Therborn, G. (2012). The killing fields of inequality. *International Journal of Health Services*, *42*(4), 579–589. doi:10.2190/HS.42.4.a PMID:23367794

UNAIDS. (2011). *Report on the global AIDS epidemic 2010*. UN.

UNESCO/COMEST. (2005). *The Precautionary Principle*. Paris: UNESCO.

UNICEF. (2006). *Relatório sobre Nutrição Infantil*. UN.

UNICEF. (2007). *Um Mundo para as Crianças*. UN.

Welch, H. G. (2016). *Less Medicine, More Health. 7 Assumptions that drive too much medical care*. Beacon Press.

WHO. (2015). *World Report on Ageing and Health*. Luxembourg: World Health Organization.

Zheng, H. (2015). Losing confidence in medicine in an era of medical expansion? *Social Science Research*, *52*, 701–715. doi:10.1016/j.ssresearch.2014.10.009 PMID:26004490

ENDNOTES

1   Female genital mutilation, in particular, is a designation adopted by the WHO in the 1990s to translate an ancestral practice. In fact, it is a concept that is surrounded by ideological and conceptual controversy, much influenced by the feminist movements, and which seeks above all to distinguish itself from the concept of circumcision and the religious connotations that it entails. Under the same name, however, there are very different practices that continue to take place in many geographical and cultural contexts in different parts of the world.

2   The "social death" of the leper, through his imprisonment in leprosy calls, is even accompanied, in some contexts, by the symbolism of a real death, for example with the performance of a present body mass.

3   This concept referred to the study of health generation in counterpoint to the notion of pathogenesis, the study of the origins of the disease. By observing, in particular, the health of women who survived the Nazi concentration camps, Antonovsky stressed the existence of people who achieve and maintain good health even though they are or have been subjected to potentially disease-causing factors, both physical and psychological. This manifestation of resilience would be associated with observations made with personality traits constituting what the author called the Sense of Coherence (SOC) and which is structured in comprehensibility (to better understand his situation and his life), manageability that it is possible for each person to influence this same situation) and experiencing meaningfulness of life, the most powerful factor of resilience. SOC is a health-enhancing factor.

320

Compilation of References

Abbott, A. (1988). *The System of Professions. An essay on the division of expert labor.* Chicago: The University of Chicago Press. doi:10.7208/chicago/9780226189666.001.0001

Abubaker, H.; Dugger, J. C. & Lee, H. (2015). Manufacturing Control, Asset Tracking, and Asset Maintenance: Assessing the impact of RFID technology adoption. *Journal of international information and technology management, 24*(2), 35-54.

Agamben, G. (1995). *Moyens sans fins. Notes sur la politique.* Paris: Rivages.

Agamben, G. (1998). *Homo Sacer: Sovereign Power and Bare Life.* Stanford University Press.

Aiello, Schfanella, & State. (2014). "How Yahoo Research Labs studies culture as a formal computational concept"--reading the source code of social ties. *MIT Technology Review.* Retrieved August 1, 2014 from http://www.technologyreview.com/view/529521/how-yahoo-research-labs-studies-culture-as-a-formal-computational-concept

Akbar, H. (2003). Knowledge Levels and their Transformation: Towards the Integration of Knowledge Creation and Individual Learning. *Journal of Management Studies, 40*(8), 1997–2021. doi:10.1046/j.1467-6486.2003.00409.x

Alarcón, T. A., & Montalvo, J. I. G. (1998). La Escala Socio-Familiar de Gijón, instrumento útil en el hospital general. *Revista Espanola de Geriatria y Gerontologia, 33*(3), 127–192. Retrieved from http://www.elsevier.es/es-revista-revista-espanola-geriatria-gerontologia-124-articulo-la-escala-socio-familiar-gijon-instrumento-13006000

Albuquerque, C. (2016). Social Care and Life Quality of Frail or Dependent Elderly: The Contribution of Technologies. *International Journal of Privacy and Health Information Management, 4*(1), 12–22. doi:10.4018/IJPHIM.2016010102

Albuquerque, C. P. (2011). Legitimidade e reconhecimento da prática de serviço social. *Serviço Social Em Revista, 13*(2), 104–118. doi:10.5433/1679-4842.2011v13n2p104

Albuquerque, C. P., & Amaro da Luz, M. H. (2018). The Potentialities of Local Innovation Ecosystems to Tackle Wicked Problems: The Case of Aging. *Technology Transfer and Entrepreneurship, 5*(2), 67–82. doi:10.2174/2213809906666181214 141821

Allen, J. F. (1981). An interval-based representation of temporal knowledge. *In International Conference of Artificial Intelligence*. Morgan Kaufmann.

Allen, J. F. (1983). Maintaining knowledge about temporal intervals. *Communications of the ACM, 26*(11), 832–843. doi:10.1145/182.358434

Allen, J. F. (1984). Towards a general theory of action and time. *Artificial Intelligence, 23*(2), 123–154. doi:10.1016/0004-3702(84)90008-0

Allen, J. F., & Ferguson, G. (1994). Actions and events in interval temporal logic. *Journal of Logic and Computation, 4*(5), 531–579. doi:10.1093/logcom/4.5.531

Almeida, F., & Albuquerque, C. P. (2018). Ciência e Responsabilidade Social. In Ética Aplicada: Investigação Científica (pp. 321-342). Lisboa: Edições 70/Livraria Almedina (publicação simultânea em Portugal e no Brasil).

Amaro, M. I. (2012). *Urgências e emergências do serviço social*. Lisboa: Universidade Católica Editora.

Amaro, M. I. (2014). Um admirável mundo novo? Tecnologia e intervenção na contemporaneidade. In M. I. Carvalho & C. Pinto (Eds.), *Serviço social: Teorias e práticas* (pp. 97–111). Lisboa: Pactor.

Antonovsky, A. (1979). *Health, stress and coping*. San Francisco: Jossey-Bass.

Anunciação, P. F., & Esteves, F. M. (2019). Challenges to Business Models in the Digital Transformation context. In *Handbook of Research on Business Models in Modern Competitive Scenarios*. Hershey, US: IGI Global. doi:10.4018/978-1-5225-7265-7.ch011

Arendt, H. (1972). *La crise de la culture. Huit exercices de pensée politique*. Paris, France: Gallimard.

Armour, J. A. (2003). *Neurocardiology: Anatomical and functional principles*. Boulder Creek, CA: HeartMath Research Center, Institute of Heartmath, Pub. N.

Armour, J. A., & Ardell, J. L. (Eds.). (1994). *Neurocardiology*. New York: Oxford University Press.

Atun, R. A., & Mohan, A. (2005). *Uses and Benefits of SMS in Healthcare Delivery*. London: Imperial College.

Audi, O., Cichy, R., & Pantazis, D. (2014). Where and when the brain recognizes, categorizes an object. *Nature Neuroscience, 26*. Retrieved from http://www.kurzweilai.net/where-and-when-the-brain-recognizes-categorizes-an-object

Auffray, C., Charron, D., & Hood, L. (2010). Predictive, preventive, personalized and participatory medicine: Back to the future. *Genome Medicine, 2*(8), 57. doi:10.1186/gm178 PMID:20804580

Ausloos, G. (1996). *A Competência das Famílias – Tempo, caos e processo*. Lisboa: Climepsi Editores.

Avram, G., Bannon, L., Bowers, J., Sheehan, A., & Sullivan, D. (2009). Bridging, Patching and Keeping the Work Flowing: Defect Resolution in Distributed Software Development. *Computer Supported Cooperative Work, 18*(5-6), 477–507. doi:10.100710606-009-9099-6

Azevedo, I. S. (2013). A relação teoria/método/instrumentais: uma leitura a partir da concepção de profissão. *Textos & Contextos, 12*(2), 325–333. Retrieved from http://revistaseletronicas.pucrs.br/fass/ojs/index.php/fass/article/view/15323

Baars, B. J. (1997). In the theatre of consciousness: Global workspace theory, a rigorous scientific theory of consciousness. *Journal of Consciousness Studies, 4*, 292–309.

Bailey, R. (2004). Transhumanism: The most dangerous idea? *Reason*.

Balasubramaniam, S. (2018). Artificial Intelligence. DAWN. *Journal for Contemporary Research in Management, 5*(1), 12–18.

Barrios-Choplin, McCraty, & Cryer. (1997). An inner quality approach to reducing stress and improving physical and emotional wellbeing at work. In US Naval Postgraduate School of Systems Management & Institute of Heartmath. John Wiley & Sons, Ltd.

Bateson, G. (1972). *Steps to An Ecology of Mind: Collected Essays in Anthropology, Psychiatry, Evolution, and Epistemology*. University Of Chicago Press.

Beard, J. R., & Bloom, D. E. (2015). Towards a comprehensive public health response to population ageing. *Lancet, 14*. Retrieved from https://www.ncbi.nlm.nih.gov/pmc/articles/PMC4663973/ PMID:25468151

Beaudoin, S. (2018). *Être gouverné. Entre science et politique* (Unpublished doctoral dissertation). Université Laval, Québec, Canada.

Beck, U. (1992). *Risk Society: Towards a New Modernity*. New Delhi: Sage.

Beck, U. (2003). *La société du risque. Sur la voie d'une autre modernité*. Paris, France: Flammarion.

Beck, U., Giddens, A., & Lash, S. (1995). *Modernização Reflexiva. Política, Tradição e Estética na ordem social moderna*. São Paulo: Editora UNESP.

Bell, J., Masaoka, J., & Zimmerman, S. (2010). *Nonprofit Sustainability. Making strategic decisions for financial viability*. San Francisco: Jossey-Bass Books.

Bergman, H., Ferrucci, L., Guralnik, J., Hogan, D. B., Hummel, S., Karunananthan, S., & Wolfson, C. (2007). Frailty: An emerging research and clinical paradigm–issues and controversies. *The Journals of Gerontology. Series A, Biological Sciences and Medical Sciences, 62*(7), 731–737. doi:10.1093/gerona/62.7.731 PMID:17634320

Berkman, L. F., Blumenthal, J., Burg, M., Carney, R. M., Catellier, D., Cowan, M. J., & Schneiderman, N. (2003). Effects of Treating Depression and Low Perceived Social Support on Clinical Events After Myocardial Infarction. *Journal of the American Medical Association, 289*(23), 3106. doi:10.1001/jama.289.23.3106 PMID:12813116

Bernstein, J., & La Valle, R. (2015). Because of Science You Also Die. *International Journal of Health Policy and Management, 4*(9), 615–616. doi:10.15171/ijhpm.2015.102 PMID:26340492

Beswick, A. D., Rees, K., Dieppe, P., Ayis, S., Gooberman-Hill, R., Horwood, J., & Ebrahim, S. (2008). Complex interventions to improve physical function and maintain independent living in elderly people: A systematic review and meta-analysis. *Lancet, 371*(9614), 725–735. doi:10.1016/S0140-6736(08)60342-6 PMID:18313501

Bhat, V. (2005). Institutional arrangements and efficiency of health care delivery systems. *The European Journal of Health Economics, 6*(3), 215–222. doi:10.100710198-005-0294-1 PMID:15864675

Bhunia, G. Kesari, S., Chatterjee, N., & Kumar, V, Das. P. (2013). Spatial and temporal variation and hotspot detection of kala-azar disease in Vaishali district (Bihar), India. *BMC infectious diseases*, *13*(1), 64. doi:.doi:10.1186/1471-2334-13-64

Bhutta, Z. A., Yakoob, M. Y., Lawn, J. E., Rizvi, A., Friberg, I. K., Weissman, E., ... Goldenberg, R. L. (2011). Stillbirths: What difference can we make and at what cost? *Lancet*, *377*(9776), 1523–1538. doi:10.1016/S0140-6736(10)62269-6 PMID:21496906

Bianic, T. (2003). Bringing the State back in the study of professions. Some peculiarities of the French model of professionalization. In the *6th ESA Conference, Research Network Sociology of Professions*, University of de Murcia. Retrieved from https://www.um.es/ESA/papers/Rn15_28.pdf

Bird, C., Nagappan, N., Devanbu, P., Gall, H., & Murphy, B. (2008). Does distribute development affect software quality? an empirical case study of Windows Vista. *Communications of the ACM*, *52*(8), 85–93. doi:10.1145/1536616.1536639

Blane, D. (2006). The life course perspective, the social gradient, and health. In M. Marmot & R. Wilkinson (Eds.), *Social Determinants of Health* (pp. 54–77). Oxford: Oxford University Press.

Blaya, J. A., Fraser, H. S., & Holt, B. (2010). E-health technologies show promise in developing countries. *Health Affairs (Project Hope)*, *29*(2), 244–250. doi:10.1377/hlthaff.2009.0894 PMID:20348068

Blumenberg, H. (2010). Care Crosses the River. Stanford, CA: Stanford University Press.

Bôas, M. L. C. V., Shimizu, H. E., & Sanchez, M. N. (2016). Creation of complexity assessment tool for patients receiving home care. *Revista Da Escola de Enfermagem*, *50*(3), 433–439. doi:10.1590/S0080-623420160000400009 PMID:27556714

Boehler, C., Abadie, F., & Sabes-Figuera, R. (2014). Monitoring and Assessment Framework for the European Innovation Partnership on Active and Healthy Ageing (MAFEIP). Second report on outcome indicators. *JRC Science and Policy Report*.

Boltanski, L., & Thévenot, L. (2006). *On justification: Economies of worth*. Princeton, NJ: Princeton University Press. (Original work published 1991)

Boncea, R., Petre, I., Smada, D., & Zamfiroiu, A. (2017). A Maturity Analysis of Big Data technologies. *Informações Econômicas*, *21*(1), 60–71. doi:10.12948/issn14531305/21.1.2017.05

Boorse, C. (1977). Health as a theoretical concept. *Philosophy of Science*, *44*(4), 542–573. doi:10.1086/288768

Boudon, R. (2003). *Raison, Bonnes raisons*. Paris: PUF.

Bowling, C. B., Sawyer, P., Campbell, R. C., Ahmed, A., & Allman, R. M. (2011). Impact of chronic kidney disease on activities of daily living in community-dwelling older adults. *Journals of Gerontology - Series A Biological Sciences and Medical Sciences*, *66*(6), 689–694. doi:10.1093/gerona/glr043

Boyd, F. (2015). Immersive media: to the holodeck and beyond. *Knowledge Transfer Network*. Retrieved May 6, 2015 from http://www.ktn-uk.co.uk/immersive-media-to-the-holodeck-and-beyond/

Boyd, C. M., Xue, Q. L., Simpson, C. F., Guralnik, J. M., & Fried, L. P. (2005). Frailty, hospitalization, and progression of disability in a cohort of disabled older women. *The American Journal of Medicine*, *118*(11), 1225–1231. doi:10.1016/j.amjmed.2005.01.062 PMID:16271906

Bradley, R. T. (2006). The psychophysiology of entrepreneurial intuition: a quantum holographic theory. *Institute of Whole Social Science & Institute of Heartmath: Proceedings of the Third AGSE International Entrepreneurship Research Exchange*.

Bragazzi, N. L., & Del Puente, G. (2013). Why P6 medicine needs clinical psychology and a trans-cultural approach. *Health Psychology Review*, *1*(e5), 21–22. PMID:26973894

Braun, L. A., Sood, V., Hogue, S., Lieberman, B., & Copley-Merriman, C. (2012). High burden and unmet patient needs in chronic kidney disease. *International Journal of Nephrology and Renovascular Disease*, *5*, 151–163. doi:10.2147/IJNRD.S37766 PMID:23293534

Braveman, P., Egerter, S., & Williams, D. R. (2011). The social determinants of health: Coming of age. *Annual Review of Public Health*, *32*(1), 381–398. doi:10.1146/annurev-publhealth-031210-101218 PMID:21091195

Breviglieri, M. (2008). L'individu, le proche et l'institution. Travail social et politique de l'autonomie. *The Information Society*, *145*, 92–101.

Brock, D. M., & Saks, M. (2016). Professions and organizations: A European perspective. *European Management Journal*, *34*(1), 1–6. doi:10.1016/j.emj.2015.11.003

Brodnik, M. S., Rinehart-Thompson, L. A., & Reynolds, R. (2012). *Fundamentals of Law for Health Informatics and Information Management*. Chicago: AHIMA - American Health Information Management Association.

Broom, A., & Kirby, E. (2012). The end of life and the family: Hospice patient's views on dying as relational. *Sociology of Health & Illness*, *35*(4), 499–513. doi:10.1111/j.1467-9566.2012.01497.x PMID:22742736

Browne, T., Peace, L., & Perry, D. (2014). *Standards of practice for nephrology social work* (6th ed.). Council of Nephrology Social Workers, National Kidney Foundation, Inc. Retrieved from http://www2.kidney.org/members/source/Custom/CNSW/pdf/CNSW-SOP_6thEd-FINAL_July2014.pdf

Brown, L., & Moore, M. (2001). Accountability, Strategy, and International Non-Governmental Organizations. *Nonprofit and Voluntary Sector Quarterly*, *30*(3), 569–587. doi:10.1177/0899764001303012

Brown, L., Moore, M., & Honan, J. (2004). Building Strategic Accountability Systems for International NGOs. *Accounting Forum*, *1*(2), 31–43.

Brown, S. A., Tyrer, F. C., Clarke, A. L., Lloyd-Davies, L. H., Stein, A. G., Tarrant, C., ... Smith, A. C. (2017). Symptom burden in patients with chronic kidney disease not requiring renal replacement therapy. *Clinical Kidney Journal*, *10*(6), 788–796. doi:10.1093/ckjfx057 PMID:29225808

Bryant, L. L., Corbett, K. K., & Kutner, J. S. (2001). In their own words: A model of healthy aging. *Social Science & Medicine*, *53*(7), 927–941. doi:10.1016/S0277-9536(00)00392-0 PMID:11522138

Brynjolfsson, E., & McAfee, A. (2016). *The second machine age: work, progress, and prosperity in a time of brilliant technologies*. New York: W.W. Norton & Company.

Buch, V. H., Ahmed, I., & Maruthappu, M. (2018). Artificial intelligence in medicine: Current trends and future possibilities. *The British Journal Of General Practice: The Journal Of The Royal College Of General Practitioners*, *68*(668), 143–144. doi:10.3399/bjgp18X695213 PMID:29472224

Burton, J., & Broek, D. (2009). Accountable and Countable: Information Management Systems and the Bureaucratization of Social Work. *British Journal of Social Work*, *39*(7), 1326–1342. doi:10.1093/bjsw/bcn027

Calder, A., & Banning, J. (2000). The ECB renal patient questionnaire: An assessment tool to determine renal patients' needs for immediate social work. *Advances in Renal Replacement Therapy, 7*(2), 184–191. doi:10.1053/rr.2000.5274 PMID:10782737

Campanini, A. (2006). *La valutazione nel servizio sociale: Proposte e strumenti per la qualità dell'intervento professionale.* Roma: Carocci Faber.

Campbell, J. (1949). The hero with a thousand faces. Bollingen/Princeton University Press.

Canguilhem, G. (1989). *The normal and the pathological.* Cambridge, MA: The MIT Press, Zone Books. (Original work published 1943)

Cao, L., Zhang, C., & Liu, J. (2006). Ontology-based integration of business intelligence. *Web Intelligence and Agent Systems. International Journal (Toronto, Ont.), 4,* 313–325.

Cappellin, R., & Wink, R. (2009). *International Knowledge and Innovation Networks: Knowledge Creation and Innovation in Medium-technology Clusters.* Cheltenham, UK: Edward Elgar Publishing Limited. doi:10.4337/9781848449084

Carman, J. M., Shortell, S. M., Foster, R. W., Hughes, E. F. X., Boerstler, H., O'Brien, J. L., & O'Connor, E. J. (2010). Keys for successful implementation of total quality management in hospitals. *Health Care Management Review, 35*(4), 283–293. doi:10.1097/HMR.0b013e3181f5fc4a PMID:20844354

Carroll, N., Kennedy, C., & Richardson, I. (2016). Challenges towards a connected community healthcare ecosystem for managing long-term conditions. *Gerontechnology (Valkenswaard), 14*(2), 64–77. doi:10.4017/gt.2016.14.2.003.00

Carvalho, T., & Santiago, R. (Eds.). (2015). *Professionalism, Managerialism and Reform in Higher Education and the Health Services. The european welfare state and the rise of the knowledge society.* Londres: Palgrave Macmillan.

Castells, M. (2012). *Era da Informação II: Economia, Sociedade e Cultura* (4th ed.). Lisboa, Portugal: Fundação Calouste Gulbenkian.

Castells, M., & Cardoso, G. (Eds.). (2005). *The Network Society: From Knowledge to Policy.* Washington, DC: Johns Hopkins Center for Transatlantic Relations.

Celaschi, F. (2017, May-August). Advanced design-driven approaches for an Industry 4.0 framework: The human-centered dimension of the digital industrial Revolution. *Strategic Design Research Journal, 10*(2), 97–104. doi:10.4013drj.2017.102.02

Cesari, M., Gambassi, G., van Kan, G. A., & Vellas, B. (2014). The frailty phenotype and the frailty index: Different instruments for different purposes. *Age and Ageing, 43*(1), 10–12. doi:10.1093/ageing/aft160 PMID:24132852

Chandrasekharan, S., & Nersessian, N. (2011). Building cognition: the construction of external representations for discovery. *Proceedings of the Cognitive Science Society, 33.*

Chau, M., & Xu, J. (2012). Business intelligence in blogs: Understanding consumer interactions and communities. *Management Information Systems Quarterly, 36*(4), 1189–1216.

Checkland, K., Marshall, M., & Harrison, S. (2004). Re-thinking accountability: Trust versus confidence in medical practice. *Quality & Safety in Health Care, 13*(2), 130–135. doi:10.1136/qshc.2003.009720 PMID:15069221

Cherry, K. (2015a). What is Flow? *AboutEducation.* Retrieved November 6, 2015 from http://psychology.about.com/od/PositivePsychology/a/flow.htm

Cherry, K. (2015b). What are peak experiences? *About Education.* Retrieved November 12, 2015 from http://psychology.about.com/od/humanist-personality/f/peak-experiences.htm

Childre, D., & Rozman, D. (2005). *Transforming Stress: The HeartMath Solution to Relieving Worry, Fatigue, and Tension.* Oakland, CA: New Harbinger Publications.

Chomsky, N. (1957). *Syntactic structures.* The Hague: Mouton.

Choo, C. W. (1996). The knowing organization: How organizations use information to construct meaning, create knowledge and make decisions. *International Journal of Information Management, 16*(5), 329–340. doi:10.1016/0268-4012(96)00020-5

Choo, C. W. (2005). *The knowing organization: how organizations use information to construct meaning, create knowledge and make decisions (2nd ed.).* Oxford: Ed. Oxford University Press. doi:10.1093/acprof:oso/9780195176780.001.0001

Chopra, D. (1995). *Body, mind & soul.* PBS Home Video.

Christensen, R., & Ebrahim, A. (2006). How does Accountability Affect Mission? The Case of a Nonprofit Serving Immigrants and Refugees. *Nonprofit Management & Leadership, 17*(2), 195–209. doi:10.1002/nml.143

Clark, T. D. Jr, Jones, M. C., & Armstrong, C. P. (2007). The dynamic structure of management support systems: Theory development, research, focus and direction. *Management Information Systems Quarterly, 31*(3), 579–615. doi:10.2307/25148808

Cocco, G., & Negri, A. (2005). *Glob(Al). Biopoder e lutas em uma américa latina globalizada*. Rio de Janeiro: Record.

Cockburn, M., Mills, P., Zhang, X., Zadnick, J., Goldberg, D., & Ritz, B. (2011). Prostate cancer and ambient pesticide exposure in agriculturally intensive areas in California. *American Journal of Epidemiology, 173*(11), 1280–1288.

Collste, G., Duquenoy, P., George, C., Hedström, K., Kimppa, K., & Mordini, E. (2006). *ICT in Medicine and Health Care: Assessing Social, Ethical and Legal Issues*. Retrieved from https://www.researchgate.net/publication/31597715

Connick, R. M., Connick, P., Klotsas, A. E., Tsagkaraki, P. A., & Gkrania-Klotsas, E. (2009). Procedural confidence in hospital based practitioners: Implications for the training and practice of doctors at all grades. *BMC Medical Education, 9*(1), 2. doi:10.1186/1472-6920-9-2 PMID:19138395

Conrad, P. (2007). *The medicalization of society: on the transformation of human conditions into treatable disorders*. Baltimore, MD: The Johns Hopkins University Press.

Conrad, P., & Leiter, V. (2004). Medicalization, Markets and Consumers. *Journal of Health and Social Behavior, 45*, 158–176. PMID:15779472

Cooper, P. W. (PwC) & Global System Mobile Association (GSMA). (2012). Touching Lives through Mobile Health: Assessment of the Global Market Opportunity. Retrieved from https://www.pwc.in/assets/pdfs/publications-2012/touching-lives-through-mobile-health-february-2012.pdf

Copeland, B. (2018, October 22). What's ahead for the health care ecosystem? *The Wall Street Journal*. Retrieved from http://www.deloitte.wsj.com

Couch, D., Han, G. S., Robinson, P., & Komesaroff, P. (2015). Public health surveillance and the media: A dyad of panoptic and synoptic social control. *Health Psychology and Behavioral Medicine, 3*(1), 128–141. doi:10.1080/21642850.2015.1049539

Coyle, D., & Meier, P. (2009). *New Technologies in Emergencies and Conflicts: The Role of Information and Social Networks*. Washington, DC and London, UK: UN Foundation-Vodafone Foundation Partnership.

Crack, A. (2013). Language, listening and learning: Critically reflective accountability for INGOs. *International Review of Administrative Sciences, 79*(4), 809–828. doi:10.1177/0020852313500599

Creating massive virtual worlds for training. (2015). Halldale Group. Retrieved August 26, 2015 from http://halldale.com/news/defence/simthetiq-releases-122000-km2-correlated-vbs3-openflight-training-environment#.Veh2xdJRGUl

Crotty, B., & Mostaghimi, A. (2011). Professionalism in the Digital Age. *Annals of Internal Medicine, 154*(8), 560–562. doi:10.7326/0003-4819-154-8-201104190-00008 PMID:21502653

Curioso, W. H., & Michael, P. N. (2010). Enhancing 'M-health' with South-to-South Collaborations. *Health Affairs (Project Hope), 29*(2), 264–267. doi:10.1377/hlthaff.2009.1057 PMID:20348071

Curtis, A. (2002). The century of self. *BBC*. Retrieved from http://topdocumentaryfilms.com/the-century-of-the-self/

Davenport, T. H., & Prusak, L. (2000). *Working knowledge: how organizations manage what they know* (2nd ed.). Harvard Business Press.

Davies, H. (1999). Falling public trust in health services: Implications for accountability. *Journal of Health Services Research & Policy, 4*(4), 193–194. doi:10.1177/135581969900400401 PMID:10623032

Dionisio, J. D. N., Burns, W. G., III, & Gilbert, R. (2013). 3D Virtual Worlds and the Metaverse: Current Status and Future Possibilities. *Computer Science Faculty Works*. Retrieved from http://digitalcommons.lmu.edu/cs_fac/8

Donaldson, L. J. (2001). Professional accountability in a changing world. *Postgraduate Medical Journal, 77*(904), 65–67. doi:10.1136/pmj.77.904.65 PMID:11161069

Doneria, K., & Vinodani, S. (2017). Marketing Emerging Technologies: A Business to Business Perspective Strategic Overview, Opportunities and Challenges. *Amity Global Business Review, 12*(2), 15-19. Retrieved from http://search.ebscohost.com/login.aspx?direct=true&db=bsu&AN=128325994&lang=pt-br&site=ehost-live

Dooley, R. (2015a). The TMI Effect for Pictures Can Reduce Your Sales. *Neuromarketing*. Retrieved November14, 2015 from http://www.neurosciencemarketing.com/blog/articles/tmi-effect-pictures.htm

Dooley, R. (2015b). The Brainfluence podcast, episode #81: The brain lady, a.k.a. Susan Weinschenk. *Neuromarketing*. Retrieved November 6, 2015 from http://www.rogerdooley.com/wp-content/uploads/2015/10/EP081-BrainfluencePodcastTranscript.pdf

Drèze, J., & Sen, A. (Eds.). (1997). *Indian Development: Selected Regional Perspectives*. New Delhi: Oxford University Press. doi:10.1093/acprof:o so/9780198292043.001.0001

Drucker, P. (1985). *Innovation and Entrepreneurship*. Harper & Row Publish, Inc.

Duffy, J., & Holland, M. (2009). *The digital hospital of tomorrow: the time has come today*. A white paper by Health Industry Insights, an IDC company. Retrieved from http://www.healthindustry-insights.com

Dustin, D. (2007). *The McDonaldization of social work*. Hampshire: Ashgate Publishing Limited.

Ebrahim, A. (2003). Making Sense of Accountability: Conceptual Perspectives for Northern and Southern Nonprofits. *Nonprofit Management & Leadership, 14*(2), 191–212. doi:10.1002/nml.29

EC – European Commission (2015). *Innovation for Active & Healthy Ageing. European Summit on Innovation for Active and Healthy Ageing*. Brussels, 9-10 March 2015. Final Report.

EC – European Commission. (2016). *European Innovation Partnership on Active and Healthy Ageing*. Action Group A3, Renovated Action Plan 2016–2018. Retrieved from https://ec.europa.eu/eip/ageing/library/action-plan-2016-2018-a3_en

EC- European Commission, Information Society and Media. (2010). i2010: Information Society and the media working towards growth and jobs. Brussels.

Ehrenberg, A. (2000). *La fatigue d'être soi. Dépression et Société*. Paris: Odile Jacob.

Ekedahl, M., & Wengstrom, Y. (2008). Coping processes in a multidisciplinary healthcare team— A comparison of nurses in cancer care and hospital chaplains. *European Journal of Cancer Care, 17*(1), 42–48. doi:10.1111/j.1365-2354.2007.00801.x PMID:18181890

El-Bashir, M. Z., Collier, P., & Sutton, S. G. (2011). The Role of Organizational Absorptive Capacity in Strategic Use of Business Intelligence to Support Integrated Management Control Systems. *The Accounting Review, 86*(1), 155–184. doi:10.2308/accr.00000010

El-Gayar, O., & Timsina, P. (2014). Opportunities for Business Intelligence and Big Data Analytics In Evidence Based Medicine. In *Annals of 47th Hawaii International Conference on System Science*. IEEE. 10.1109/HICSS.2014.100

Elkaïm, M. (1985). From general laws to singularities. *Family Process, 24*(2), 151–164. doi:10.1111/j.1545-5300.1985.00151.x PMID:4018238

Ellaway, R. H. (2014). Panoptic, synoptic, and omnoptic surveillance. *Medical Teacher, 36*(6), 547–549. doi:10.3109/0142159X.2014.914680 PMID:24873680

Ellaway, R. H., Coral, J., Topps, D., & Topps, M. (2015). Exploring digital professionalism. *Medical Teacher, 37*(9), 844–849. doi:10.3109/014215 9X.2015.1044956 PMID:26030375

EmWave Technology. (2015). *Institute of HeartMath.* Retrieved November 14, 2015 from http://www.heartmath.com/emwave-technology/

Esteva, A., Kuprel, B., Novoa, R. A., Ko, J., Swetter, S. M., Blau, H. M., & Thrun, S. (2017). Dermatologist-level classification of skin cancer with deep neural networks. *Nature, 542*(7639), 115–118. doi:10.1038/nature21056 PMID:28117445

Etchegoyen, A. (1995). *A era dos responsáveis.* Linda-a-Velha: Diffel.

Eurofound. (2018). *Automation, digitalisation and platforms: Implications for work and employment.* Luxembourg: Publications Office of the European Union. Retrieved from http://eurofound.link/ef18002

Europe's Information Society. (2011). ICT for Better Healthcare in Europe. *Europa.* Retrieved April 27, 2011 from http://ec.europa.eu/information_society/activities/health/index_en.htm

European Commission (EC). (2018). Innovation Partnership on Active and Healthy Ageing (EIP on AHA) (2018-2020). Brussels: EC.

European Economy 2. (2009). *2009 Ageing Report: Economic and budgetary projections for the EU-27 Member States (2008-2060).* Joint Report prepared by the European Commission (DG ECFIN) and the Economic Policy Committee (AWG). Luxembourg: European Commission - Directorate-General for Economic and Financial Affairs.

European Union. (2016). Regulation (EU) 2016/679 of the European Parliament and of the Council of 27 April 2016 on the protection of natural persons with regard to the processing of personal data and on the free movement of such data, and repealing Directive 95/46/EC (General Data Protection Regulation). *Official Journal of the European Union.*

Evans, R. S. (2016). Electronic Health Records: Then, Now, and in the Future. *Yearbook of medical informatics, 25*(S 01), S48-S61. doi:10.15265/IYS-2016-s006

Evetts, J. (2012a), Professionalism in turbulent times: changes, challenges and opportunities. *Sociologia, Problemas e Práticas, 88,* 43-59. Retrieved from https://revistas.rcaap.pt/sociologiapp/article/view/14797

Evetts, J. (2012b). Sociological Analysis of the New Professionalism: Knowledge and Expertise in Organizations. In T. Carvalho, R. Santiago, & T. Caria (Eds.), *Grupos Profissionais, Profissionalismo e Sociedade do Conhecimento* (pp. 13–27). Porto: Edições Afrontamento.

Evetts, J. (2014). The Concept of Professionalism: Professional Work, Professional Practice and Learning. In S. Billett, C. Harteis, & H. Gruber (Eds.), *International Handbook of Research in Professional and Practice-based Learning* (pp. 29–56). Dordrecht, Sweden: Springer. doi:10.1007/978-94-017-8902-8_2

Exley, C. (2004). Review article: The sociology of dying, death and bereavement. *Sociology of Health & Illness, 26*(1), 110–122. doi:10.1111/j.1467-9566.2004.00382.x PMID:15027994

Fagot-Largeault, A. (2010). *Médecine et philosophie*. Paris, France: Presses Universitaires de France. doi:10.3917/puf.fagot.2010.01

FAO. (2010). *The State of Food Insecurity in the World. Addressing food insecurity in protracted crises*. Rome: FAO UN.

FAO. (2012). *The State of World Fisheries and Aquaculture*. Rome: FAO UN.

Faulconbridge, J. R., & Muzio, D. (2008). Organizational professionalism in globalizing law firms. *Work, Employment and Society, 22*(1), 7–25. doi:10.1177/0950017007087413

Ferrel, O. C., & Hartline, M. (2010). *Marketing Strategy*. South Western College Publications.

Fineber, I. (2005). Preparing professionals for family conferences in palliative care: Evaluation results of na interdisciplinary approach. *Journal of Palliative Medicine, 8*(4), 857–866. doi:10.1089/jpm.2005.8.857 PMID:16128661

Flenady, V., Wojcieszek, A. M., Middleton, P., Ellwood, D., Erwich, J. J., Coory, M., ... Goldenberg, R. L. (2016). Stillbirths: Recall to action in high-income countries. *Lancet, 387*(10019), 681–702. doi:10.1016/S0140-6736(15)01020-X PMID:26794070

Fonseca, A. (2006). *O envelhecimento. Uma abordagem psicológica*. Lisboa: Universidade Católica Editora.

Fook, J. (2002). *Social Work: Critical theory and practice*. London: Sage.

Foster, D. (1985). *The philosophical scientists*. New York: Dorset Press.

Foucault, M. (1997). Il faut défendre la société. Cours au Collège de France (1975-1976). Paris: Gallimard.

Foucault, M. (1975). *Surveiller et punir. Naissance de la prison*. Paris, France: Gallimard.

Foucault, M. (1976). *Histoire de la sexualité: La volonté de savoir* (Vol. 1). Paris: Les Éditions Gallimard.

Foucault, M. (1976). Histoire de la sexualité: Vol. 1. *La volonté de savoir*. Paris: Gallimard.

Foucault, M. (1976). *La volonté de savoir. Histoire de la sexualité 1*. Paris, France: Gallimard.

Foucault, M. (2001a). Crise de la médecine ou crise de l'antimédecine. In M. Foucault (Ed.), *Dits et écrits II. 1976-1988* (pp. 40–58). Paris, France: Gallimard.

Foucault, M. (2001b). Un système fini face à une demande infinie. In M. Foucault (Ed.), *Dits et écrits II. 1976-1988* (pp. 1186–1202). Paris, France: Gallimard.

Freedberg, S. J., Jr. (2015). Marines explore augmented reality. *Breaking Defense*. Retrieved September 1, 2015 from http://breakingdefense.com/2015/09/marines-explore-augmented-reality-training/

Freidson, E. (2004). *Professionalism: The Third Logic*. Cambridge, UK: Polity Press.

Fried, L. P., Tangen, C. M., Walston, J., Newman, A. B., Hirsch, C., Gottdiener, J., ... McBurnie, M. A. (2001). Frailty in older adults: Evidence for a phenotype. *The Journals of Gerontology. Series A, Biological Sciences and Medical Sciences, 56*(3), M146–M156. doi:10.1093/gerona/56.3.M146 PMID:11253156

Frysinger, R. C., & Harper, R. M. (1990). Cardiac and respiratory correlations with unit discharge in epileptic humantemporal lobe. *Epilepsia, 31*(2), 162–171. doi:10.1111/j.1528-1167.1990.tb06301.x PMID:2318169

Fukuyama, F. (1996). *Confiança, Valores sociais & criação de prosperidade*. Lisboa: Gradiva.

Gaggioli, A., Riva, G., Peters, D., & Calvo, R. A. (2017). Positive Technology, Computing, and Design: Shaping a Future in Which Technology Promotes Psychological Well-Being. In M. Jeon (Ed.), Emotions and Affect in Human Factors and Human-Computer Interaction (pp. 477–502). Academic Press; doi:10.1016/B978-0-12-801851-4.00018-5

Galeon, D. (2016). An AI was taught to hunt & kill humans in a video game. *Futurism*. Retrieved 7/11/2017 from http://futurism.com/scientists-taught-an-ai-to-hunt-and-kill-humans-in-a-video-game/

Gallos, P., Minou, J., Routsis, F., & Mantas, J. (2017). Investigating the Perceived Innovation of the Big Data Technology in Healthcare. *Studies in Health Technology and Informatics*, *238*, 151–153. Retrieved from http://search.ebscohost.com/login.aspx?direct=true&db=mdc&AN=28679910&lang=pt-br&site=ehost-live PMID:28679910

Gartner. (2012). *Forecast: Mobile Advertising, Worldwide, 2009-2016*. Retrieved from http://www.gartner.com/resId=2247015

Gaßner, K., & Conrad, M. (2010). *ICT enabled independent living for elderly. A status-quo analysis on products and the research landscape in the field of Ambient Assisted Living (AAL) in EU-27*. Berlin: Institute for Innovation and Technology.

Geere, D. (2015). A robot just passed the self-awareness test. *Techradar*. Retrieved July 16, 2015 from http://www.techradar.com/news/world-of-tech/uh-oh-this-robot-just-passed-the-self-awareness-test-1299362

Gholami-Kordkheili, F., Wild, V., & Strech, D. (2013). The Impact of Social Media on Medical Professionalism: A Systematic Qualitative Review of Challenges and Opportunities. *Journal of Medical Internet Research*, *15*(8), 1-8. Retrieved from https://www.jmir.org/2013/8/e184/

Giddens, A. (2000). *Conversas com Anthony Giddens: O sentido da Modernidade*. Rio de Janeiro: FGV.

Giles, R. (2012). *Envisioning the digital hospital: the future of healthcare*. Hewlett Packard Development Company. Retrieved from http://www.hp.com/go/healthcare

Gillin, Lapira, McCraty, Bradley, Atkinson, Simpson, & Scicluna (n.d.). Before cognition: the active contribution of the heart/ANS to intuitive decision making as measured in repeat entrepreneurs in the Cambridge TECHNOPOL. *Heartmath Institute Research Library*. Retrieved November 6, 2015 from https://www.heartmath.org/assets/uploads/2015/01/language-of-entrepreneurship.pdf

Gill, T. M., Baker, D. I., Gottschalk, M., Peduzzi, P. N., Allore, H., & Byers, A. (2002). A program to prevent functional decline in physically frail, elderly persons who live at home. *The New England Journal of Medicine*, *347*(14), 1068–1074. doi:10.1056/NEJMoa020423 PMID:12362007

Ginsberg, J. P., Berry, M. E., & Powell, D. A. (2010). Cardiac Coherence and PTSD in Combat Veterans. Alternative Therapies in Health and Medicine, 16(4).

Giorgi, E., Diggle, P., Snow, R., & Noor, A. (2018). Geostatistical methods for disease mapping and visualization using data from spatio-temporally referenced prevalence surveys. *International Statistical Review*, *86*(3), 571–597. doi:10.1111/insr.12268

Glaser, B., & Strauss, A. (2007). *Time for dying*. Aldine Transaction.

Glaser, B., & Strauss, A. (2009). *Awareness of dying*. Aldine Transaction.

Glassner, A. (2004). *Interactive storytelling*. Natick, MA: A.K. Peters.

Global System Mobile Association. (2017). GSMA Connected Society & Connected Women Dalberg Global Development Advisors. Accelerating affordable smartphone ownership in emerging markets. Retrieved from https://www.gsma.com/mobilefordevelopment/wp-content/uploads/2017/07/accelerating-affordable-smartphone-ownership-emerging-markets-2017.pdf

Glover, J. (2017). Questions de vie ou de mort. Genève: Labor et Fides.

Goh, Z. S., & Griva, K. (2018). Anxiety and depression in patients with end-stage renal disease: Impact and management challenges - a narrative review. *International Journal of Nephrology and Renovascular Disease*, *11*, 93–102. doi:10.2147/IJNRD.S126615 PMID:29559806

González, A. M., Fuentes, F. C., & García, M. M. (1988). *Psicologia comunitaria*. Madrid: Visor.

González, J., Palacios, E., García, A., González, D., Calcoya, A., & Sanchez, A. (1999). Evaluación de la fiabilidad y validez de una escala de valoración social en el anciano. *Atencion Primaria*, *23*(7), 434–440. Retrieved from http://www.elsevier.es/es-revista-atencion-primaria-27-articulo-evaluacion-fiabilidad-validez-una-escala-14810 PMID:10363397

Goodman, B., Dretzen, R., Rushkoff, D., Soenens, M., & Fanning, D. (2004). *The Persuaders. Frontline. WGBH Educational Foundation distributed by PBS Home Video, a department of the Public Broadcasting Service*.

Grammar, T. (2007). In *Wikipedia*. Retrieved April 27 from http://en.wikipedia.org/wiki/Minimalist_Program

Greenwood, E. (1955). Social science and social work: A theory of their relationship. *The Social Service Review, 29*(1), 20–33. doi:10.1086/639761

Greenyear, F. (2015). Simthetiq Releases 122,000 km2 Correlated VBS3 & Openflight Training Environment. *Halldale Group*. retrieved November 14, 2015 from http://halldale.com/news/defence/simthetiq-releases-122000-km2-correlated-vbs3-openflight-training-environment#.VkYlJ9JdHnO

Griffin, D. (2012). *Hospitals: What They Are and How They Work*. Burlington: Jones & Bartlett Learning.

Grunwald, A. (2011). Responsible Innovation: Bringing together Technology Assessment, Applied Ethics, and STS research. *Enterprise and Work Innovation Studies, 7*, 9–31.

Guadalupe, S. (2017). *As redes de suporte social informal em Serviço Social: as redes sociais pessoais de idosos portugueses nos processos de avaliação diagnóstica em respostas sociais*. Unpublished doctoral dissertation, ISCTE – Instituto Universitário de Lisboa, Escola de Sociologia e Políticas Públicas e CIES, Centro de Investigação e Estudos de Sociologia, Lisboa, Portugal. Retrieved from http://hdl.handle.net/10071/16706

Guadalupe, S. (2012). A intervenção do serviço social na saúde com famílias e em redes de suporte social. In *M. I. Carvalho (coord.), Serviço Social na Saúde* (pp. 183–217). Lisboa: Pactor.

Guadalupe, S. (2016). *Intervenção em rede: Serviço social, sistémica e redes de suporte social* (2nd ed.). Coimbra: Imprensa da Universidade de Coimbra. doi:10.14195/978-989-26-0866-2

Guerra, J. (2017). *Serviço Social, Profissão e Professionalismo no Contexto do Estado-Providência em Portugal. Os assistentes sociais nos hospitais do Serviço Nacional de Saúde*. Unpublished doctoral dissertation, Catholic University of Portugal, Lisbon, Portugal.

Guerra, Y. (2000). Instrumentalidade do processo de trabalho do serviço social. *Serviço Social & Sociedade, 62*(XX), 5–34.

Guerra, Y. (2012). A Dimensão técnico-operativa do exercício profissional. In C. M. dos Santos, S. Backx, & Y. Guerra (Eds.), *A dimensão técnico-operativa no Serviço Social: desafios contemporâneos* (pp. 39–68). Juiz de Fora: UFRJE.

Hacking, I. (1982). Biopower and the avalanche of printed numbers. *Humanity & Society*, 5(3-4), 279–295.

Hacking, I. (1990). *The Taming of Chance*. Cambridge, UK: Cambridge University Press. doi:10.1017/CBO9780511819766

Hacking, I. (2003). "Vrai", les valeurs et les sciences. In J.-P. Changeux (Ed.), *La vérité dans les sciences* (pp. 201–214). Paris, France: Odile Jacob.

Hacking, I. (2007). Kinds of People: Moving Targets. *Proceedings of the British Academy*, 151, 285–318.

Hall, M. P. (2003). *The secret teachings of all ages*. New York: Jeremy P. Tarcher/Penguin.

Hameroff, S., & Penrose, S. R. (2014). Discovery of quantum vibrations in "microtubules" corroborates theory of consciousness. *PhysOrg*. Retrieved January 16, 2014 from http://phys.org/news/2014-01--discovery-quantum-vibrations--microtubules-corroborates.html

Hamilton, G. (1958). *Teoria e prática do serviço social de casos*. Rio de Janeiro, Brazil: Agir.

Hardesty, L. (2015). System automatically converts 2-D video to 3-D: Exploiting video game software yields broadcast quality 3-D video of soccer game in real time. *MIT News*. Retrieved November 4, 2015 from http://news.mit.edu/2015/software-converts-2-d-3-d-video-1104#.VjsetvPiDfc.linkedin

Hardey, M., & Loader, B. (2009). The Informatization of Welfare: Older People and the Role of Digital Services. *British Journal of Social Work*, 39(4), 657–669. doi:10.1093/bjsw/bcp024

Harding, A., & Preker, A. S. (2000). *Understanding organizational reforms: the corporatization of public hospitals*. Retrieved from http://siteresources.worldbank.org/HEALTHNUTRITIONANDPOPULATION/Resources/281627-1095698140167/Harding-UnderstandingOrganizational-whole.pdf

Harfouche, A. P. (2008). *Hospitais Transformados em Empresas. Análise do impacto na eficiência: estudo comparativo*. Lisboa, Portugal: Instituto Superior de Ciências Sociais e Políticas da Universidade Técnica de Lisboa.

Hargens-Esbjörn, S. (2009). *An overview of integral theory – An all-inclusive framework for the 21st century*. Integral Institute, Resource Paper. Disponível em: http://integraleurope.org/wp-content/uploads/2013/05/IT_3-2-2009.pdf

Harrison, S., & Smith, C. (2004). Trust and moral motivation: Redundant resources in health and social care? *Policy and Politics, 2*(3), 371–386. doi:10.1332/0305573041223726

Heidegger, M. (1958). Essais et conférences. Paris, France: Gallimard.

He, W., Goodkind, D., & Kowal, P. (2016). *An Aging World. International Population Reports*. Washington: U.S. Government Publishing Office.

Hill, A., & Shaw, I. (2011). *Social Work and ICT*. London, UK: Sage Publication.

Hoffman, L. (2013, April). Looking back at the big data. *Communications of the ACM, 56*(4), 21–23. doi:10.1145/2436256.2436263

Hollis, F. (1970). The psychosocial approach to casework practice. In R. W. Roberts & R. H. Nee (Eds.), *Theories of Social Casework* (pp. 33–46). Chicago, IL: University of Chicago Press.

Holmgren, D., & Mollison, B. (1978). *Permaculture one. A perennial agriculture for human settlements*. Melbourne: Transworld.

Homan, R. (1991). *The Ethics of Social Research*. Londres: Longman.

Hood, L., & Auffray, C. (2013). Participatory medicine: A driving force for revolutionizing healthcare. *Genome Medicine, 4*(110). PMID:24360023

Hopkins, R. (2008). *The Transition Handbook. From the oil dependency to local resilience*. Chelsea Green Publishing.

How Yahoo Research Labs studies culture as a formal computational concept. (2014). *MIT Technology Review*. Retrieved January 25, 2015 from http://www.technologyreview.com/view/529521/how-yahoo-research-labs-studies-culture

Howe, D. (1992). Child abuse and the bureaucratisation of social work. *The Sociological Review, 40*(3), 491–508. doi:10.1111/j.1467-954X.1992.tb00399.x

Huber, M. A. S. (2014). *Towards a new, dynamic concept of Health. Its operationalisation and use in public health and healthcare, and in evaluating health effects of food* (Unpublished Doctoral dissertation). School for Public Health and Primary Care CAPHRI, Maastricht University, Maastricht.

Huber, G. P. (1990). A theory of the effects of advanced information technologies on organizational design, intelligence and decision making. *Academy of Management Review, 15*(1), 47–71. doi:10.5465/amr.1990.4308227

Hughes, J. (2004). *Citizen Cyborg: Why Democratic Societies Must Respond to the Redesigned Human of the Future*. Westview Press.

Hull, R. F. C. (1974). *Dreams*. New York: Princeton University Press.

Hussain, A., Ali, S., Ahmed, M., & Hussain, S. (2018). The Anti-vaccination Movement: A Regression in Modern Medicine. *Cureus, 10*(7), e2919. doi:10.7759/cureus.2919 PMID:30186724

Hutchins, E. (2005). Material anchors for conceptual blends. *Journal of Pragmatics, 37*(10), 1555–1577. doi:10.1016/j.pragma.2004.06.008

Huxley, J. S. (1957). *(Transhumanisme) New Bottles for New Wine*. Londres: Chatto & Windus.

IA Institute – Information Architecture Institute. (2014) *Recommended reading*. Retrieved from http://iainstitute.org/en/learn/education/recommended_reading.php

ICATT. (2010). *Computer-based Learning Program for Health Professionals in Developing Countries*. Basel: Novartis Foundation for Sustainable Development. Retrieved from novartisfoundation.org

Ikeda, E., Stewart, T., Garrett, N., Egli, V., Mandic, S., Hosking, J., ... & Moore, A. (2018). Built environment associates of active school travel in New Zealand children and youth: A systematic meta-analysis using individual participant data. Journal of Transport & Health. doi:10.1016/j.jth.2018.04.007

Illario, M., Vollenbroek-Hutten, M. M. R., Molloy, W., Menditto, E., Iaccarino, G., & Eklund, P. (2016). Active and Healthy Ageing and Independent Living. *Journal of Aging Research, 2016*, 8062079. doi:10.1155/2016/8062079 PMID:27818798

Illich, I. (1975). The medicalization of life. *Journal of Medical Ethics, I*(2), 73–77. doi:10.1136/jme.1.2.73 PMID:809583

Inamdar, N., Kaplan, R. S., & Bower, M. (2002). Applying the balanced scorecard in healthcare provider organizations. *Journal of Healthcare Management*, *47*(3), 179–195. doi:10.1097/00115514-200205000-00008 PMID:12055900

Inmon, B., Strauss, D., & Neushloss, G. (2008). *DW 2.0: The Architecture for the Next Generation of Data Warehousing*. Morgan Kaufmann.

Innerarity, D. (2010). *O Novo Espaço Público*. Lisboa, Portugal: Teorema.

Institute of Heartmath. (2007). New research project: global coherence monitoring system. *IHM Summer 2007 Newsletter*. Retrieved May 1, 2009 from http://www.heartmath.org/templates/ihm/e-newsletteer/2007/Summer-2007/summer_2007_newsletter.htm

Instituto de Arquitetos do Brasil (IAB). (2014). Retrieved from http://www.iab.org

Israel, M., & Hay, I. (2006). *Research Ethics for Social Scientists*. Londres: Sage. doi:10.4135/9781849209779

Ivatury, G., Moore, J., & Bloch, A. (2009). A Doctor in your Pocket: Health Hotlines in Developing Countries. *Innovations: Technology, Governance, Globalization*, *4*(1), 119–153. doi:10.1162/itgg.2009.4.1.119

Iyer, R., & Eastman, J. K. (2006). The Elderly and Their Attitudes toward the Internet: The Impact on Internet Use, Purchase and Comparison Shopping. *Journal of Marketing Theory and Practice*, *14*(1), 57–67. doi:10.2753/MTP1069-6679140104

Jacobi, J. (1973). *The psychology of CG Jung*. London: Yale University Press.

Jambroes, M., Nederland, T., Kaljouw, M., van Vliet, K., Essink-Bot, M.-L., & Ruwaard, D. (2016). Implications of health as 'the ability to adapt and self-manage' for public health policy: A qualitative study. *European Journal of Public Health*, *26*(3), 412–416. doi:10.1093/eurpub/ckv206 PMID:26705568

Jamil, G. L. (2001). *Repensando a TI na empresa moderna*. Rio de Janeiro: Axcel Books do Brasil.

Jamil, G. L. (2005). *Gestão da Informação e do conhecimento em empresas brasileiras: estudo de múltiplos casos*. Belo Horizonte: Ed. Con / Art.

Jamil, G. L. (2018). *Market intelligence as an information system element: delivering knowledge for decisions in a continuous process in Handbook of Research on Expanding Business Opportunities with information systems and analytics*. Hershey, PA: IGI Global.

Jamil, G. L., & Berwanger, S. G. (2019). Choosing a Business Model: Entrepreneurship, Strategy and Competition. In *Handbook of Research on Business Models in Modern Competitive Scenarios*. Hershey, PA: IGI Global. doi:10.4018/978-1-5225-7265-7.ch001

Jamil, G. L., Jamil, L. C., Vieira, A. A. P., & Xavier, A. J. D. (2015). Challenges in modelling Healthcare services: A study case of information architecture perspectives. In G. L. Jamil, J. P. Rascão, A. M. Silva, & F. Ribeiro (Eds.), *Handbook of Research on Information Architecture and Management in Modern Organizations*. Hershey, PA: IGI Global.

Jamil, G. L., & Magalhães, L. F. C. (2015). Perspectives for big data analysis for knowledge generation in project management contexts. In G. L. Jamil, *S.M. Lopes, A.M. Silva et al.* (Ed.), *Handbook of research on effective project management research through the integration of knowledge and innovation*. Hershey, PA: IGI Global. doi:10.4018/978-1-4666-7536-0.ch001

Jamil, G. L., Santos, L. H. R., Lindgren, M. A., Furbino, L., Santiago, R., & Loyola, S. A. (2011). Design Framework for a Market Intelligence System for Healthcare Sector: A Support Decision Tool in an Emergent Economy. In M. M. Cruz-Cunha, I. S. Miranda, & P. Gonçalves (Eds.), *Handbook of Research on ICTs and Management Systems for Improving Efficiency in Healthcare and Social Care*. Hershey, PA: IGI Global.

Jamison, D. T., Summers, L. H., Alleyne, G., Arrow, K. J., Berkley, S., Binagwaho, A., ... Yamey, G. (2013). Global health 2035: A world converging within a generation. *Lancet*, *382*(9908), 1898–1955. doi:10.1016/S0140-6736(13)62105-4 PMID:24309475

Jayanthi, G., & Uma, V. (2018). Modeling Spatial Evolution: Review of Methods and Its Significance. In C. Pshenichny, P. Diviacco, & D. Mouromtsev (Eds.), *Dynamic Knowledge Representation in Scientific Domains* (pp. 235–259). Hershey, PA: IGI Global. doi:10.4018/978-1-5225-5261-1.ch010

Jha, V., Wang, A. Y. M., & Wang, H. (2012). The impact of CKD identification in large countries: The burden of illness. *Nephrology, Dialysis, Transplantation*, *27*(Suppl. 3), 32–38. doi:10.1093/ndt/gfs113 PMID:23115140

Johnson, J. E. (2012). Big data + Big Analytics + Big opportunity. Financial & Executive, (July/August), 51-53.

Jonas, H. (1995). *El principio de responsabilidad. Ensayo de una ética para la civilización tecnológica.* Barcelona: Editorial Herder. (Original work published 1979)

Jotheeswaran, A. T., Bryce, R., Prina, M., Acosta, D., Ferri, C. P., Guerra, M., & ... (2015). Frailty and the prediction of dependence and mortality in low- and middle-income countries: A 10/66 population-based cohort study. *BMC Medicine*, *13*(138), 1–12. PMID:25563062

Jung, C. G. (1933). *Modern man in search of a soul.* Harcourt Brace & Company.

Kaethler, Y., Molnar, F., Mitchell, S., Soucie, P., & Manson-hing, M. (2003). Defining the concept of frailty: A survey of multi-disciplinary health professionals. *Geriatrics Today: Journal of the Canadian Geriatrics Society*, *6*, 26–31.

Kahana, E., Kahana, B., & Kercher, K. (2003). Emerging lifestyles and proactive options for successful ageing. *Ageing International*, *28*(2), 155–180. doi:10.100712126-003-1022-8

Kanaher, L. (1998). *Competitive Intelligence: How to gather, analyse, and use Information to move your business to the top.* New York: Touchstone Books.

Kaplan, W. A. (2006). Can the Ubiquitous Power of Mobile Phones be used to improve Health Outcomes in Developing Countries? *Globalization and Health*, *2*(9), 21. PMID:16719925

Kaplesky, B. (2007b). *The imago effect—notes on presentation by Harvey Smith of Midway Games.* Retrieved November 14, 2015 from http://www.secretlair.com/index.php?/clickableculture/entry/notes_the_imago_effect_avatar_psychology/

Karavides, M. K., Leehrer, P. M., & Vaschillo, V. (2007). Preliminary reports of an open label study of heartrate variability biofeedback for treatment of major depression. *Applied Psychophysiology and Biofeedback*, *32*(1), 19–30. doi:10.100710484-006-9029-z PMID:17333315

Kearns, G. S., & Lederer, A. L. (2003). A resource based view of IT alignment: How knowledge sharing creates a competitive advantage. *Decision Sciences*, *34*(1), 1–29. doi:10.1111/1540-5915.02289

Kearns, K. (1994). The Strategic Management of Accountability in Nonprofit Organizations: An Analytical Framework. *Public Administration Review*, *54*(2), 185–192. doi:10.2307/976528

Keating, M. (2002), Working Together – Integrated Governance. *United Nations.* Retrieved from http://unpan1.un.org/intradoc/groups/public/documents/apcity/unpan007118.pdf

Keplesky, B. (2007a). The Imago Effect: Avatar Psychology. *Behind the Door SXSW07.* Retrieved November 14, 2015 from https://doornumber3.wordpress.com/2007/03/14/the-imago-effect-avatar-psychology/

Khatri, N., Baveja, A., Boren, S. A., & Mammo, A. (2006). Medical errors and quality of care: From control to commitment. *California Management Review*, *48*(3), 115–141. doi:10.2307/41166353

Khodarahimi, S. (2009). Dreams in Jungian psychology: The use of dreams as an instrument for research diagnosis and treatment of social phobia. *The Malaysian Journal of Medical Sciences: MJMS, 16*(4), 42–49. PMID:22135511

Khokhar, A. (2009). Short text messages (SMS) as a reminder system for making working women from Delhi breast aware. *Asian Pacific Journal of Cancer Prevention, 10*, 319–322. PMID:19537904

Kimball, R., & Ross, M. (2010). *Relentlessly Practical Tools for Data Warehousing and Business Intelligence.* John Wiley and sons.

Kirby, R. S., Delmelle, E., & Eberth, J. M. (2017). Advances in spatial epidemiology and geographic information systems. *Annals of Epidemiology, 27*(1), 1–9. doi:10.1016/j.annepidem.2016.12.001 PMID:28081893

Kirk, T. (2014). Superconducting spintronics pave way for next-generation computing. *PhysOrg.* Retrieved January 15, 2014 from http://phys.org/news/2014-01-superconducting-spintronics-pave-next-generation.html

Kleinman, A., Eisenberg, L., & Good, B. (1978). Culture, illness, and care: Clinical lessons from anthropologic and cross-cultural research. *Annals of Internal Medicine, 88*(2), 251–258. doi:10.7326/0003-4819-88-2-251 PMID:626456

Knight, W. (2015). A new tool for analyzing academic papers uses cutting-edge AI to find meaning in billions of words. *MIT Technology Review.* Retrieved from http://www.technologyreview.com/news/542981/academic-search-engine-grasps-for-meaning/

Knox, Lentini, & Alton. (2012). Effects of game-based relaxation training on attention problems in anxious children. *Priory.com.*

Kobusingye, O. C. (2005). Emergency Medical Systems in Low and Middle Income Countries: Recommendations for Action. *Bulletin of the World Health Organization*, *83*(8), 626–631. PMID:16184282

Kosslyn, S. M. (1994). *Image and Brain*. Massachusetts Institute of Technology.

Kotler, P., & Keller, K. (2005). *Marketing Management* (12th ed.). Prentice Hall.

Kowal, E. (2015). *Computer simulations improve lethality*. Retrieved May 19, 2015 from http://htl.li/N8e9W

Krishna, S., Boren, S. A., & Balas, E. A. (2009). Healthcare Via Cell Phones: A Systemic Review. *Telemedicine Journal and e-Health*, *15*(3), 231–240. doi:10.1089/tmj.2008.0099 PMID:19382860

Kvedar, J., Coye, M. J., & Everett, W. (2014). Connected health: A review of technologies and strategies to improve patient care with telemedicine and telehealth. *Health Affairs*, *33*(2), 194–199. doi:10.1377/hlthaff.2013.0992 PMID:24493760

Lacerda, L. E. (2014). Exercício profissional do assistente social: Da imediaticidade às possibilidades históricas. *Serviço Social & Sociedade*, *117*(117), 22–44. doi:10.1590/S0101-66282014000100003

Lakoff, George, & Narayanan. (2010). Toward a computational model of narrative. *International Computer Science Institute and University of California at Berkeley*. Retrieved from http://www1.icsi.berkeley.edu/~snarayan/narrative-aaai-fs2010.pdf

Lakoff, G. (2002). *Moral politics*. Chicago: University of Chicago Press. doi:10.7208/chicago/9780226471006.001.0001

Lakoff, G. (2008). *The political mind*. Viking Penguin.

Lapão, L. V. (2016). The Future Impact of Healthcare Services Digitalization on Health Workforce: The Increasing Role of Medical Informatics. *Studies in Health Technology and Informatics*, *228*, 675–679. PMID:27577470

Laudon, K., & Laudon, L. (2009). *Management Information Systems* (11th ed.). Prentice Hall.

Lautrette, A., Ciroldi, M., Ksibi, H., & Azoulay, E. (2006). End-of-life family conferences: Rooted in the evidence. *Critical Care Medicine*, *34*(Suppl), S364–S372. doi:10.1097/01.CCM.0000237049.44246.8C PMID:17057600

346

Lawn, J. (2011). *Stillbirths –An Executive Summary for The Lancet's Series*. Retrieved from https://www.thelancet.com/series/stillbirth

Leal, A.S.L., & Bogi, A. (2014). Network for the Market uptake of ICT for Ageing Well. In *Good Practices Handbook*. Project co-funded by the European Commission within the ICT Policy Support Programme.

Lee, D. (2015). Facebook set to share AI advances. *BBC News*. Retrieved November 5, 2015 from http://www.bbc.com/news/technology-34717958?post_id=10206805 820649209_10208064398872878

Lee, P., Lan, W., & Yen, T. (2011). Aging successfully: A four-factor model. *Educational Gerontology*, *37*(3), 210–227. doi:10.1080/03601277.2010.487759

Lehrer, P., Vaschillo, E., Lu, S. E., Eckberg, D., Vaschillo, B., Scardella, A., & Habib, R. (2006). Heart rate variability biofeedback: Effects of age on heart rate variability, baroreflex gain, and athsma. *Chest*, *129*(2), 278–284. doi:10.1378/chest.129.2.278 PMID:16478842

Leidner, D., & Elam, J. J. (1995). The impact of executive information systems on organizational design, intelligence and decision making. *Organization Science*, *6*(6), 645–664. doi:10.1287/orsc.6.6.645

Levinas, E. (1993). *Entre nous. Essais sur le penser-à-l'autre*. Paris: Grasset.

Levin, Z. D., & Bertschi, I. (2018). Media health literacy, eHealth literacy, and the role of the social environment in context. *International Journal of Environmental Research and Public Health*, *15*(8), 16–43. doi:10.3390/ijerph15081643 PMID:30081465

Lindmark, S., Wiklund, U., Bjerle, P., & Eriksson, J. W. (2003). Does the autonomic nervous system play a role in the development of insulin resistance? A study on heartrate variability in first degree relatives of Type 2 diabetes patients and control subjects. *Diabetic Medicine*, *20*(5), 399–405. doi:10.1046/j.1464-5491.2003.00920.x PMID:12752490

Lindquist, A. M., Johansson, P. E., Peterson, G. I., Saveman, B. I., & Nilsson, G. C. (2008). The Use of Personal Digital Assistant (PDA) among Personnel and Students in Healthcare: A Review. *Journal of Medical Internet Research*, *10*(4), 31. doi:10.2196/jmir.1038 PMID:18957381

Lindström, B., & Eriksson, M. (2005). Salutogenesis. *Journal of Epidemiology and Community Health*, *59*(6), 440–442. doi:10.1136/jech.2005.034777 PMID:15911636

Lipovetsky, G., & Serroy, J. (2011). *Cultura-Mundo. A cultura-mundo, respostas a uma sociedade desorientada*. São Paulo, Brazil: Companhia das Letras.

Liukkonen, M. (2015). RFID technology in manufacturing and supply chain. *International Journal of Computer Integrated Manufacturing*, 28(8), 861–880. do i:10.1080/0951192X.2014.941406

Lopes, J. M., Fukushima, R. L. M., Inouye, K., Pavarini, S. C. I., Orlandi, F. de S., Lopes, J. M., & Orlandi, F. de S. (2014). Quality of life related to the health of chronic renal failure patients on dialysis. *Acta Paulista de Enfermagem*, 27(3), 230–236. doi:10.1590/1982-0194201400039

Lorenz, W. (2004). Towards a European paradigm of social work - Studies in the history of modes of social work and social policy in Europe. Retrieved from http://webdoc.sub.gwdg.de/ebook/dissts/Dresden/Lorenz2005.pdf

Lorenz, W. (2006). *Perspectives on European Social Work: From the Birth of the Nation State to the Impact of Globalisation*. Opladen: Barbara Budrich Publishers.

Lucas, H. C. Jr. (2005). *Information technology: strategic decision making for managers*. Hoboken, NJ: John Wiley and Sons.

Ludlow, P. (2007). Noam Chomsky (1928). In Encyclopedia of the Philosophy of Science. Routledge.

Lunin, L. F., & Smith, L. C. (1984). Artificial Intelligence: Concepts, Techniques, Applications, Promise. *Journal of the American Society for Information Science*, 35(5), 277–279. doi:10.1002/asi.4630350504

Luppi, F., & Campanini, A. (1991). *Servicio Social y modelo sistemico: una nueva perspectiva para la practica cotidiana*. Barcelona, Spain: Paidós Ibérica.

Luskin, R., & Newell, Q. (2002). A controlled pilot study of stress management training of elderly patients with congestive heart failure. *Preventive Cardiology*, 5(4), 168–172, 176. doi:10.1111/j.1520.037X.2002.01029.x PMID:12417824

Macy, J. (2014). *Coming back to life. The Updated Guide to the Work That Reconnects*. New Society Publishers.

Malik, J. (2017). What Led Computer Vision to Deep Learning? *Communications of the ACM*, 60(6), 82–83. doi:10.1145/3065384

Manavalan, M., Majumdar, A., Harichandra Kumar, K., & Priyamvada, P. (2017). Assessment of health-related quality of life and its determinants in patients with chronic kidney disease. *Indian Journal of Nephrology, 27*(1), 37. doi:10.4103/0971-4065.179205 PMID:28182041

Mangematin, V., & Thuderoz, C. (2003). *Des mondes de confiance. Un concept à l'épreuve de la réalité sociale.* Paris: CNRS-Éditions.

Marchand, D., & Davenport, T. (Eds.). (2000). *Mastering Information Management.* New York: Financial Times Prentice Hall.

Marchand, D., Kettinger, W., & Rollins, J. (2001). *Making the invisible visible: how companies win the right information, people and IT.* Wiley.

Marjanovic, S., Ghiga, L., & Knack, A. (2018). Understanding value in health data ecosystems: A review of current evidence and ways forward. *Rand Hand Quarterly, 7*(2), 3. PMID:29416943

Markovitch, D. G., Steckel, J. H., & Yeung, B. (2005). Using Capital Markets as Market Intelligence: Evidence from the Pharmaceutical Industry. *Management Science, 51*(10), 1467–1480. doi:10.1287/mnsc.1050.0401

Marmot, M., & Bell, R. (2012). Fair society, healthy lives. *Public Health, 126*(Suppl. 1), S4–S10. doi:10.1016/j.puhe.2012.05.014 PMID:22784581

Marmot, M., & Wilkinson, R. (2006). *Social Determinants of Health* (2nd ed.). Strasbourg: Oxford University Press.

Martinelli, M. L. (2007). O exercício profissional do assistente social na área da saúde: algumas reflexões éticas. *Serviço Social & Saúde, 6*(6), 21–34. Retrieved from www.bibliotecadigital.unicamp.br/document/?down=46133%5Cn

Martins, A. (2018). Viver e morrer no hospital: retratos sociológicos do desacordo nas relações familiares dos idosos em cuidados paliativos. In J. Resende & C. Delaunay (Orgs.), Democracia, promessas, utopias e (des)ilusões: Dilemas e disputas nas arenas públicas (pp. 123-139). Carviçais: Lema de Origem.

Martins, A. (2015). Building paths towards death: sociological portraits of discord in family relations of the elderly in palliative care. In J. M. Resende & A. C. Martins (Eds.), *The making of the common in social relations* (pp. 6–21). Newcastle Upon Tyne, UK: Cambridge Scholars Publishing.

Marx, K. (1970). Bénéfices secondaires du crime (Translated from the German, circa 1861-1863). In D. Szabo (Ed.), *Déviance et criminalité* (pp. 83–85). Paris, France: Armand Colin.

Mason, E., McDougall, L., Lawn, J. E., Gupta, A., Claeson, M., Pillay, Y., ... Chopra, M. (2014). From evidence to action to deliver a healthy start for the next generation. *Lancet, 384*(9941), 455–467. doi:10.1016/S0140-6736(14)60750-9 PMID:24853599

Mattedi, A., & Butzke, I. (2001). A relação entre o social e o natural nas abordagens de hazards e de desastres. *Ambiente & Sociedade, 9*(9), 93–114. doi:10.1590/S1414-753X2001000900006

Maturo, A. (2012). Medicalization: Current concept and future directions in bionic society. *Mens Sana Monographs, 10*(1), 122–133. doi:10.4103/0973-1229.91587 PMID:22654387

Max-Neef, M. (1991). *Human Scale Development. Conception, application and further reflections*. New York: Apex Press.

McAfee, A., & Brynjolfsson, E. (2012). Big data: The management revolution. *Harvard Business Review, 90*(10), 60–68. PMID:23074865

McCraty, R., & Childre, D. (2010). Coherence: bridging personal, social, and global health. *Alternative Therapies, 16*(4). Retrieved November 6, 2015 from https://www.heartmath.org/assets/uploads/2015/01/coherence-bridging-personal-social-global-health.pdf

McCraty, R., Atkinson, M., Stolc, V., Alabdulgader, A. A., Vainoras, A., & Ragulskis, M. (2017). Synchronization of human autonomic nervous system rhythms with geomagnetic activity in human subjects. *IEJRPH*. Retrieved from http://www.mdpi.com/1660-4601/14/7/770/htm

McCraty, R. (2002a). Heart rhythm coherence: And emerging area of biofeedback. *Biofeedback, 30*(1), 17–19.

McCraty, R. (2002b). Influence of cardiac afferent influence on heart-brain synchronization and cognitive performance. *International Journal of Psychophysiology, 45*(1-2), 72–73.

McCraty, R. (2005). *Enhancing emotional, social, and academic learning with heart rhythm coherence feedback*. Heartmath Research Center, Institute of Heartmath.

McCraty, R., & Tomasino, D. (2006). Coherence-building techniques and heart rhythm coherence feedback: New tools for stress reduction, disease prevention, and rehabilitation. In E. Molinari, A. Compare, & G. Parati (Eds.), *Clinical Psychology and Heart Disease*. Milan, Italy: Springer-Verlag. doi:10.1007/978-88-470-0378-1_26

McKinlay, J. B., & Marceau, L. D. (2002). The end of the golden age of doctoring. *International Journal of Health Services*, *32*(2), 379–416. doi:10.2190/JL1D-21BG-PK2N-J0KD PMID:12067037

McLean, A. (2011). Ethical frontiers of ICT and older users: Cultural, pragmatic and ethical issues. *Ethics and Information Technology*, *13*(4), 313–326. doi:10.100710676-011-9276-4

Mechael, P. N., Batavia, H., Kaonga, N., Searle, S., Kwan, A., Fu, L., & Ossman, J. (2010). *Barriers and Gaps Affecting mHealth in Low and Middle Income Countries.* Policy White Paper. Columbia: Center for Global Health and Economic Development, Earth Institute, Columbia University.

Mehry, E. (2002). *Saúde: A cartografia do Trabalho vivo*. São Paulo: Editora Hucitec.

Meliker, J. R., & Sloan, C. D. (2011). Spatio-temporal epidemiology: Principles and opportunities. *Spatial and Spatio-temporal Epidemiology*, *2*(1), 1–9. doi:10.1016/j.sste.2010.10.001 PMID:22749546

Messu, M. (2018). *L'Ere De La Victimisation*. La Tour d'Aigues: Éditions de l'Aube.

Messu, M. (2008). Le temps social fractal. In V. Châtel (Ed.), *Les Temps des Politiques Sociales* (pp. 49–71). Fribourg: Academic Press.

Messu, M. (2017). Confiance et vitimisation. In M. Messu & C. Albuquerque (Eds.), *Confiance et Barbarie. Pour une anthropologie renouvelée de l'action* (pp. 95–150). Paris: L'Harmattan.

Michel, J. P., Dreux, C., & Vacheron, A. (2016). Healthy ageing: Evidence that improvement is possible at every age. *European Geriatric Medicine*, *7*(4), 298–305. doi:10.1016/j.eurger.2016.04.014

Miller, S. (2002). Competitive Intelligence - an overview. *Competitive Intelligence Magazine*, *14*(3), 43-55. Retrieved from http://www.sci.org/library/overview.pdf

Miskelly, F. (2005). Electronic tracking of patients with dementia and wandering using mobile phone technology. *Age and Ageing*, *34*(5), 497–499. doi:10.1093/ageing/afi145 PMID:16107453

Mittelmark, M. B., Sagy, S., Eriksson, M., Bauer, G., Pelikan, J. M., Lindström, B., & Espnes, G. A. (Eds.). (2017). The Handbook of Salutogenesis. Cham: Springer. doi:10.1007/978-3-319-04600-6

Mollenkopf, H., & Walker, A. (2007). Quality of Life in old age. Synthesis and future perspective. In H. Mollenkopf & A. Walker (Eds.), *Quality of Life in Old Age* (pp. 235–248). Springer. doi:10.1007/978-1-4020-5682-6_14

Moraes, E. N., Lanna, F. M., Santos, R. R., Bicalho, M. A. C., Machado, C. J., & Romero, D. E. (2012). A new proposal for the clinical functional categorization of the elderly visual scale of frailty. *The Journal of Aging Research & Clinical Practice.* Retrieved from http://www.jarcp.com/1808-a-new-proposal-for-the-clinical-functional-categorization-of-the-elderly-visual-scale-of-frailty-vs-frailty.html

Morris, S. M. (2010). Achieving collective coherence: Group effects on heart rate variability coherence and heart rhythm synchronization. Alternative Therapies, 16(4).

Moulaert, F., Martinelli, F., Swyngedouw, E., & Gonzalez, S. (2005). Towards Alternative Model(s) of Local Innovation. *Urban Studies, 42*(11), 969-90.

Moulaert, F. (2009). Social Innovation: Institutionally Embedded, Territorially (Re) Produced. In D. MacCallum, F. Moulaert, J. Hilier, & S. Haddock (Eds.), *Social Innovation and Territorial Development*. Ashgate.

Mullan, Z., & Horton, R. (2011). Bringing stillbirths out of the shadows. *Lancet, 377*(9774), 1291–1292. doi:10.1016/S0140-6736(11)60098-6 PMID:21496920

Muñoz, M. M., Barandalla, M. F. M., & Aldalur, A. V. (1996). *Manual indicadores para el diagnóstico social.* Bilbao: Colegios Oficiales de Diplomados en Trabajo Social y Asistentes Sociales de la Comunidad Autónoma Vasca. Retrieved from https://www.cgtrabajosocial.es/files/51786ad45be4d/Manual_de_indicadores_para_el_diagnstico_social.pdf

Mutheneni, S. R., Mopuri, R., Naish, S., Gunti, D., & Upadhyayula, S. M. (2018). Spatial distribution and cluster analysis of dengue using self-organizing maps in Andhra Pradesh, India, 2011–2013. *Parasite Epidemiology and Control, 3*(1), 52–61. doi:10.1016/j.parepi.2016.11.001 PMID:29774299

Nahar, P., Kannuri, N. K., Mikkilineni, S., Murthy, G. V. S., & Phillimore, P. (2017). mHealth and the management of chronic conditions in rural areas: A note of caution from Southern India. *Anthropology & Medicine, 24*(1), 1–16. doi:10.1080/136484 70.2016.1263824 PMID:28292206

Nair, P., & Bhaskaran, H. (2015). The Emerging Interface of Healthcare System and Mobile Communication Technologies. *Health and Technology, 4*(4), 337–343. doi:10.100712553-014-0091-x

NAS - National Academies of Sciences, Engineering, and Medicine. (2017). *Human Genome Editing: Science, Ethics, and Governance.* Washington, DC: The National Academies Press. doi:10.17226/24623

National Health Policy, Government of India. (2017). Retrieved from http://pib.nic.in/newsite/PrintRelease.aspx?relid=159376

Negri, A., & Hart, M. (2002). *Império.* Barcelona: Paidós.

Ngai, E. W. T. (2010). RFID technology and applications in production and supply chain management. *International Journal of Production Research, 48*(9), 2481–2483. doi:10.1080/00207540903564892

NIC. (2012). *Global Trends 2030: Alternative Worlds.* National Intelligence Council.

Niklas, L. (1979). *Trust and Power.* John Wiley & Sons, Ltd.

Noll, H. H. (2007). Monitoring the Quality of Life of the Elderly in European Societies. A social indicators' approach. In B. Marin & A. Zaidi (Eds.), *Mainstream Ageing: Indicators to monitor sustainable policies* (pp. 329–358). Aldershot: Ashgate.

Nonaka, I. (2008). *The knowledge creating company.* Harvard Business Review Classics.

Noordegraaf, M. (2006). Professional Management of Professionals: Hybrid Organizations and Professional Management in Care and Welfare. In J. W. Duyvendak, T. Knijn, & M. Kremer (Eds.), *Policy, People and the New Professional: De-professionalisation and Re-professionalisation in Care and Welfare* (pp. 181–193). Amsterdam, The Netherlands: Amsterdam University Press.

Noordegraaf, M. (2007). From "Pure" to "Hybrid" Professionalism: Present-Day Professionalism in Ambiguous Public Domains. *Administration & Society, 39*(6), 761–785. doi:10.1177/0095399707304434

Norris, P. (2001). *Digital divide: Civic engagement, information poverty and the internet worldwide.* Cambridge: Cambridge University Press. doi:10.1017/CBO9781139164887

O'Brien, K., & Hochachka, G. (n.d.). Integral adaptation to climate change. *Journal of Integral Theory and Practice, 5*(1), 89–102.

O'Sullivan, T. (2011). *Decision making in Social Work*. New York: Palgrave-Macmillan. doi:10.1007/978-1-137-28540-9

OECD. (2013). *ICTs and the Health Sector.Towards Smarter Health and Wellness Models*. Paris: OECD Publishing; doi:10.1787/9789264202863-

OECD. (2014). *Recommendation of the Council on Digital Government Strategies*. Retrieved from http://www.oecd.org/gov/digital-government/Recommendation-digital-government-strategies.pdf

OECD. (2017). *Health at a Glance 2017: OECD Indicators*. Paris: OECD Publishing; doi:10.1787/health_glance-2017-

OECD. (2017). *New Health Technologies: Managing Access, Value and Sustainability*. doi:10.1787/9789264266438-

Ogren, E. H., Norris-Shortle, C., & Showalter, A. (1979). Typologies in social work practice. *Social Work in Health Care*, 4(3), 319–330. doi:10.1300/J010v04n03_07 PMID:472982

Ohata, M. & Kumar, A. (2012). Big Data: A Boom for Business Intelligence. *Financial Executive*, (September).

Okpala, P. (2018). Balancing quality healthcare services and costs through collaborative leadership. *Journal of Healthcare Management*, 63(6), e148–e157. doi:10.1097/JHM-D-18-00020 PMID:30418376

Oosterlynck, S., van den Broek, J., Albrechts, L., Moulaert, F., & Verhetsel, A. (2010). *Bridging the Gap between Planning and Implementation: Turning Transformative Visions into Strategic Projects*. Routledge.

Orme-Johnson, D. W. (n.d.). Maharishi Effect. *Global Good News*. Retrieved November 12, 2015 from maharishi-programmes.globalgoodnews.com/maharishi-effect

Ortega, Y., & Gasset, J. (1987). *El tema de nuestro tiempo*. Madrid: Alianza Editorial.

Øvrum, A., Gustavsen, G. W., & Rickertsen, K. (2014). Age and socioeconomic inequalities in health: Examining the role of lifestyle choices. *Advances in Life Course Research*, 19, 1–13. doi:10.1016/j.alcr.2013.10.002 PMID:24796874

Parkin, S. (2015). Virtual reality startups look back to the future. *MIT Technology Review*. Retrieved March 7, 2014 from https://www.linkedin.com/grp/post/1039687-6003159104225366019

Parrott, L., & Madoc-Jones, L. (2008). Reclaiming information & communication technologies for empowering social work practice. *Journal of Social Work, 8*(2), 181–197. doi:10.1177/1468017307084739

Particle based simulations. (2014). Particle based simulations (physX flex). *NVIDIA*. Retrieved December 9, 2014 from https://www.youtube.com/watch?v=1o0Nuq71 gI4&feature=share

Parton, N. (2000). *Social Theory, Social Change and Social Work (The State of Welfare)*. London, UK: Routledge.

Parton, N. (2008). Changes in the Form of Knowledge in Social Work: From the 'Social' to the 'Informational'? *British Journal of Social Work, 38*(2), 253–269. doi:10.1093/bjsw/bcl337

Patnaik, S., Brunskill, E., & Thies, W. (2009). Evaluating the Accuracy of Data Collection on Mobile Phones: A Study of Forms, SMS, and Voice Calls. In *Proceedings of the International Conference on Information and Communication Technologies and Development* (pp. 74-84). Retrieved from http://hdl.handle.net/1721.1/60077

Patrick, K., Griswold, W. G., Raab, F., & Intille, S. S. (2008). Health and the Mobile Phone. *American Journal of Preventive Medicine, 35*(2), 177–181. doi:10.1016/j.amepre.2008.05.001 PMID:18550322

Peña-Casas, R., Ghailani, D., & Coster, S. (2018). Digital transition in the European Union: what impacts on job quality? In B. Vanhercke, D. Ghailani & S. Sabato (Eds.), *Social policy in the European Union: state of play 2018*, Brussels, European Trade Union Institute (ETUI) and European Social Observatory (OSE). Retrieved from http://www.ose.be/EN/team/ose/ghailani.htm

Peyrefitte, A. (1995). *La société de confiance. Essai sur les origines et la nature du développement*. Paris: Éditions Odile Jacob.

Pfleeger, S., & Atlee, J. (2009). *Software Engineering: Theory and Practice* (4th ed.). Prentice Hall.

Phadke, A. (2016). Regulations of Doctors and private Hospitals in India. *Economic and Political Weekly, 51*(6), 46–55.

Pilotto, A., Panza, F., Sancarlo, D., Paroni, G., Maggi, S., & Ferrucci, L. (2012). Usefulness of the multidimensional prognostic index (MPI) in the management of older patients with chronic kidney disease. *Journal of Nephrology, 25*(Suppl. 19), 79–84. doi:10.5301/jn.5000162 PMID:22641578

Pires, S. R. A. (2007). O Instrumental Técnico na Trajetória Histórica do Serviço Social Pós-Movimento de Reconceituação. *Serviço Social Em Revista, 9*(2), 15–25. Retrieved from http://www.uel.br/revistas/ssrevista/c-v9n2_sandra.htm

Planning Commission. (2012). Retrieved from www.planningcomssion.nic.in

Pollitt, C. (2013, January). What do we know about public management reform? Concepts, models and some approximate guidelines. *Paper presented at the Workshop Towards a comprehensive reform of public governance*, Lisboa, Portugal. Retrieved from https://www.bportugal.pt/pt-pt/obancoeoeurosistema/eventos/documents/pollitt_paper.pdf

Pollitt, C., & Bouckaert, G. (2011). *Public Management Reform. A comparative analysis - New Public Management, Governance, and the Neo-Weberian State*. New York: Oxford University Press.

Ponnert, L., & Svensson, K. (2016). Standardisation – the end of professional discretion? *European Journal of Social Work, 19*(3-4), 586–599. doi:10.1080/136 91457.2015.1074551

Popper, K. (2000). *Conjecturas e refutações*. Coimbra: Almedina.

Porter, J., Morphet, J., Missen, K., & Raymond, A. (2013). Preparation for high-acuity clinical placement: Confidence levels of final-year nursing students. *Advances in Medical Education and Practice, 4*, 83–89. doi:10.2147/AMEP.S42157 PMID:23900655

Portes, L. F., & Portes, M. F. (2009). A observação e a abordagem no exercício profissional: revisitanto a dimensão técnico-operativa no serviço social. *Cadernos Da Escola de Educação e Humanidades, 1*(4), 28–35. Retrieved from http://revistas.unibrasil.com.br/cadernoseducacao/index.php/educacao/article/view/35

Portuguese Ministry of Health (PMH). (2015). National Health Plan (PNS) 2012-2016. Retrieved from https://www.dgs.pt/em-destaque/plano-nacional-de-saude-revisao-e-extensao-a-2020-aprovada-pelo-governo.aspx

Portuguese Ministry of Health (PMH). (2016). *Plano de Desenvolvimento da RNCCI 2016-2019*. Lisboa: Ministérios do Trabalho e da Solidariedade Social e da Saúde. Retrieved from https://www.sns.gov.pt/wp-content/uploads/2016/02/Plano-de-desenvolvimento-da-RNCCI.pdf

Postman, N. (1985). *Amusing ourselves to death*. Viking Penguin Inc.

Postman, N. (1992). *Technopoly: the Surrender of Culture to Technology*. New York: Vintage.

Prathap, G. (1993). *The finite element method (FEM)*. Retrieved from http://www.nal.res.in/oldhome/gages/fepace.htm

Prizzon, C. (2006). Assessment e qualità dell'azione professionale dell'assistent sociale. In A. Campanini (Ed.), *La valutazione nel servizio sociale* (pp. 115–144). Roma: Carocci Faber.

Ragnedda, M., & Muschert, G. W. (2013). *The Digital Divide: The internet and social inequality in international perspective*. Abingdon: Routledge. doi:10.4324/9780203069769

RAIC – Raic Canada. (2014). Raic / Irac Architecture Canada. Retrieved from https://www.raic.org/

Rajagopal, D. (2018, August 26). Not all is well with India's corporate hospital chains. *The Economic Times*. Retrieved from https://economictimes.indiatimes.com/industry/healthcare/biotech/healthcare/not-all-is-well-with-indias-corporate-hospital-chains/articleshow/65545784.cms

Randell, D. A., Cui, Z., & Cohn, A. G. (1992). A spatial logic based on regions and connection. *KR*, *92*, 165–176.

Rascanu, R., & Radu, S. M. (2014). Psycho-social assessment of patients with chronic renal diseases undergoing dialysis. *Procedia: Social and Behavioral Sciences*, *127*, 379–385. doi:10.1016/j.sbspro.2014.03.275

Ray, P. K. (2017). An integrated approach for healthcare systems management inIndia. In P. Mandal & J. Vang (Eds.), *Entrepreneurship in Technology for ASEAN*. Singapore: Springer; doi:10.1007/978-981-10-2281-4_6

Reamer, F. G. (2013). Social Work in a Digital Age: Ethical and Risk Management Challenges. *Social Work*, *58*(2), 163–172. doi:10.1093wwt003 PMID:23724579

Reeves, B., & Nass, C. (1996). The media equation. Cambridge University Press.

Rein, A. (1995). The physiological and psychological effects of compassion & anger. *Journal of Advancement in Medicine*, *8*(2).

Restrepo, O. L. V. (2003). *Reconfigurando el trabajo social – Perspetivas y tendencias contemporâneas*. Buenos Aires: Espacio.

Revel, J. (2005). *Michel Foucault: Expériences de la pensée*. Paris: Bordas.

Rey, Y., & Prieur, B. (1991). Systèmes, éthique, perspectives en thérapie familiale. Paris: EME Editions Sociales Françaises (ESF).

Ribeiro, J. L. (1994). A importância da qualidade de vida para a psicologia da saúde. *Análise Psicológica, XII*(2–3), 179–191. doi:10.1177/1089253207311685

Rockwood, K., Song, X., MacKnight, C., Bergman, H., Hogan, D. B., McDowell, I., & Mitnitski, A. (2005). A global clinical measure of fitness and frailty in elderly people. *Canadian Medical Association Journal, 173*(5), 489–495. doi:10.1503/cmaj.050051 PMID:16129869

Rodrigues, M. J. (2005). The European Way to a Knowledge-Intensive Economy—The Lisbon Strategy. In M. Castells & G. Cardoso (Eds.), *The Network Society: From Knowledge to Policy* (pp. 405–424). Washington, DC: Johns Hopkins Center for Transatlantic Relations.

Rodrigues, M. L. (2012). *Profissões. Lições e Ensaios*. Coimbra: Almedina.

Rolland, J. S. (2000). *Famílias, enfermedad y discapacidad – Una propuesta desde la terapia sistémica*. Barcelona: Gedisa.

Rollet, C. (1998). Lorsque la mort devint mortalité. In C. Le Grand-Sébille, M. F. Morel, & F. Zonabend (Eds.), *Le fœtus, le nourrisson et la mort* (pp. 105–126). Paris, France: L'Harmattan.

Roque Amaro, R. (2009). A Economia Solidária da Macaronésia – Um Novo Conceito. *Revista de Economia Solidária, 1*, 11–29.

Roque Amaro, R. (2011). Projeto ECOS. *Revista de Economia Solidária, 3*, 157–171.

Rose, N. (2006). *The Politics of Life Itself: Biomedicine, Power, and Subjectivity in the Twenty-First Century*. Princeton, NJ: Princeton University Press.

Rose, N. (2007). Beyond medicalization. *Lancet, 369*(9562), 700–702. doi:10.1016/S0140-6736(07)60319-5 PMID:17321317

Rowe, J. W., & Kahn, R. L. (1997). Successful Aging. *The Gerontologist, 37*(4), 433–440. doi:10.1093/geront/37.4.433 PMID:9279031

Royal Institute of British Architects (RIBA). (2014). Retrieved from http://www.architecture.com/Explore/Home.aspx

Russel, S., & Norvig, P. (2009). *Artificial intelligence: A modern approach* (3rd ed.). Prentice Hall.

Saffell, N. (2015). *On the origin of robot species: robots building robots by "natural selection".* University of Cambridge. Retrieved August 12, 2015 from http://www.cam.ac.uk/research/news/on-the-origin-of-robot-species?sthash.zMSyp5OS.mjjo

Samarasekera, U. (2016). *Ending preventable stillbirths –An Executive Summary for The Lancet's Series.* Retrieved from https://www.thelancet.com/series/ending-preventable-stillbirths

Samarasekera, U., & Horton, R. (2014). The world we want for every newborn child. *Lancet, 384*(9938), 107–109. doi:10.1016/S0140-6736(14)60837-0 PMID:24853598

Santos, F. (2009). *A positive theory of social entrepreneurship.* Working paper, INSEAD, Faculty & Research.

Santos, C. M. (2012). *Na prática a teoria e outra? Mitos e dilemas na relação entre teoria, pratica, instrumentos e técnicas no serviço social.* Rio de Janeiro: Lumen Juris.

Santos, C. M., Filho, R. S., & Backx, S. (2012). Dimensão técnico-operativa no Serviço Social. In C. M. dos Santos, S. Backx, & Y. Guerra (Eds.), *Dimensão técnico-operativa no Serviço Social: desafios contemporâneos* (pp. 15–38). Juiz de Fora: Editora UFJF.

Sapir-Whorf Hypothesis. (2007). In *Wikipedia.* retrieved April 27, 2011 from http://en.wikipedia.org/wiki/Sapir-Whorf_hypothesis

Sarmento, H. B. de M. (2012). Instrumental técnico e o Serviço Social. In C. M. dos Santos, S. Backx, & Y. Guerra (Eds.), *Dimensão técnico-operativa no Serviço Social: desafios contemporâneos* (pp. 103–121). Juiz de Fora: Editora UFJF.

SAS. (2014). *SAS Enterprise Miner – SEMMA.* Retrieved from http://www.sas.com/technologies/analytics/datamining/miner/semma.html

SAS. (2017). *What is Analytics?* Retrieved from https://www.sas.com/en_us/insights/analytics/what-is-analytics.html

Schafer, E. (2003). *Digital Technology.* Retrieved from http://www.encyclopedia.com/doc/1G2-3401801216.html

Schafer, S. (2007). Premise: The key to interactive storytelling. *Game Career Guide.* Retrieved April, 3, 2007 from http://www.gamecareerguide.com/features/357/premise_the_key_to_interactive_.php?page=1

Schafer, S. (2011). Articulating the paradigm shift: Serious games for psychological healing of the collective persona. In *Business Social Networking: Organizational, Managerial, and Technological Dimensions*. IGI Global. Retrieved from http://www. igi-global.com/book/handbook-research-serious-games-educational/5

Schafer, S. (2012). Optimizing Cognitive Coherence, Learning, and Psychological Healing with Drama-based Games. In *Video Game Play and Consciousness*. Nova Science Publishers. Retrieved from http://www.facebook.com/insights/?sk =po_261980910540561#!/pages/Video-Game-Play-and-Consciousness/2619809 10540561?sk=wall

Schafer, S. (Ed.). (2017). *Exploring the collective unconscious in a digital age*. Hershey, PA: IGIG Global.

Schafer, S. B. (2018). *Generating a superconductive culture of conscience*. Beau Bassin, Mauritius: LAP LAMBERT Academic Publishing.

Schafer, S., & Yu, G. (2011). *Meaningful video games: drama-based video games as transformational experience*. Hershey, PA: IGI Global. doi:10.4018/978-1-60960-567-4.ch019

Scheler, M. (1936). *Le sens de la souffrance*. Paris: Aubier.

Schieber, A. C., Delpierre, C., Lepage, B., Afrite, A., Chantal, J. P., & Lombrail, P. (2014). Do gender differences affect the doctor–patient interaction during consultations in general practice? Results from the INTERMEDE study. *Family Practice*, *31*(6), 706–713. doi:10.1093/fampra/cmu057 PMID:25214508

Schieppati, A., & Remuzzi, G. (2005). Chronic renal diseases as a public health problem: Epidemiology, social, and economic implications. *Kidney International. Supplement*, *68*(98), 7–10. doi:10.1111/j.1523-1755.2005.09801.x PMID:16108976

Schiffman, L., & Kanuk, L. (2010). *Consumer behavior*. Prentice Hall.

Schmidt, L., & Valente, S. (2004). Factos e opiniões: uma abordagem transnacional ao desenvolvimento sustentável. In L. Lima, M. Cabral, M. & Vala, J. (Eds.), Atitudes Sociais dos Portugueses – Ambiente e desenvolvimento. Lisboa: Imprensa de Ciências Sociais.

Schön, D. (1994). *Le Praticien Réflexif. À la recherche du savoir caché dans l'agir professionnel*. Montréal: Les Éditions Logiques Inc. (Original publication 1983)

Schulz, J., Decamp, M., & Berkowitz, S. A. (2018). Spending patterns among medicare ACOS that have reduced costs. *Journal of Healthcare Management, 63*(6), 374–381. doi:10.1097/JHM-D-17-00178 PMID:30418364

SCIP. (2011). Strategic and Competitive Intelligence Professionals. *What is competitive intelligence,* Retrieved from http://www.scip.org/content.cfm

Seligman, B., Tuljapurkar, S., & Rehkopf, D. (2018). Machine learning approaches to the social determinants of health in the health and retirement study. *Social Science and Medicine Population Health., 4,* 95–99. doi:10.1016/j.ssmph.2017.11.008 PMID:29349278

Sen, A. (1993). Capability and Well-being. In M. Nussbaum & A. Sen (Eds.), *The Quality of Life* (pp. 30–53). Oxford: Clarendon Press. doi:10.1093/0198287976.003.0003

Sen, A. (2009). *The Idea of Justice.* UK: Penguin Press.

Senellart, M. (2004). Situation des cours. In M. Foucault (Ed.), Sécurité, territoire, population. Cours au Collège de France (1977-1978) (pp. 379-411). Paris: Gallimard.

Serafim, M. do R., & Santo, M. I. E. (2012). Criação e validação de uma escala de complexidade da intervenção social com adultos em contexto hospitalar (ECISACH). *Intervenção Social, 39,* 45–87. Retrieved from http://revistas.lis.ulusiada.pt/index.php/is/article/viewFile/1186/1297

Serres, M. (1991). *Le Tiers-Instruit.* Paris, France: Gallimard.

Shankar, P., Balasubramanian, D., Gurusimer, J., Verma, R., Kumar, D., Bahuguna, P., ... Kumar, R. (2017). Cost of delivering secondary-level health care services through public sector district hospitals in India. *The Indian Journal of Medical Research, 146*(3), 354–361. PMID:29355142

Sheppard, M. (1995). Social work, social science and practice wisdom. *British Journal of Social Work, 25*(3), 265–293. doi:10.1093/oxfordjournals.bjsw.a056180

Shetty, B. (2018, May 10). Improving the healthcare ecosystem. *Business World.* Retrieved from http://www.businessworld.com

Shirazian, S., Aina, O., Park, Y., Chowdhury, N., Leger, K., Hou, L., & Mathur, V. S. (2017). Chronic kidney disease-associated pruritus: Impact on quality of life and current management challenges. *International Journal of Nephrology and Renovascular Disease, 10,* 11–26. doi:10.2147/IJNRD.S108045 PMID:28176969

Shumpeter, J. (1911). *The theory of Economic Development*. Boston: Harvard University Press.

Silva, J. F. S. (2013). Serviço Social: Razão ontológica ou instrumental? *Katalysis, 16*(1), 72–81. doi:10.1590/S1414-49802013000100008

Simões, J. (2004). *Retrato Político da Saúde. Dependência do percurso e inovação em saúde: da ideologia ao desempenho*. Coimbra: Almedina.

Simonite, T. (2015). A better way to design brain inspired chips. *MIT Technology Review*. Retrieved May 6, 2015 from http://www.technologyreview.com/news/537211/a-better-way-to-build-brain-inspired-chips/

Singh, R. (2016). Integrated Healthcare in India – A Conceptual Framework. *Annals of Neurosciences, 23*(4), 197–198. doi:10.1159/000449479 PMID:27780986

Siune, K. (2009). *Challenging Futures of Science in Society. Report of the MASIS Expert Group*. European Commission.

Skansi, S. (2018). *Introduction to Deep Learning: from logical calculus to artificial intelligence*. New York: Springer-Verlag. doi:10.1007/978-3-319-73004-2

Skillmark, M., & Oscarsson, L. (2018). Applying standardisation tools in social work practice from the perspectives of social workers, managers, and politicians: A Swedish case study. *European Journal of Social Work*, 1–12. doi:10.1080/1369 1457.2018.1540409

Smith, G. C. S., & Fretts, R. C. (2007). Stillbirth. *Lancet, 370*(9600), 1715–1725. doi:10.1016/S0140-6736(07)61723-1 PMID:18022035

Sommerville, I. (2010). *Software Engineering* (9th ed.). Addison Wesley.

Somvanshi, K. K. (2018, July 27). Five Paradoxes of Indian Healthcare. *The Economic Times*. Retrieved from https://economictimes.indiatimes.com/industry/healthcare/biotech/healthcare/five-paradoxes-of-indian-healthcare/articleshow/65159929.cms

Sourbati, M. (2004). *Internet use in sheltered housing. Older people's access to new media and online service delivery*. London: Goldsmiths College, University of London.

Sousa, C. T. (2008). A prática do assistente social: Conhecimento, instrumentalidade e intervenção profissional. *Emancipação, 8*(1), 119–132. doi:10.5212/Emancipacao.v.8i1.119132

362

Sowar, A., Tobiasz-Adamczyk, B., Topór-Mądry, R., Poscia, A., & La Milia, D. I. (2016). Predictors of healthy ageing: public health policy targets. *BMC Health Services Research*, *16*(Suppl. 5), 289.

Stair, R., & Reynolds, G. (2009). *Principles of information systems.* Course Technology.

Stathopoulos, C. (2013). *DELIVERABLE D6.3 - Ethical and Social Best Practices on e-Accessibility. Value Aging.* TECNALIA. Retrieved from http://va.annabianco. it/wp-content/uploads/2014/09/07AGE03_D6.3_FINAL.pdf

Steyaert, J., & Gould, N. (2009). Social work and the changing face of the digital divide. *British Journal of Social Work*, *39*(4), 740–753. doi:10.1093/bjsw/bcp022

Streeter, C. L., & Franklin, C. (1992). Defining and measuring social support: Guidelines for social work practitioners. *Research on Social Work Practice*, *2*(1), 81–98. doi:10.1177/104973159200200107

Sun, Y., Yan, H., Lu, C., Bie, R., & Thomas, P. (2012). A holistic approach to visualizing business models for the internet of things. *Communications in Mobile Computing*, *1*(1), 1–7. doi:10.1186/2192-1121-1-4

Swarte, V., & Stephan, C. (2002). *European Senior Watch Observatory and Inventory. A market study about the specific IST needs of older and disabled people to guide industry, RDT and policy. Case Studies.* Society and Technology Programme.

Tadeu, H. F. B., Duarte, A. L. C., Chade, C. T., & Jamil, G. L. (2018). *Digital Transformation: Digital Maturity Applied to Study Brazilian Perspective for Industry 4.0. In J.L.G. Alcaraz et al. (Eds.), Best Practices in Manufacturing: Experiences from Latin America.* Cham, Switzerland: Springer Nature AG.

Taylor, A. (2017). Social work and digitalisation: Bridging the knowledge gaps. *Social Work Education*, *36*(8), 869–879. doi:10.1080/02615479.2017.1361924

Telecom Regulatory Authority of India. (2018). Report on Indian Telecom Services Performance Indicators, Quarterly Report - July-September. Retrieved from Retrieved from https://www.trai.gov.in/sites/default/files/PRNo114Eng28112018_0.pdf

Thakur, R., Hsu, S., & Fontenot, G. (2012). Innovation in healthcare: Issues and future trends. *Journal of Business Research*, *65*(4), 562–569. doi:10.1016/j. jbusres.2011.02.022

The Bengal Chamber (BCC) & Price Water Cooper (PWC). (2018). *Reimaging the possible in the Indian healthcare ecosystem with emerging technologies*. Retrieved from https://www.pwc.in/assets/pdfs/publications/2018/reimagining-the-possible-in-the-indian-healthcare-ecosystem-with-emerging-technologies.pdf

The curious evolution of artificial life. (2014). When it comes to research into Artificial Life, commercial projects have begun to outpace academic ones. *MIT Technology Review*. Retrieved July 30, 2014 from https://www.linkedin.com/grp/post/1039687-5900533809526378496

The emerging science of human-data interaction. (2015). *MIT Technology Review*. Retrieved January 11, 2015 from http://www.technologyreview.com/view/533901/the-emerging-science-of-human-data-interaction

The emerging science of human-data interaction—simulation of living systems. (2014). *MIT Technology Review*. Retrieved July 31, 2014 from https://www.linkedin.com/grp/post/1039687-5900533809526378496

The Lancet. (2016). *The best science for better lives*. Retrieved from https://www.thelancet.com/about-us

Therborn, G. (2012). The killing fields of inequality. *International Journal of Health Services*, *42*(4), 579–589. doi:10.2190/HS.42.4.a PMID:23367794

Thévenot, L. (1997). Un gouvernement par les normes. Pratiques et politiques des formats d'information. In B. Conein & L. Thévenot (Eds), Cognition et information en société (pp. 205-241). Paris: Éditions de l'EHESS (Raisons pratiques 8).

Thévenot, L. (1986). Les investissements de formes. In L. Thévenot (Ed.), *Conventions économiques* (pp. 21–71). Paris: Presses Universitaires de France.

Thévenot, L. (1990). L'action qui convient. In P. Pharo & L. Quéré (Eds.), *Les formes de l'action. Sémantique et Sociologie* (pp. 39–69). Paris: EHESS.

Thévenot, L. (1998). Pragmatiques de la connaissance. In A. Borzeix, A. Bouvier, & P. Pharo (Eds.), *Sociologie et connaissance. Nouvelles approches cognitives* (pp. 101–139). Paris: Éditions du CNRS.

Thévenot, L. (2001). Pragmatic regimes governing the engagement with the world. In T. Schatzki, K. Knorr-Cetina, & E. von Savigny (Eds.), *The practice turn in contemporary theory* (pp. 56–73). Brighton, UK: Psychology Press.

Thévenot, L. (2006). *L'action au pluriel. Sociologie des régimes d'engagement.* Paris: Éditions La Découverte.

Thévenot, L. (2009). Governing Life by Standards: A View from Engagements. *Social Studies of Science, 39*(5), 793–813. doi:10.1177/0306312709338767

Tobiasz-Adamczyk, B., & Brzyski, P. (2005). Psychosocial work conditions as predictors of quality of life at the beginning of older age. *International Journal of Occupational Medicine and Environmental Health, 18*(1), 43–52. PMID:16052890

Trafton, A. (2014). New brain-scanning technique allows scientists to see when and where the brain processes visual information. *Medical Press.* Retrieved January 27, 2014 from http://medicalxpress.com/news/2014-01-brain-scanning-technique-scientists-brain-visual.html

Tuomi, I. (2000). Data is more than knowledge: Implications of the reversed knowledge hierarchy for knowledge management and organizational memory. *Journal of Management Systems, 16*(3), 103–117.

Turban, E., Mc Lean, E., & Wetherbe, J. (2002). *Information technology for management: transforming business in the digital economy* (3rd ed.). Hoboken, NJ: John Wiley and Sons.

Turban, E., Rainer, R. K. Jr, & Potter, R. E. (2007). *Introduction to information systems.* Hoboken, NJ: John Wiley and Sons.

Turber, S., & Smiela, C. (2014). A business model type for the internet of things. In *22nd European Conference on Information Systems (ECIS 2014), Tel Aviv, Israel.*

Turchetti, G., Bellelli, S., Amato, M., Bianchi, S., Conti, P., Cupisti, A., & Scatena, A. (2017). The social cost of chronic kidney disease in Italy. *The European Journal of Health Economics, 18*(7), 847–858. doi:10.100710198-016-0830-1 PMID:27699568

UNAIDS. (2011). *Report on the global AIDS epidemic 2010.* UN.

UNESCO/COMEST. (2005). *The Precautionary Principle.* Paris: UNESCO.

UNICEF. (2006). *Relatório sobre Nutrição Infantil.* UN.

UNICEF. (2007). *Um Mundo para as Crianças.* UN.

United Nations Population Fund. (2017). *Delivering a world where every pregnancy is wanted, every childbirth is safe and every young person's potential is fulfilled.* Retrieved from https://www.unfpa.org/about-us

United Nations Secretary-General. (2015). *The Global Strategy for Women's, Children's and Adolescents' Health (2016-2030)*. New York: United Nations.

Urban, T. (2015). AI revolution—road to superintelligence. *But Wait Why*. Retrieved November 5, 2015 from http://www.technologyreview.com/news/525301/virtual-reality-startups-look-back-to-the-future/

Vago, S. (2004). *Social Change* (5th ed.). New Jersey: Pearson Education, Inc.

Varshney, U. (2007). Pervasive Healthcare and Wireless Health Monitoring. *Mobile Networks and Applications, 12*(2-3), 113–127. doi:10.100711036-007-0017-1

Vayena, E., Blasimme, A., & Cohen, I. G. (2018). Machine learning in medicine: Addressing ethical challenges. *PLoS Medicine, 15*(11), 1–4. doi:10.1371/journal.pmed.1002689 PMID:30399149

Vourlekis, B. S., & Rivera-Mizzoni, R. A. (1997). Psychosocial problem assessment and end-stage renal disease patient outcomes. *Advances in Renal Replacement Therapy, 4*(2), 136–144. Retrieved from http://www.ncbi.nlm.nih.gov/pubmed/9113229. doi:10.1016/S1073-4449(97)70040-2 PMID:9113229

Waldman, J. D., Kelly, F., Aurora, S., & Smith, H. (2004). The shocking cost of turnover in health care. *Health Care Management Review, 43*(3), 181. PMID:14992479

Watzlawick, P. (1991). *A Realidade é Real?* Lisboa: Relógio D'Água.

Weiss, S. M., & Verma, N. K. (2002). A System for Real-time Competitive Market Intelligence. In *Proceedings of the eighth ACM SIGKDD international conference on Knowledge discovery and data mining* (pp. 360-365). 10.1145/775047.775100

Welch, H. G. (2016). *Less Medicine, More Health. 7 Assumptions that drive too much medical care*. Beacon Press.

WHO. (2015). *World Health Statistics 2015*. Global Health Observatory (GHO) data.

WHO. (2015). *World Report on Ageing and Health*. Luxembourg: World Health Organization.

WHO. (2016). *Global strategy and action plan on ageing and health (2016-2020)*.

World Health Organization. (1948). *Constitution of the World Health Organization*. Geneva: World Health Organization.

World Health Organization. (2014). Every newborn. An Action Plan To End Preventable Deaths. Geneva: World Health Organization; United Nations International Children's Fund; Committing to Child Survival.

Worsfold, A. (2011). *Information for social care: A framework for improving quality in social care through better use of information and information technology.* Retrieved from http://www.differ.freeuk.com/learning/health/socialcareinfo.html

Yaoguang, H., & Rao, W. (2008). Research on collaborative design software integration on SOA. *Journal of Advanced Manufacturing Systems, 7*(1), 91–99. doi:10.1142/S0219686708001152

Yohn, D. L. (2015). The Secret Behind Retail Customer Experience Success is Brain Science. *Neuromarketing.* Retrieved November 20, 2015 from http://www.neurosciencemarketing.com/blog/articles/retail-customer-experience.htm

Yonce, C.; Taylor, J.; Kelly, N. & Gnau, S. (2017). BI Experts´ perspective: Are you ready for what´s coming in Analytics. *Business Intelligence Journal, 22*(3), 36-42.

Yu, G., Yang, R., Wei, Y., Yu, D., Zhai, W., Cai, J., & Qin, J. (2018). Spatial, temporal, and spatiotemporal analysis of mumps in Guangxi Province, China, 2005–2016. *BMC Infectious Diseases, 18*(1), 360. doi:10.118612879-018-3240-4 PMID:30068308

Yunbiao, S. (n.d.). Internet of Things: Wireless Sensor Networks. *IEC White Paper.* Retrieved from http://www.iec.ch/whitepaper/pdf/iecWP-internetofthings-LR-en.pdf

Zaltman, G., & Zaltman, L. (2008). *Marketing Metaphoria.* Harvard Business Press.

Zayyad, M. A., & Toycan, M. (2018). Factors affecting sustainable adoption of e-Health technology in developing countries: An exploratory survey of Nigerian hospitals from the perspective of healthcare professionals. *PeerJ, 6,* e4436. doi:10.7717/peerj.4436 PMID:29507830

Zheng, H. (2015). Losing confidence in medicine in an era of medical expansion? *Social Science Research, 52,* 701–715. doi:10.1016/j.ssresearch.2014.10.009 PMID:26004490

Zola, I. K. (1982). *Missing Pieces: A Chronicle of Living with a Disability.* Philadelphia, PA: Temple University Press.

Zucker, T. L., Samuelson, K. W., Muench, F., Greenberg, M. A., & Gevirtz, R. N. (2009). The effects of respiratory sinus arrhythmia biofeedback on heart rate variability and posttraumatic stress disorder symptoms: A pilot study. *Applied Psychophysiology and Biofeedback, 34*(2), 135–143. doi:10.100710484-009-9085-2 PMID:19396540

About the Contributors

Cristina Albuquerque has a PhD in Humanities (Specialty in Social Work and Social Policy) by the University of Fribourg, Switzerland (2004). Actually she is Professor of social policy and social entrepreneurship at the Faculty of Psychology and Educational Sciences of the University of Coimbra (PT).

* * *

Samuel Beaudoin is lecturer at Université Laval, Québec, Canada, since 2009, he received his Ph. D. in anthropology in 2018 from the same institution. He is currently working on a book about the relations between science, ethics and politics.

Luís Carrasco is a Social Worker in the area of Nephrology in Diaverum, Portugal. He is a Master in Social Policy.

Fernanda Daniel is an Assistant Professor in Instituto Superior Miguel Torga (Coimbra, Portugal). She is a PhD in Psychology and PhD in Social Work. Currently, she is a Researcher in the Center for Health Studies and Research of the University of Coimbra, Portugal, being her main research interests on aging, health and gender.

Sónia Guadalupe is a Social Worker and an Assistant Professor in Instituto Superior Miguel Torga (Coimbra, Portugal). She is a PhD in Social Work (2017, ISCTE-IUL, Lisbon) and a PhD in Mental Health (2009, University of Oporto). Currently she is the Coordinator of the Degree Course in Social Work of ISMT and Editor-in-Chief of the Portuguese Journal of Behavioral and Social Research. She is also a Researcher in CEISUC (Coimbra, Portugal), being her main research interests about families and social support networks for vulnerable populations and social work in the health field.

Joana Guerra is an Invited Assistant Professor at the Faculty of Psychology and Educational Sciences, University of Coimbra. She received her Ph.D. in Social Work at the Catholic University of Portugal in Lisbon with a focus on professionalism in health care professions under new public management reforms and received her Master's in Public Health at Faculty of Medicine at University of Coimbra. She teaches Social Policy, Social Work, Territory and Population with publications and work developed in Health, Education and Territorial Governance in policy. She is a researcher on the European project ISOTIS - Inclusive Education and Social Support to Tackle Inequalities in Society - H2020, which is contributing to effective policy and practice development to combat early arising and persisting educational inequalities. She is also a researcher at the Center for Interdisciplinary Studies of the 20th Century at the University of Coimbra (CEIS20).

George Jamil is a professor of several post-graduation courses from Minas Gerais, Brazil. He has two post-doctoral titles (from Universidade do Porto, Portugal - market intelligence and from Univsersidad Politecnica de Cartagena, Spain - Entrepreneurship). PhD in Information Science from the Federal University of Minas Gerais (UFMG), Masters degree in Computer Science (UFMG) and under-graduated in Electric Engineering (UFMG). He got a pos-doctorate certificate at FLUP – Communication School at University of Porto, Portugal, in 2014. He wrote more than thirty books in the information technology and strategic management areas, with more than ten works in books as co-author and Editor. He works also as a business consultant and as an active ecossystem actor in business innovation and startups front in several countries. His main research interests are information systems management, strategy, knowledge management, software engineering, marketing and IT adoption in business contexts.

Liliane Jamil is a Medical Doctor and Independent researcher. Currently she is a MsC Student in Plastic Surgery with a Medical specialty in Plastic Surgery.

G. Jayanthi has completed M. Tech Computer Science and Engineering in the year 2016 from Pondicherry Central University, Puducherry, India. She was awarded Pondicherry University Gold Medal in the year 2017. She has an interdisciplinary postgraduate degree in Remote Sensing completed in the year 2007 from Anna University, India. She is the university rank holder both in graduate and under graduate engineering studies. She has 9 years of teaching experience in engineering education (Computer Science and Engineering and Civil Engineering). Presently, she is pursuing research at Anna University, Chennai, India under faculty of Information and Communication Engineering. She has presented papers in international (IEEE) conference. She has authored a paper published in International Journal of Artificial Intelligence and Soft Computing, Inderscience, indexed in ACM digital library. Her research interests include Artificial Intelligence, Knowledge Engineering, Statistical & Machine Learning, Spatial Analytics, Spatio temporal Network Modeling and Analysis.

Alexandre Cotovio Martins has a PhD. in Sociology (New University of Lisbon, 2011) and is a Professor at the Polytechnic Institute of Portalegre and Integrated Researcher at CICS.NOVA (Portugal). He is member of the editorial board of Cambridge Scholars Publishing. He has coordinated several research projects in the field of Sociology of Health, namely two projects funded by the Portuguese Science and Technology Foundation, which were evaluated by panels of international experts. He won a distinction as a reviewer for his refereeing work in the field of palliative care.

Pradeep Nair is presently working as Professor of New Media and Dean of School of Journalism, Mass Communication and New Media at the Central University of Himachal Pradesh, Dharamshala, India. He also holds the post of Director, Computer Centre at the University. Dr. Nair obtained his PhD in Development Communication with an emphasis on Health Communication from the University of Lucknow. He has been involved in communication research for over 15 years. Trained in the qualitative aspects of communication research, is research interests focus on New Communication Technologies, Communication Research, Development Communication, ICT based Health Governance, and Humanities and Social Science Interface with New Media He worked as Senior Scientist (Communication Research) at Anwar Jamal Kidwai Mass Communication Research Centre (AJK-MCRC), Jamia Millia Islamia before joining the Central University of Himachal Pradesh, where he coordinated the Doctoral Program (Ph.D.) and Post-Graduate Program in Development Communication. Dr. Nair has been recognized for his teaching and mentoring and had worked on a number of health projects funded by WHO, World Bank and other international funding and policy agencies. He is presently in the Editorial Board of International Peer Reviewed Journals – Pedagogy in Health Promotion (PHP) published by SAGE and Society for Public Health Education (SOPHE), Washington DC and Asia Pacific Media Educator (APME) published by SAGE and University of Wollongong, Australia. As a Review Editor he is reviewing for journals – Frontiers in Public Health and Inquiry published by SAGE and John Hopkins University, USA.

Marta Olim has a Social work degree and a Master in Social Work. Currently she is the Director of Social Work Department, Social Responsability Office and the Head of Communications is Diaverum, Portugal.

Joana Pimenta is a Social Worker in the field of Nephrology in Diaverum, Portugal.

Augusto Pinho Vieira is a Medical Doctor and Independent researcher. He is PhD Student in Ophthalmology Surgery and has a Medical specialty in Ophthalmology.

Leandro Santos is a Professor, consultant and entrepreneur of Market Intelligence. He has a MSc in Management, a BSc in Communication Sciences, and an MBA in Marketing management. He has authorship in several IGI Book's Chapters and Journals.

Stephen Brock Schafer's interest is on communications research relating to media influence on cultural transformation. He has been developing an analog between cognitive models and video game structure based on a multidimensional common denominator—narrative-metaphorical linguistic structure—that operates as an affective transducer between conscious and unconscious cognitive dimensions. Accordingly, a genre of psychology-based video games (PEG) may be used to access robust data relative to collective unconscious cognitive states. His current project is to generate a Global Humanitarian Advocacy Organism. Prof Schafer is Past Chairman of the Humanities & Social Sciences Department at Digipen Institute of Technology where he taught for fifteen years. In addition to teaching at several colleges and universities, he has twenty-five years of experience that includes senior management in both the public and private sectors, social and environmental activism, marketing, and journalism. The unusual breadth and depth of his practical experience supports his research on the media dynamics of cultural evolution.

Alexandre Gomes da Silva is a Coordinator Professor in Coimbra Business School ISCAC, Instituto Politécnico de Coimbra, and a researcher in the Centre for Health Studies and Research of the University of Coimbra, Portugal. He is Graduated in Mathematics, MSc in Statistics by the University College Dublin. PhD in Statistics by the University of Reading, He is also the UK Coordinator of the Master's program in Data Analysis and Decision Support Systems.

Uma V. received the M.Tech, and PhD degrees in computer science from Pondicherry University in 2007 and 2014 respectively. She was awarded the Pondicherry University gold medal for M.Tech. degree in Distributed Computing Systems. She has more than 10 years of teaching experience at PG level. Her research interest includes Data mining, knowledge representation and reasoning (spatial and temporal knowledge) and sentiment analysis. She has authored and co-authored more than 20 peer-reviewed journal papers, which includes publications in Springer and Inderscience. She has also authored 3 chapters in various books published by IGI Global. She has also authored a book on temporal knowledge representation and reasoning. She received the Best Paper Award in International Conference on Digital Factory in the year 2008.

Index

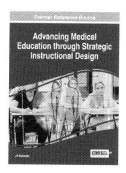
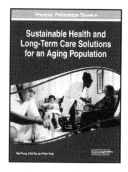
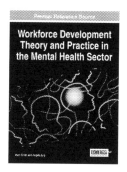
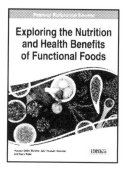
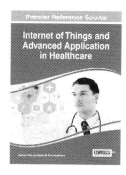
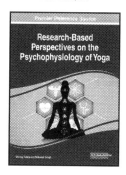
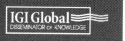

Ensure Quality Research is Introduced to the Academic Community

Become an IGI Global Reviewer for Authored Book Projects

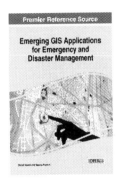

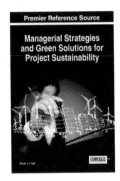

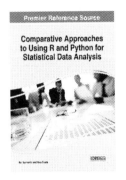

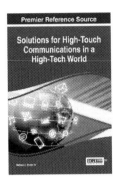

The overall success of an authored book project is dependent on quality and timely reviews.

In this competitive age of scholarly publishing, constructive and timely feedback significantly expedites the turnaround time of manuscripts from submission to acceptance, allowing the publication and discovery of forward-thinking research at a much more expeditious rate. Several IGI Global authored book projects are currently seeking highly qualified experts in the field to fill vacancies on their respective editorial review boards:

Applications may be sent to:
development@igi-global.com

Applicants must have a doctorate (or an equivalent degree) as well as publishing and reviewing experience. Reviewers are asked to write reviews in a timely, collegial, and constructive manner. All reviewers will begin their role on an ad-hoc basis for a period of one year, and upon successful completion of this term can be considered for full editorial review board status, with the potential for a subsequent promotion to Associate Editor.

If you have a colleague that may be interested in this opportunity, we encourage you to share this information with them.

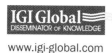

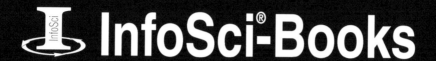
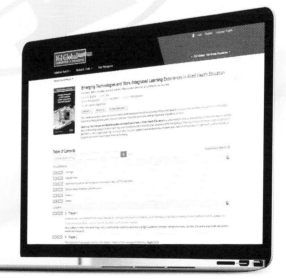

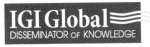
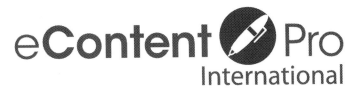
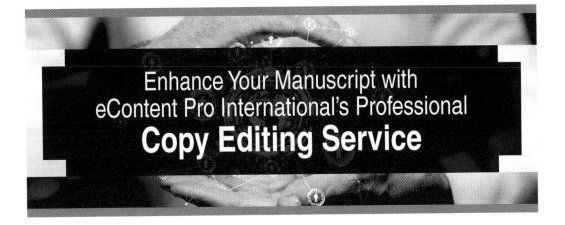

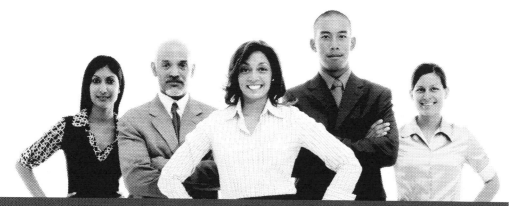

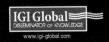
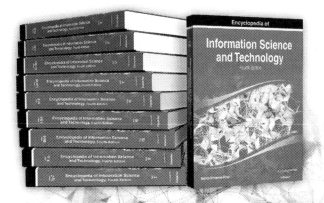
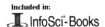

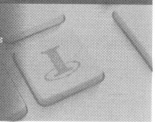
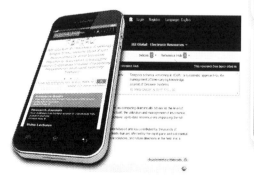

Printed in the United States
By Bookmasters